A Little,
Brown
Nursing # Critical Care Fact Finder

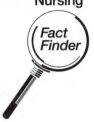

Manual of Critical Care Nursing

Jennifer Hebra, R.N., M.S.N., M.B.A., C.C.R.N.

Nurse Manager, Special Projects, and
Business Manager, Clinical Centers, Medical
University of South Carolina Medical Center,
Charleston, South Carolina; Former Critical
Care Instructor, Department of Nursing Staff
Development, Hospital of the University of
Pennsylvania, Philadelphia

Merrily A. Kuhn, R.N., M.S.N., Ph.D.

Associate Professor, Daemen College, Buffalo,
New York; President, Educational Services,
Hamburg, New York

1837

Little, Brown and Company
Boston   New York   Toronto   London

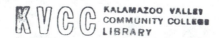

Library of Congress Cataloging-in-Publication Data
Hebra, Jennifer.
     Manual of critical care nursing / Jennifer Hebra, Merrily
Kuhn.
        p.   cm.
     Includes index.
     ISBN 0-316-35596-8
     1. Intensive care nursing—Handbooks, manuals, etc.   I.
Mathewson
  Kuhn, Merrily, 1945-   . II. Title.
  RT120.I5H43   1996
  610.73'61—dc20
  DNLM/DLC
  for Library of Congress   95-31696
                                                        CIP

Printed in the United States of America

SEM

Editorial: Evan R. Schnittman, Suzanne Jeans
Production Supervisor: Michael A. Granger
Designer: Linda Däna Willis
Cover Designer: Martucci Studio

Contents

Appendixes

X ▼ Contents

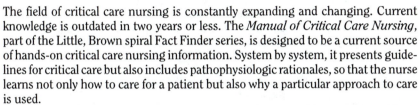

The field of critical care nursing is constantly expanding and changing. Current knowledge is outdated in two years or less. The *Manual of Critical Care Nursing*, part of the Little, Brown spiral Fact Finder series, is designed to be a current source of hands-on critical care nursing information. System by system, it presents guidelines for critical care but also includes pathophysiologic rationales, so that the nurse learns not only how to care for a patient but also why a particular approach to care is used.

Part I, "Methods and Approaches in Critical Care," addresses the problems that are experienced by many critical care patients—infection, psychosocial issues, and changes in nutritional requirements. A special chapter on trauma is also included.

Part II, "Disorders in the Patient in Critical Care," examines critical care requirements by body system. For each condition addressed, the condition is defined, and etiology, assessment, patient management, and discharge planning are discussed.

The assessment sections identify the signs and symptoms of a particular condition and list the required lab tests with their pathophysiologic rationales. Abnormal lab results are indicated as being above or below the normal value; normal values are included in Appendix D, "Laboratory Values."

The patient management sections include only the most important nursing diagnoses. For each diagnosis, a "problem" is presented. It is the problem that leads to the nursing diagnosis, and the goal of all nursing interventions should be to improve, eliminate, or treat the specific problem. Both medical and nursing interventions are included for each nursing diagnosis, and they are given in order of priority. Desired outcomes are also identified. Discharge planning concludes each discussion; however, discharge planning should start on admission to keep pace with the increase in shortened hospital stays.

Medications commonly administered for each condition are identified in drug boxes that include the drug's action, administration guidelines, and any special considerations. The drug information presented here should serve as a guide for the nurse, and it is suggested that other drug source books be consulted for additional information. For intravenous drugs, see the *Manual of Intravenous Medications*, another book in the Little, Brown Fact Finder series.

A variety of helpful appendixes are also included. Appendix A covers modalities used in critical care and addresses special procedures, such as ventilator use, hemodynamic lines, and renal therapies, that are common to multiple conditions.

Procedures specific to a particular condition are discussed with the condition. In addition, Advanced Cardiac Life Support algorithms, a body surface area nomogram, scoring systems (Apache III, Glasgow Coma Scale, trauma), and information on dysrhythmias are included.

We assembled a group of noted experts and scholars for participation in the preparation of this book. We thank the authors and reviewers who contributed their time and expertise so that this source book might be used to administer and improve patient care. In this technological age, we must be careful not to lose sight of the importance of the patient. As health care providers, we should strive to assist the patient back to his or her maximal state of health or, as the case may be, to a comfortable, compassionate, peaceful death.

We thank Evan Schnittman, Medical Editor, and Suzanne Jeans, Editorial Assistant, for allowing this dream to become a reality.

J.H.
M.A.K.

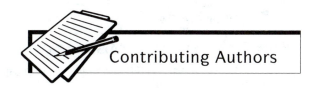

Contributing Authors

Dan Brennan, R.N., M.S.N.
Regional Managed Care Coordinator, University of Pennsylvania Health System, Philadelphia

Susan Davidoff, R.N., M.S.N., F.N.P.
Clinician, Planned Parenthood of Southeastern Pennsylvania, Philadelphia

Nancy Dodd, R.N., M.S.N., C.C.R.N.
Nursing Coordinator/Evening Administrator, Hospital of the University of Pennsylvania, Philadelphia

Nancy Evans, R.N., M.S.N.
Clinical Nurse Specialist, Nutrition Support/Parenteral Infusion Therapy, University of Pennsylvania Medical Center, Philadelphia

Jennifer Hebra, R.N., M.S.N., M.B.A., C.C.R.N.
Nurse Manager, Special Projects, and Business Manager, Clinical Centers, Medical University of South Carolina Medical Center, Charleston, South Carolina; Former Critical Care Instructor, Department of Nursing Staff Development, Hospital of the University of Pennsylvania, Philadelphia

Susan Krupnick, R.N., M.S.N., C.A.R.N., C.S.
Psychiatric Consultation Liaison, Comprehensive Behavioral Health Home Care Program, Skilled Nursing, Inc., Flourtown, Pennsylvania

Merrily A. Kuhn, R.N., M.S.N., Ph.D.
Associate Professor, Daemen College, Buffalo, New York; President, Educational Services, Hamburg, New York

Mary Clark Robinson, R.N.C., M.S.
Coordinator of Education and Research, Harris Methodist Hospital, Fort Worth, Texas

Diane Schwenker, R.N., M.S.N., C.C.R.N., C.N.R.N.

Neurosurgical Clinical Nurse Specialist, Hospital of the University of Pennsylvania, Philadelphia

Brenda Shelton, R.N., M.S.N., C.C.R.N., O.C.N.

Critical Care Clinics, The Johns Hopkins Oncology Center, Baltimore

Laurie Zone-Smith, R.N., M.S.N.

Trauma Nurse Coordinator, Trauma Center, Medical University of South Carolina Medical Center, Charleston, South Carolina

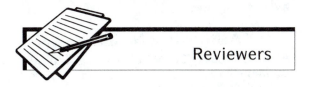

Gerald W. Bryant, R.N., B.S.N., C.C.R.N.

Critical Care Nurse Manager, Lake Charles Memorial Hospital, Lake Charles, Louisiana

Denise F. Collett, R.N.

Unit Coordinator, Department of Critical Care, Lake Charles Memorial Hospital, Lake Charles, Louisiana

Janet Courtcoul, R.N., M.S.N.

Director of Intensive Care and Surgical Services, Department of Nursing, Memorial Hospital, Midland, Texas

Jane Flynt, R.N., M.S.N., C.C.R.N.

Instructor in Nursing, McNeese State University, Lake Charles, Louisiana; Clinical Nurse Specialist, West Calcasieu-Cameron Hospital, Sulphur, Louisiana

Rose M. Hogg, R.N., M.S.N.

Assistant Professor of Nursing, Columbus College, Columbus, Georgia

Allison Lertora, R.N., M.S.N., C.C.R.N., O.C.N.

Associate Faculty, School of Nursing, Johns Hopkins University; Clinical Nurse, Department of Oncology, Johns Hopkins Hospital, Baltimore

Eileen Markman, R.N.

Inpatient Transplant Coordinator, Hospital of the University of Pennsylvania, Philadelphia

Anne M. Moraca-Sawicki, R.N., M.S.N.

Instructor, Health Science Division, Niagara Community College, Sanborn, New York; Clinical Nurse Specialist/Surgery Coordinator, Private Practice, Niagara Falls and Lewiston, New York

Cheryl A. Nicosia, R.N., M.S.N., C.C.R.N.

Adjunct Faculty, School of Nursing, State University of New York at Buffalo; Surgical Critical Care Nurse Clinician, Erie County Medical Center, Buffalo, New York

Karen S. Romano, R.N., C.C.R.N., C.E.T.N.

Clinical Instructor, School of Nursing, State University of New York at Buffalo; Trauma Nurse Coordinator, Department of Surgery, Erie County Medical Center, Buffalo, New York

Mary Elizabeth Rommel, R.N., M.S., C.C.R.N.

Adjunct Faculty, School of Nursing, State University of New York at Buffalo; Critical Care Instructor, Department of Nursing, Veterans Administration Medical Center, Buffalo, New York

Phyllis A. Schiavone-Gatto, R.N., M.S.N.

Clinical Nurse Specialist, Hospital of the University of Pennsylvania, Philadelphia

Cameron L. Schmidt, R.N., M.S.

Clinical Instructor, Critical Care Education, Critical Care Nursing Service, Erie County Medical Center, Buffalo, New York

Sally Ann Shimmel, R.N., M.S.

Adjunct Faculty, School of Nursing, State University of New York at Buffalo; Respiratory Clinical Nurse Specialist, Veterans Administration Medical Center, Buffalo, New York

Frances B. Walker, R.N., M.S.N., O.C.N.

Clinical Preceptor in Nursing, University of Pennsylvania, Philadelphia; Clinical Nurse Specialist, Department of Nursing, Hematology/Oncology/Bone Marrow Therapy, Hospital of the University of Pennsylvania, Philadelphia

Lee Ann Watson Duplechain, R.N.

Inservice/Patient Educator, Department of Nursing Education, Lake Charles Memorial Hospital, Lake Charles, Louisiana

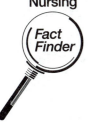

A Little, Brown Nursing

Fact Finder

Critical Care Fact Finder

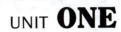

UNIT **ONE**

Methods and Approaches in Critical Care

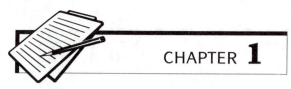

CHAPTER **1**

Infection Control in the Critical Care Unit

Susan Davidoff and Jennifer Hebra

An individual in the critical care environment is at constant risk for acquiring a nosocomial infection. Various factors lead to this enhanced susceptibility including (1) decreased body defenses from illness, immunosuppression, altered skin integrity, or stress; (2) increased exposure from the numerous interventions required such as multiple antibiotics, suctioning, etc; (3) the use of invasive devices such as central lines and catheters; and (4) depleted nutritional status that interferes with healing. Unfortunately, the most frequent source of contamination is cross-infection by health care providers. Nurses have very frequent interactions with patients and must take responsibility for a portion of these cross-contaminations.

Nosocomial infections complicate the hospitalization and increase the length of stay. Although universal precautions have improved basic infection control practices, they are designed to protect the health care provider, not the patient. Nurses must continue to be very aggressive in controlling cross-contamination to protect the critically ill patient. The most effective way is to *wash hands before and after every patient contact, whether or not gloves are worn.*

In this chapter, basic infection control issues are discussed to protect both the patient and the nurse from infectious diseases. For an in-depth discussion of the primary diseases, refer to the appropriate chapter.

I. Nosocomial infection

A. Definition: an infection acquired in the hospital
B. Types of transmissions
    1. Infectious diseases transmitted directly from infected person to susceptible person
    2. Infectious disease transmitted indirectly from infected person to susceptible person by a carrier (ie, nurse, physician, other health care worker)
    3. Normal flora that invade and colonize other systems in the same person
    4. Normally nonpathogenic organisms that invade and colonize susceptible patients
    5. Infections passed from an infected mother to her newborn
C. Extent
    1. 5%–7% of patients admitted to a general hospital

2. Approximately 25% of all nosocomial infections occur within the intensive care unit (ICU)
3. As many as one third of all ICU admissions will experience a nosocomial infection.

D. Common sites (in decreasing order of frequency)
1. Urinary tract
2. Surgical wounds
3. Lower respiratory tract
4. Blood (primary bacteremias)
5. Skin

E. Common pathogens
1. *Escherichia coli*
2. *Pseudomonas aeruginosa*
3. Enterococci
4. *Staphylococcus aureus*

F. Risk factors
1. Impaired host defenses from effects of critical illness
2. Disease-altered immune function (ie, diabetes, cirrhosis, renal failure, malignancy)
3. Immunosuppression (ie, organ transplantation, corticosteroid therapy)
4. Prolonged and frequent exposure to pathogens, resistant organisms in particular in the ICU environment
5. Invasive devices
6. Poor nutritional status

G. Nursing interventions for infection control
1. General guidelines
   a. *Wash hands* before contact with patients to prevent cross-infection and after removing gloves, since leaks and tears are not always apparent and wrists may be contaminated.
   b. Adhere to universal precautions (Table 1.1)[1].
   c. Adhere to isolation procedures in suggested categories (Table 1.2).

Table 1.1 Centers for Disease Control Recommendations: Universal Precautions

1. All health-care workers should routinely use appropriate barrier precautions to prevent skin and mucous-membrane exposure when contact with blood or other body fluids of any patient is anticipated. Gloves should be worn for touching blood and body fluids, mucous membranes, or nonintact skin of all patients, for handling items or surfaces soiled with blood or body fluids, and for performing venipuncture and other vascular access procedures. Gloves should be changed after contact with each patient. Masks and protective eyewear or face shields should be worn during procedures that are likely to generate droplets of blood or other body fluids to prevent exposure of mucous membranes of the mouth, nose, and eyes. Gowns or aprons should be worn during procedures that are likely to generate splashes of blood or other body fluids.
2. Hands and other skin surfaces should be washed immediately and thoroughly if contaminated with blood or other body fluids. Hands should be washed immediately after gloves are removed.

Table 1.1 *Continued*

3. All health-care workers should take precautions to prevent injuries caused by needles, scalpels, and other sharp instruments or devices during procedures; when cleaning used instruments; during disposal of used needles; and when handling sharp instruments after procedures. To prevent needlestick injuries, needles should not be recapped, purposely bent or broken by hand, removed from disposable syringes, or otherwise manipulated by hand. After they are used, disposable syringes and needles, scalpel blades, and other sharp items should be placed in puncture-resistant containers for disposal; the puncture-resistant containers should be located as close as practical to the use area. Large-bore reusable needles should be placed in a puncture-resistant container for transport to the reprocessing area.

4. Although saliva has not been implicated in HIV transmission, to minimize the need for emergency mouth-to-mouth resuscitation, mouthpieces, resuscitation bags, or other ventilation devices should be available for use in areas in which the need for resuscitation is predictable.

5. Health-care workers who have exudative lesions or weeping dermatitis should refrain from all direct patient care and from handling patient-care equipment until the condition resolves.

6. Pregnant health-care workers are not known to be at greater risk of contracting HIV infection than health-care workers who are not pregnant; however, if a health-care worker develops HIV infection during pregnancy, the infant is at risk of infection resulting from perinatal transmission. Because of this risk, pregnant health-care workers should be especially familiar with and strictly adhere to precautions to minimize the risk of HIV transmission.

7. All health-care workers who participate in invasive procedures must routinely use appropriate barrier precautions to prevent skin and mucous membrane contact with blood and other body fluids of all patients. Gloves and surgical masks must be worn for procedures that commonly result in the generation of droplets, splashing of blood or other body fluids, or the generation of bone chips. Gowns or aprons made of materials that provide an effective barrier should be worn during invasive procedures that are likely to result in the splashing of blood or other body fluids. All health-care workers who perform or assist in vaginal or cesarean deliveries should wear gloves and gowns when handling the placenta or the infant until blood and amniotic fluid have been removed from the infant's skin and should wear gloves during post-delivery care of the umbilical cord.

8. If a glove is torn or a needlestick or other injury occurs, the glove should be removed and a new glove used as promptly as patient safety permits; the needle or instrument involved in the incident should also be removed from the sterile field.

From the Centers for Disease Control. Recommendations for prevention of HIV transmission in health-care settings. *Morb. Mortal. Wkly. Rep.* 36:(suppl. 2S):6S–7S, 1987.

    d. Wear gloves whenever contact with bodily secretions is anticipated.

    e. Change gloves *immediately* after contamination occurs, even when one is completing tasks on the same patient.

    f. Keep gloved hands away from face area (ie, do not wipe nose or mouth).

    g. Use aseptic technique when one is opening sterile packages and during insertion of invasive devices.

    h. Use aseptic technique during dressing changes.

Table 1.2 Isolation Categories

Isolation Categories	Single Room?	Gowns	Masks[a]	Wash Hands	Gloves	Comments
Strict Door closed at all times	Yes, negative pressure	Yes, at all times	Yes, at all times and on patient while in transit	Yes	Yes, at all times	Disinfect objects in room
Enteric	No	Yes, if contact with excreta	No	Yes	Yes, if contact with excreta or non-intact skin	Disinfect objects in room
Respiratory Door closed at all times	Yes, negative pressure	Yes, if direct contact	Yes, while in room or on patient while in transit	Yes	Yes, if direct contact with nonintact skin	Disinfect objects in room
Special respiratory (TB) Door closed	Yes, negative pressure	Not necessary	Yes, as above submicron mask required[b]	Yes	Yes, if direct contact with nonintact skin	Disinfect objects in room
Neutropenic	Yes, if granulo-cyte count < 1000	Not necessary	Yes, if visitor has a respiratory infection	Yes	Yes, if direct contact with nonintact skin	No rectal temperatures
Skin and wound	Desirable	During contact	Yes, for large wound infections	Yes	Yes, if direct contact with nonintact skin	Disinfect objects in room
Blood and body fluid	Not necessary	Yes, if splashing likely	Yes, if splashing likely	Yes	Yes, if contact with body fluid	Disinfect items contaminated

Table 1.2 *Continued*

Isolation Categories	Single Room?	Gowns	Masks[a]	Wash Hands	Gloves	Comments
Secretion and excretion	Not necessary	Yes, if contact with secretions or excretions likely	Not necessary, unless splashing likely	Yes	Yes, if contact with fluids, membranes, nonintact skin	Disinfect items contaminated

This table demonstrates the various types of isolation categories. Protective eyewear or faceshields should be worn anytime splashing is likely.

[a]Masks should be worn when one is suctioning *all* patients unless closed tracheal suction is used.

[b]Patients who are AFB smear positive (TB) should leave their room only for *essential* procedures prior to 14 days of effective therapy.

  i. Keep surfaces and equipment in patient's room clean.
  j. Disinfect surfaces and equipment if contaminated by infectious blood or body fluids; disinfection solutions are regulated and vary by hospital; any tuberculocidal solution is acceptable to disinfect areas contaminated with bodily secretions (Centers for Disease Control, telephone communication, September 3, 1994).
  k. Follow sterilization procedures for reusable equipment.
  l. Administer antibiotic therapy at prescribed times and adhere to schedule to maintain adequate drug levels.
2. IV catheters
  a. Wash and glove hands before venipuncture.
  b. Use antiseptic preparation before venipuncture.
  c. Use sterile needles for IV infusions.
  d. Secure catheter and apply sterile dressing.
  e. Inspect catheter site daily.
  f. Insert new cannula every 48–72 hours.
  g. Change dressing and possibly apply antibiotic ointment every 48 hours or in accordance with nursing practice guidelines.
  h. Change IV tubing every 48 hours and after blood product or lipid emulsion infusions.
  i. Avoid using IV catheters for irrigations or blood draws.
3. Ventilators
  a. Use sterile, disinfected, or disposable mouthpieces (tubing, cannula).
  b. Replace circuitry every 24–48 hours.
  c. Remove fluid buildup in tubing.
  d. Change, sterilize, or disinfect aerosol-producing equipment every 24 hours and between patients.
  e. Use sterile solutions in fluid reservoirs; discard unused portions after 24 hours.
  f. Use sterile catheter and sterile gloves when one is suctioning if open catheter system is used.

    g. Change suction catheter after each use.

    h. If closed tracheal suctioning apparatus used, change entire setup every 24 hours.

4. Waste disposal

    a. Recommendations based on The Occupational Safety and Health Administration's Blood Borne Pathogen Standard

        i. Sharps

- Do not recap, bend, or break disposable needles; if recapping is unavoidable, place cap on flat surface and thread needle into cap using only one hand.
- Do not remove needles from disposable syringes.
- Place contaminated disposable sharps in container specifically designed for sharps disposal immediately after use.
- Place contaminated reusable sharps in a puncture-resistant, leak-proof (on sides and bottom), color-coded or labeled container.
- Containers for contaminated sharps must be easily accessible, stand upright throughout use, and replaced before allowed to overfill.
- Close containers of contaminated sharps before removing or replacing.
- If leakage occurs or is possible, place container within a secondary container that is closable, leak-proof, and color coded.

        ii. Specimens and other regulated waste

- Wear gloves when one is handling specimens and all waste materials.
- Place in containers that are closable, leak-proof, color coded or labeled, and contain all contents without leakage or protrusion.

5. Contaminated laundry

    a. Wear gloves and any other appropriate personal protective wear when one is handling contaminated laundry.

    b. Handle as infrequently as possible.

    c. Bag or contain at site of use.

    d. Do not rinse or sort at site of use.

    e. Place wet laundry in containers that prevent soaking through.

    f. Use labeled or color-coded bags.

II. Isolation procedures

A. Purpose: to prevent the transmission of microorganisms among patients, personnel, and visitors

B. Universal blood and body fluid precautions: In 1987 the Centers for Disease Control (CDC) published guidelines to prevent the transmission of human immunodeficiency virus (HIV) and other bloodborne pathogens. These universal precautions (see Table 1.1) are to be used consistently by all personnel who come in contact with blood and body fluids, regardless of patient history/diagnosis.

C. Other isolation categories: See Table 1.2 for other suggested isolation categories. Institutions usually develop their own isolation categories, and they should be followed consistently.

III. Special considerations

A. Tuberculosis

  1. Definition: Tuberculosis (TB) is an infectious disease caused by the tubercle bacillus, *Mycobacterium tuberculosis*. Pathologic characteristics include inflammatory infiltrations, formation of tubercles, caseation, necrosis, abscesses, fibrosis, and calcification. Infection may occur in the respiratory system (most common), GI and genitourinary tracts, bones, joints, nervous system, lymph nodes, and skin. The incidence of TB has increased in recent years, and the emergence of resistant strains have been identified. TB occurs in several stages as described below.

    a. Stages

      i. *Primary TB* infection is characterized by the presence of *M tuberculosis* organisms in the host that multiply and create inflammatory lesions. This phase is generally without clinical symptoms.

      ii. *The latent phase* is the time between the primary infection and the development of active disease. This time period is variable (up to 50 years) depending upon the host's immune system; active TB can occur at anytime after exposure, usually when the patient is under stress or otherwise immunocompromised. Although the patient is not contagious in the latent period, there will be a positive TB skin test reaction if patient is not immunosuppressed.

      iii. *TB (active TB)* is characterized by pathologic and functional symptoms indicating destruction of host tissue by mycobacteria. The skin test and chest radiograph are positive. Transmission to others can occur.

  2. Transmission/Communicability

    a. Inhalation of dried droplet nuclei each containing a single tubercle bacillus; droplet nuclei are dispelled from the patient through coughing, sneezing, laughing, and singing.

    b. Ingestion or skin penetration, although rare

    c. Communicable for as long as bacilli are in sputum; may be years for some

  3. Incubation

    a. 4–12 weeks after exposure

    b. Anytime disease is in latent stage

  4. Risk factors

    a. Close contacts of person with infectious TB, especially if person is at high risk for any infection

    b. HIV infection

    c. Medical conditions known to increase the risk of active TB (ie, immunosuppression, diabetes, leukemia, and Hodgkin's disease)

    d. Medically underserved, low-income populations

    e. Foreign-born person from a country with high incidence of TB or living in areas with high incidence of immigration from such countries

    f. Chronic illness

    g. Malnourishment

h. Being a resident of a long-term care facility (elderly, incarcerated, mentally ill)

i. Alcoholic addiction or user of IV drugs

j. Working with silicone or asbestos

5. Postexposure precautions

    a. Skin test: Once TB bacilli enter the body, antibodies are usually produced that result in a positive skin test within 2–3 weeks; does not indicate active disease; it is possible to have a TB infection with a negative skin test

    b. Chest x-ray: may show calcification at infection site; possible pleural effusion

    c. Collaborate with occupational health to evaluate need for preventative treatment if exposure to TB is realized or new infection develops.

Isoniazid

Action Antibiotic that acts against actively growing tubercle bacilli.

Administration Guidelines 300 mg/day in a single dose for an average of 9–12 months. Preventative therapy protects most infected individuals from developing active TB.

Special Considerations Severe and fatal hepatitis has been associated with isoniazid therapy; monitor liver function tests closely.

---

    d. Multiple resistant strains of TB require treatment with two or more drugs.

6. Nursing interventions for infection control

    a. Acid-fast bacilli (AFB) sputum smears on patients with pulmonary symptoms who are at risk for TB

    b. AFB isolation until sputum smear results are known

    c. AFB (special respiratory) isolation for patients with active infection (see Table 1.2)

    d. AFB isolation may be discontinued after patient demonstrates evidence of response to therapy such as decreased cough, decreased maximum daily temperature, resolution of night sweats, and improved general health with increased appetite and weight gain; usually improvement is seen after approximately 2 weeks of continuous antibiotic therapy.

    e. Secretion precautions on patients with external TB lesions

    f. Skin tests on close contacts of infectious TB patients who do not have a documented history of positive test results

    g. Negative pressure room until there are no organisms on smear

    h. Observe ingestion of TB medications.

    i. Teach patient to cover nose and mouth while coughing, wear mask properly when out of room, limit excursions from room, and take medications appropriately and complete medication course.

    j. Report new cases of TB to public health department.

    k. Mask patients when in transit out of room.

    l. TB skin testing of nurses upon employment and every 6–12 months depending on prevalence of TB in the unit

    m. Chest radiograph for nurses with a documented history of positive skin test or active disease at employment and yearly thereafter

B. HIV and acquired immune deficiency syndrome (AIDS)

  1. Definition: Infection with HIV is characterized by a gradual and accelerating destruction of the immune system. This degeneration occurs in five phases and results in AIDS. Criteria for diagnosing AIDS have been established by the CDC. For a diagnosis of AIDS, a patient must have either a T4 lymphocyte cell count less than $200/mm^3$ or certain AIDS indicator conditions (see Chap. 9).

    a. Five phases of infection [2] (transmission may occur during all phases)

      i. *First* (also called window period): lasts 4 weeks to 6 months after infection; no detectable antibodies and no symptoms

      ii. *Second* (also called acute primary HIV infection): lasts 1–2 weeks; antibodies may be detected; flulike symptoms, skin rash

      iii. *Third* (also called asymptomatic HIV infection): lasts 1–15 or more years; antibodies are detectable; no symptoms

      iv. *Fourth:* lasts up to 3 years; although symptomatic, does not meet CDC criteria for AIDS diagnosis; antibodies are detectable; symptoms include fever, night sweats, diarrhea, weight loss, fatigue, neuropathy, lymphadenopathy, oral lesions, and cognitive slowing

      v. *Fifth* (AIDS): variable length, may survive 1–5 years from first AIDS-defining condition; antibodies are detectable; symptoms include severe opportunistic infections, tumors in any body system, and neurologic deficits

  2. Transmission/Communicability

    a. Contact with contaminated blood (needlestick, transfusion, open skin wounds, ocular and oral mucous membranes)

    b. Oral, anal, vaginal intercourse

    c. Perinatal (transplacental, exposure to infected blood at birth, breast milk)

    d. Communicable from presence of HIV in sera until death

  3. Incubation

    a. Variable: Time from exposure to seroconversion is 4 weeks to 6 months, and time from symptomatic immune suppression to AIDS can be 20 years

  4. Risk factors

    a. Risk of HIV transmission with a typical needlestick from a HIV-positive source is 0.4% [3]

    b. Individuals participating in unprotected sexual activities with HIV-positive persons

    c. Multiple sex partners

    d. IV drug use

    e. Persons receiving blood transfusions

    f. Persons with hemophilia or coagulation disorders

    g. Infant born to HIV-positive mother

Table 1.3 Issues Related to Occupational Exposure to HIV

Definitions

Exposure: needlestick, cut, or contact with mucous membrane or nonintact skin with body fluid

Body fluid: blood, cerebrospinal fluid, synovial fluid, pleural fluid, peritoneal fluid, pericardial fluid, and amniotic fluid; although saliva, urine, and stool are considered body fluids, they are not considered potential sources of HIV

Source: The source of body fluid must be evaluated for HBV and HIV; if source has AIDS, is known seropositive, or refuses testing, the worker is evaluated clinically and serologically

Precautions: During follow-up, worker should refrain from donating blood or sperm, sexual intercourse, and should take actions to prevent transmission

Zidovudine prophylaxis: *inclusion criteria*

Zidovudine prophylaxis is controversial and is associated with significant side effects; workers should consider the option carefully

1. Body-fluid exposure of blood, semen, vaginal secretions, and other fluids that are bloody or blood tinged; tissue that has not been inactivated; blood or tissue containing HIV in research labs
2. Contact with fluids by needlestick or cut; contact with mucous membranes or nonintact skin
3. Source has AIDS, positive HIV serology, or culture; individuals with unknown serostatus and high risk: IV drug user, homosexual male, hemophiliac, regular sex partner with HIV-positive person, persons with multiple sex partners, prostitutes
4. Women must not be pregnant or breast-feeding
5. Must be willing to use effective birth control during treatment and for 4 weeks thereafter
6. Treatment must be started within 72 hours; 45 minutes to 6 hours is preferred
7. Informed consent to include counseling to minimize sexual contacts, lack of documented efficacy of this treatment, possibility treatment will delay seroconversion, side effects, and cost of drug

Adapted from Guidelines for Preventing the Transmission of Tuberculosis in Health-Care Settings, with Special Focus on HIV-Related Issues. *Morb. Mortal. Wkly. Rep.* 39:1, 1990, and Bartlett, J. *Pocketbook of Infectious Disease Therapy.* Baltimore: Williams & Wilkins, 1993.

5. Postexposure precautions
   a. Report immediately to employee or occupational health services to plan postexposure treatment and to determine need for zidovudine prophylaxis, formally known as azidothymidine (AZT); see Table 1.3 [3,4] for issues related to occupational exposures to HIV.

> ### *Zidovudine*
> *Action* Antiviral drug active against HIV.
> *Administration Guidelines* See Table 1.4.
> *Special considerations* Associated with hematologic toxicity including granulocytopenia and severe anemia requiring transfusions; monitor CBC and SMA-12 at 2, 4, and 6 weeks.

Table 1.4 Medication Administration Guidelines

Drug	Administration Guidelines
Zidovudine (Retrovir), formally known as azidothymidine (AZT)	200 mg 6 times per day for 3 days (1200 mg/day), then 100 mg or 200 mg 5 times per day for 25 days (500 or 1000 mg/day)
Hepatitis B immune globulin	0.06 mL/kg IM within 7 days after exposure; repeat 28 days after exposure
Hepatitis B vaccine (Recombivax HB, Engerix-B)	Regimen for either brand: *1st dose:* baseline *2nd dose:* 1 month after 1st dose *3rd dose:* 6 months after 1st dose Each dose: 10 μg (1.0 mL) (green vial) 20 μg (1.0 mL)

   b. Obtain HIV serology at baseline (exposure), 6 weeks, 3 months, and 6 months (also at 12 months if zidovudine therapy initiated as seroconversion is delayed by therapy).
  6. Nursing interventions for infection control
   a. Universal precautions (see Table 1.1)
   b. Wear face mask, protective eyewear, apron, and gloves when at risk for splash contamination.
   c. Follow sterilization procedures for ventilators.
   d. Clean contaminated surfaces and equipment with disinfectant.
   e. Flush mucous membranes with water if contact with blood or other infectious material occurs.
   f. Do not eat, drink, or apply makeup or contact lenses in areas where infectious materials are present.
   g. Report new cases of AIDS to Public Health department; HIV reporting varies by state.
 C. Hepatitis B virus
  1. *Definition:* Infection with the hepatitis B virus (HBV) causes damage in the liver including inflammation, mononuclear cell infiltration in the parenchyma and portal ducts, hepatic cell necrosis, proliferation of Kupffer cells, and cellular collapse. Bilirubin excretion becomes impaired resulting in jaundice. Infection with HBV can be acute or chronic, and clinical severity may range from subclinical infection to acute fulminating disease.
  2. Transmission/Communicability
   a. Contact with infectious blood through needlesticks, transfusions, open skin wounds, or mucosa of eye and mouth; contact with environmental surfaces containing contaminated blood. HBV virus can survive 1 week or longer on surfaces.
   b. Sexual contact (saliva, semen, vaginal secretions)
   c. Perinatal (transplacental or exposure to infected maternal blood at birth)

    d. Communicable during incubation and throughout clinical course of disease; carrier state (infectious) may persist for years

3. Incubation period: 45–180 days, average 60–90 days

4. Risk factors

    a. Male homosexual activity

    b. Female prostitution

    c. Heterosexual relations with multiple sex partners

    d. IV drug use

    e. Hemodialysis

    f. Foreign persons from areas with high HBV rates

    g. Blood contact in the health care environment

5. Postexposure precautions

    a. Report immediately to occupational or employee health for follow-up treatment.

    b. Follow postexposure immunoprophylaxis guidelines recommended by CDC for percutaneous (needlestick, laceration, bite) or permucosal (ocular, mucous membrane) exposure found in Table 1.5[5]; hepatitis B immune globulin (HBIG) may be recommended.

HBIG

Action Provides passive immunity to hepatitis B.

Administration Guidelines See Table 1.4.

Special Considerations HBIG may interfere with response to live virus vaccines, administration of other vaccines should be deferred 3 months, anaphylaxis.

---

6. Nursing interventions for infection control

    a. Universal precautions (see Table 1.1)

Table 1.5 Exposure to Hepatitis B Virus: Guide to Postexposure Immunoprophylaxis

Type of Exposure	Immunoprophylaxis
Perinatal	Vaccination + HBIG*
Sexual—acute infection	HBIG ± vaccination
Sexual—chronic carrier	Vaccination
Household contact—chronic carrier	Vaccination
Household contact—acute case	None unless known exposure
Household contact—acute case, known exposure	HBIG ± vaccination
Infant (<12 months)—acute case in primary care-giver	HBIG + vaccination
Inadvertent—percutaneous/permucosal	Vaccination ± HBIG

*HBIG = hepatitis B immune globulin.
From the Centers for Disease Control. Hepatitis B virus: A comprehensive strategy for eliminating transmission in the United States through universal childhood vaccination— Recommendations of the Immunization Practices Advisory Committee (ACIP). *Morb. Mortal. Wkly. Rep.* 40:9, 1991.

b. Hepatitis B vaccination for nurses who are not immune (pregnancy is not a contraindication for hepatitis B vaccine, although response may be blunted).

Hepatitis B Vaccine

Action Noninfectious viral vaccine that protects recipient from contracting hepatitis B only, but *not* A, C, and E (hepatitis D does not occur without hepatitis B; therefore, it is assumed that hepatitis D will be prevented with vaccination).

Administration Guidelines See Table 1.4; for a full description of the various forms of hepatitis, see Chapter 7.

Special Considerations Must be administered by IM injection; *do not administer IV or intradermally.*

---

c. Follow serologic markers: blood infectious if positive hepatitis B surface antigen (HbsAg) occurs with present infection or carrier state; positive hepatitis B e antigen (HbeAg) is associated with progression from active hepatitis to chronic hepatitis and represents a highly infectious state.

d. Clean contaminated surfaces and equipment with disinfectant.

e. Do not eat, drink, or apply makeup or contact lenses in areas where infectious materials are present.

f. Report new cases to Public Health Department.

D. Cytomegalovirus

1. Definition: Cytomegalovirus (CMV) is a member of the herpes virus group. CMV typically produces an asymptomatic mononucleosis-type infection in adults. It remains latent in body tissue and may produce recurrent infections. Congenital and acquired CMV infections in newborns can lead to irreversible central nervous system damage. Infections in the immunocompromised patient may lead to pneumonitis, hemolytic anemia, hepatitis, and pericarditis.

2. Transmission/Communicability

   a. Congenital: CMV crosses the placenta and can cause severe congenital anomalies.

   b. Perinatal: CMV is present in the cervical secretions of mothers with primary infection or reactivation of latent infection; long-term effects on neurologic development of baby are unknown.

   c. Blood transfusions

   d. Organ transplantations

   e. Close and prolonged contact with infected body secretions (CMV is found in all body secretions)

   f. Sexual contact and kissing

   g. Communicable for as long as virus is excreted in saliva and urine; may be months to years

3. Incubation

   a. Unknown, estimated to be 3–8 weeks following transfusion, 3–12 weeks in neonate following perinatal exposure

4. Risk factors
   a. Immunosuppression (HIV, transplantations)
   b. Chronic illness
   c. Fetus and neonate
5. Postexposure precautions
   a. If pregnant or immunocompromised, notify physician if exposure is suspected.
6. Nursing interventions for infection control
   a. Universal precautions (see Table 1.1)
   b. CMV is a special concern to pregnant nurses. Although universal precautions should be effective against transmission, the danger to the unborn fetus may prompt the nurse to request reassignment.
E. Antibiotic resistant organisms
   1. Definition: organisms that are resistant to multiple antibiotics. Examples include *Staphylococcus aureus* resistant to methicillin (MRSA), oxacillin, nafcillin, the cephalosporins, erythromycin, clindamycin, tetracycline, or aminoglycosides and vancomycin-resistant enterococci (VREC). Infection with resistant organisms in a critically ill patient often leads to systemic inflammatory response syndrome with multiple organ failure and death as an end result.
   2. Transmission/Communicability
      a. Direct contact with contaminated hands (ie, from sputum or dressing changes). MRSA can be carried on contaminated body surfaces (hands, wrists, nose) for more than 3 hours after inoculation.
      b. Communicable from time of infection or colonization
   3. Incubation
      a. Varies with each organism
   4. Risk factors
      a. Numerous and prolonged antibiotic therapies
      b. Prolonged hospitalization
      c. Burn injury
      d. Surgical procedure
      e. Traumatic wounds
   5. Postexposure precautions
      a. None known
   6. Nursing interventions for infection control
      a. *Hand washing before and after every patient contact*
      b. Contact isolation (gowns and gloves when in contact with patient or patient's environment) for duration of hospitalization to prevent nosocomial spread of infection
      c. Private room, or group similar resistant patients together
      d. Collaborate with physician/staff to control antibiotic therapy.
      e. Disinfect surfaces/objects regularly.
F. Epidemiologically significant organisms
   1. Definition: There are many microorganisms that cause nosocomial infections in the hospitalized patient as a result of cross-contamination. Protection of the patient can be achieved through meticulous hand washing and basic infection control measures. However, there are a

few normally nonpathogenic microorganisms that may cause disease in the compromised critical care patient. These organisms are often found in water sources such as flower arrangements and in tap water in many areas of the country. Examples of commonly detected organisms include *Pseudomonas* and *Acinetobacter,* and contamination with these organisms may cause pneumonia or central line sepsis.

2. Transmission/Communicability
   a. Direct contact with contaminated hands or items exposed to tap water (ie, ventilation bag [Ambu-bag] or suction apparatus rinsed in tap water)
   b. Communicable each time exposure occurs
3. Incubation
   a. Nonspecific
4. Risk factors
   a. Wounds
   b. Central venous catheter
   c. Artificial airway (ie, endo- or nasotracheal airway or tracheostomy)
5. Postexposure prophylaxis
   a. None known
6. Nursing interventions for infection control
   a. Universal precautions (see Table 1.1)
   b. Wash hands before and after manipulating IV lines or respiratory and suction apparatus.
   c. Use sterile water to flush suction catheters and to rinse all airway apparatus (ie, ventilation bag or suction apparatus); never rinse patient items in tap water.
   d. Never clean tracheostomy area with gauze soaked in tap water; use sterile saline or water only.
   e. Never allow tap water to come in contact with IV catheter insertion sites.
   f. Avoid handling central venous catheters unless necessary.
   g. Do not allow fresh flowers or potted plants in the patient's room, since they may harbor microorganisms in the water or soil.

References

1. Centers for Disease Control. Recommendations for prevention of HIV transmission in health-care settings. *Morb. Mortal. Wkly. Rep.* 36(suppl. 2S):6S, 1987.

2. Grimes, D. *Infectious Diseases.* St. Louis: Mosby-Year Book, 1991.

3. Bartlett, J. *Pocketbook of Infectious Disease Therapy.* Baltimore: Williams & Wilkins, 1993. P. 166.

4. Dooley, S., et al. Guidelines for Preventing the Transmission of Tuberculosis in Health-Care Settings, with Special Focus on HIV-Related Issues. *Morb. Mortal. Wkly. Rep.* 39:RR-17, 1990.

5. Centers for Disease Control. Hepatitis B virus: A comprehensive strategy for eliminating transmission in the United States through universal childhood vaccination—Recommendations of the Immunization Practices Advisory Committee. *Morb. Mortal. Wkly. Rep.* 40:9, 1991.

CHAPTER **2**

Psychosocial Issues

Susan Krupnick

Physical and emotional crises, suffering, and significant distress occur daily in the critical care environment. The stress of being critically ill, or watching a significant other be critically ill, greatly influences an individual's psychological state and emotional responses. Personality structure in conjunction with the nature of the illness interact to determine what coping strategies an individual will use to manage and decrease stress. Critical care nurses often discover that an individual's anxiety and/or coping strategies are hindering his or her health and recovery as well as the health care provider's ability to deliver effective care. Understanding the specific stressors in critical care and their impact on the patient, family, and nursing staff is of the utmost importance in the delivery of holistic nursing care while balance is maintained in the health care provider's life.

The common presentation of the dying patient in critical care is a significant stressor that impacts on all of these environments and, therefore, is addressed in this discussion of psychosocial issues. In particular, the provocative nature of suicide can produce intense emotional responses in the client, his or her family, and in the health care team. The care of the suicidal patient is specifically addressed in order to provide the critical care nurse with concrete skills and independent nursing strategies to be used in conjunction with suicide aftermath care for the client and self-care strategies for the health care providers.

Stressors in Critical Care: Impact on Patient, Family, and Nursing

I. **Definition:** Stress is a complex psychophysiologic response to the demands of a stressor. A stressor is any internal or external demand(s) that exceed the available resources of the individual. Stress is represented in a variety of responses manifested as anxiety, anger, emotional tension, frustration, an inability to adjust to a situation, or difficulty with judgment- and decision-making abilities.

Stress can be a temporary, continual, or recurrent experience. Recurrent and/or continual stress responses can produce psychologic and/or physiologic exhaustion. Stress is healthy when it produces stimulation and alertness, contributes to personal growth and development, and assists an

▲ 17

individual in meeting personal psychophysiologic needs. However, when stress becomes "distressful" to the individual, it can create feelings of helplessness, apathy, and fatigue, interfering with optimal functioning and eventually contributing to the development of illness.

II. Etiology

A. General adaptation syndrome (Fig. 2.1)
B. Stressors on critically ill patients
   1. Physical stressors
      a. Pain

Figure 2.1 General adaptation syndrome.

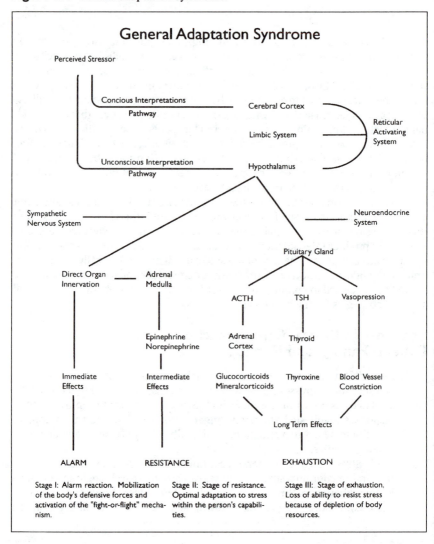

        b. Sleep deprivation
        c. Treatment side effects
    2. Psychological stressors
        a. Fear
        b. Lack of control
        c. Crowding
        d. Depersonalization
        e. Depression
        f. Loss
    3. Sensory stressors
        a. Noise
        b. Lighting
        c. Technologic overload
        d. Lack of environmental cues (lack of outside environment stimulation)
C. Stressors on families of the critically ill
    1. Loss of a "healthy" person to a critically ill patient
    2. Potential death of patient
    3. Separation from patient
    4. Recurrence of own illness
    5. Financial insecurity
    6. Changing family roles/responsibilities
    7. Strange and overwhelming hospital environment
    8. Uncertainty
D. Stressors of critical care nurses
    1. Environment
        a. Crowded work space
        b. Noisy environment
        c. Shift rotation
        d. Inadequate equipment/personnel
    2. Interpersonal (work) relationships
        a. Communication barriers/lack of communication
        b. Lack of authority
        c. Lack of reward
        d. Negative feedback
        e. Nurse/physician relationship difficulties
        f. Patient/family relations
        g. Inexperienced peers
        h. Potential aggression/violence in workplace
    3. Knowledge level
        a. Constant technologic advances
        b. Complicated ever-changing equipment/devices
    4. Patient care
        a. Crisis-laden environment
        b. Continual exposure to loss
        c. Seriousness of patient's condition
    5. Professionalism
        a. Downsizing effect in critical care units
        b. Feelings of inadequacy

III. Assessment

A. Assessment of life stress and coping responses
  1. Assess life events and stressors over last 12 months
     a. Use Holmes and Rahe Social Readjustment Rating Scale to obtain types and degree of cumulative stress that individuals have experienced over the last year.
  2. Assess how individual has coped with these stressors
     a. Problem-focused coping
     b. Emotion-focused coping
B. Assessment of psychophysiologic response to stressors
  1. Behavioral responses
     a. Anger
     b. Defensiveness
     c. "Criticalness," increased criticism of others
     d. Easily upset
     e. Emotional/Prone to outbursts
     f. Irritability
     g. Mood fluctuations
     h. Rigid thinking
     i. Sad
     j. Seeks constant reassurance
     k. Withdrawn
     l. Tearful
  2. Physical responses
     a. Cognitive disturbances
     b. Eating disturbances such as anorexia or overeating
     c. Gastrointestinal (GI) disturbances
     d. Headache
     e. Increased vulnerability to illness or injury
     f. Weight fluctuations
     g. Sleep disturbances
     h. Sympathetic nervous system activation
  3. Kinetic responses
     a. Agitation
     b. Anxiety
     c. Fatigue
     d. Frustration
     e. Restlessness
     f. Tremors
  4. Functioning/Productivity
     a. Accident proneness
     b. Decreased interest in work
     c. Decreased productivity
     d. Sense of being overwhelmed

C. Assessment of present coping measures
  1. Activity
    a. Hobbies
    b. Physical exercise
  2. Chemical mediation
    a. Stimulants
      i. Caffeine
      ii. Nicotine
      iii. Illicit drugs
    b. Depressants
      i. Alcohol
      ii. Prescription medications
      iii. Anxiolytics (antianxiety medication)
      iv. Sleeping medication
      v. Pain medication
  3. Communication
    a. Discussion of problems/conflicts with family, friends, colleagues
    b. Problem solving
  4. Escape mechanisms
    a. Avoidance
    b. Absenteeism, not visiting
    c. Alcohol
    d. Drugs to relax
  5. Mind/Body techniques
    a. Guided imagery
    b. Meditation
    c. Progressive relaxation technique
    d. Self-hypnosis
  6. Nutrition
    a. Compulsive eating behaviors
    b. Balanced eating habits

IV. Stress management strategies for patient, family, and staff members

A. Ineffective individual coping related to inability to manage stress effectively
  1. Problem: anger, agitation, hostility, and emotional instability
  2. Intervention
    a. Initiate a relationship with patient, family member, or staff person
    b. Patient/family teaching
      i. Assertive communication
      ii. Establish realistic expectations and goals
      iii. Relaxation techniques
    c. Assist patient/family in setting reasonable, achievable life-style goals
    d. Encourage patient/family to plan for changes in life-style (proper diet, exercise)

   3. Desired outcomes
       a. Identify and acknowledge sources of stress
       b. Identify and use skills, knowledge, and abilities to cope with stress
       c. No evidence of self-destructive behavior
 B. Potential fear related to life-threatening illness
   1. Problem: anxiety, agitation, fear, panic
   2. Intervention
       a. Observe patient/family for signs of fear
           i. Increased agitation
          ii. Increased heart rate, respiration, blood pressure
         iii. Diaphoresis
          iv. Panic
           v. Pupil dilation
       b. Share and clarify your observations of physical symptoms with pa-
          tient/family.
       c. Remain with patient/family during periods of fear.
       d. Assist patient in identifying source of fear.
       e. Explain all tests, procedures, and expectations to patient and family.
       f. Consultation and collaboration with medical psychiatry to determine
          appropriateness of psychopharmacologic intervention.
       g. Use mental health clinical specialist to assist in developing plan to
          manage patient, family, and staff member conflicts or strain that may
          develop.
   3. Desired outcomes
       a. Diminish and control fear
       b. Use health enhancing coping skills more effectively and frequently
       c. Verbalizations of fears related to life-threatening illness
 C. Potential alteration in family process related to life-threatening ill-
    ness
   1. Problem: family disruption, emotional outbursts, distancing of family
   2. Intervention
       a. Assess family reactions to this crisis situation
       b. Discuss with the patient and family member the impact of the crisis
       c. Assess
           i. Ability to adapt
          ii. Anticipatory grieving
         iii. Expectations of family members
          iv. Negative reactions
           v. Role adjustments
       d. Consider referral for family members to supportive therapy or spiritual
          counseling.
       e. Facilitate access to patient for family members.
   3. Desired outcome
       a. Containment and reduction of crisis and stress symptoms that con-
          tribute to ineffective coping
       b. Effective family problem solving
       c. Patient and family are able to discuss problems and concerns.

D. High risk for violence due to stress of life-threatening illness on patient and family

1. Problem: anger, hostility, verbal intimidation, physical assault

2. Interventions

    a. Assess and document degree of anger/agitation present in patient and family.

        i. Accusatory statements

        ii. Anger

        iii. Fear

        iv. Distrust

        v. Fist clenching

        vi. Pacing

        vii. Swearing

        viii. Screaming

        ix. Shouting

        x. Verbal threats of violence

        xi. Statements expressing loss of control

    b. Determine "reasons" for angry/agitated response by patient or family.

    c. Discuss methods to manage anger without loss of behavior control.

    d. Encourage patient/family to express anger, frustration, or unmet expectations.

    e. Instruct patient/family in relaxation techniques and practice with them.

    f. Collaborate with physical therapy/occupational therapy regarding patient's increased level of physical agitation to facilitate a therapeutic release of tension. This will contribute to improved functional capacity.

    g. Maintain at least an arm's length from an extremely agitated, potentially violent patient or family member.

    h. Attempt verbal engagement and de-escalation of the agitated patient.

    i. Talk *with* the patient/family in a low voice; show concern and respect.

    j. Assure the patient/family that your intention is to help them.

    k. Make certain you have an exit available in case the violence of the patient/family escalates.

    l. Use restrictive/restraining mechanisms for the protection of the patient; monitor the patient every 15 minutes to assure his or her safety.

    m. Explain to family members the reason for using restrictive/restraining devices.

    n. Collaborate with security officer(s) to facilitate the safe exit of the family if it becomes necessary to have them removed.

    o. Directly observe and monitor a potentially violent family member who is visiting a critically ill patient (especially if there has been a history of family/interpersonal violence).

3. Desired outcome

    a. The patient will not harm self, family members, or staff.

    b. Family members will remain safe and nonthreatening toward patient who is critically ill.

    c. Family members will not use threatening behaviors or violence toward staff.

E. Sensory-perceptual alteration/altered thought processes due to delirium in the critically ill patient
  1. Problem: acute confusional state, agitation (intensive care unit [ICU] psychosis, ICU delirium)
  2. Intervention: related to level of agitation (Table 2.1)
  3. Desired outcomes
    a. Patient
      i. Has reduction of hallucinatory experience
      ii. Remains unhurt during delirium
      iii. Recovers with baseline cognitive abilities
      iv. Does not harm staff

Table 2.1 Levels of Agitation

Alarm	Resistance	Exhaustion
Physical Change		
Release of norepinephrine and epinephrine causing vasoconstriction, increased blood pressure, and increased rate and force of cardiac contraction	Hormone levels readjust	Decreased immune response with suppression of T cells and atrophy of thymus
Increased hormone levels	Reduction in activity and size of cortex	Depletion of adrenal glands and hormone production
Enlargement of adrenal cortex	Lymph nodes return to normal size	Weight loss
Marked loss of body weight	Weight returns to normal	Enlargment of lymph nodes and dysfunction of lymphatic system
Shrinkage of thymus, spleen, and lymph nodes		If exposure to the stressor continues, cardiac failure, renal failure, or death may occur
Irritation of the gastric mucosa		
Psychosocial Change		
Increased level of alertness	Increased and intensified use of coping mechanisms	Defense-oriented behaviors become exaggerated
Increased level of anxiety	Tendency to rely on defense-oriented behavior	Disorganization of thinking
Task-oriented, defense-oriented, inefficient, or maladaptive behavior may occur		Disorganization of personality
		Sensory stimuli may be misperceived with appearance of illusion
		Reality contact may be reduced with appearance of delusions or hallucinations
		If exposure to the stressor continues, stupor or violence may occur

b. Family

    i. Will be provided with information about delirium and specific ways members can help the patient

    ii. Will participate in patient's care to keep family involved and feeling competent

The Suicidal Patient in the Critical Care Environment

I. Definition: Suicide is the act of voluntarily and intentionally taking one's own life. Suicide can be accomplished in ways that range from active to passive, acute to chronic, and consciously to unconsciously determined self-destructive behaviors that result in the end of life. Suicide may be methodically planned or committed on an impulse.

There can be two distinct presentations of suicidal behavior: the actively suicidal patient and the potentially suicidal patient. However, potentially suicidal behavior can quickly progress to actively suicidal behavior. Presently suicide is the fifth major cause of death in the United States.

II. Etiology: There are several theoretical explanations addressing the issue of suicide. These theories include psychophysiologic, psychodynamic, and psychosocial conceptualizations.

In the category of psychophysiologic studies, there have been several correlates reported with suicide. In review, lethal suicide attempts and successful suicides tend to be associated with a decrease in the neurotransmitter serotonin in the brain, in conjunction with a decrease in its primary metabolite, 5-hydroxyindoleacetic acid, in the cerebrospinal fluid. Additionally, the ratio of norepinephrine to epinephrine is decreased in the urine of individuals who have attempted suicide while corticotropic releasing factor (CRF) is demonstrated to be hypersecreted. These findings suggest the presence of hyperactivity in the hypothalamic–pituitary–adrenal axis in suicidal patients. Another significant biochemical finding is the dexamethasone suppression test (DST), which demonstrates high rates of nonsuppression among those who attempt or succeed in suicide.

The psychodynamic model of suicide focuses on the individual, specifically his or her personality development and ability to balance between two basic instincts—the will to live and the will to die. Some theorists characterize suicidal individuals as narcissistic and attempting to harm or hurt others by destroying themselves. Other theorists propose that under sufficient distress and conflict, the wish to die defeats the wish to live.

Finally, the psychosocial framework of suicide behavior explores the factors that influence the relationship between the individual and his or her sociocultural system. The psychosocial perspective attempts to provide meaning to the rising statistics of suicide in the United States. A specific finding is that individuals who repeat attempts at suicide tend to have histories of more frequent episodes, beginning at an earlier age. They experience more powerlessness and normlessness and suffer more feelings of externally directed hostility.

In reality the psychophysiologic, psychodynamic, and psychosocial factors interact in complex systems. Therefore, multiple interactive etiologies are involved in producing suicidal behavior.

III. Assessment
A. Mental status assessment
  1. Behavior and general appearance
      a. Verbalizes direct statements such as, "I want to die," "I wish I were dead," "the voices are telling me to hurt/kill myself"
      b. Makes indirect statements about "not being here anymore," "they will miss me," "I know the pain will be over soon"
      c. Asks about suicide methods
      d. Hides medication to ingest later
      e. Shows agitation
      f. Neglects personal hygiene and appearance
  2. Focused suicide assessment
      a. A directed interview with a focused suicide assessment must be completed by a psychiatric/mental health professional before decreasing the level of observation, transferring the patient from the critical care unit, or discharging the patient from the hospital.
      b. A focused suicide assessment includes the following questions:
          i. Have you ever felt depressed for several days at a time?
          ii. During this time, have you ever had thoughts of killing yourself?
          iii. When did these thoughts occur?
          iv. What did you think about doing to yourself?
          v. Did you act on your thoughts?
          vi. How often have these thoughts occurred?
          vii. When is the last time you had these thoughts?
          viii. Have your thoughts ever included harming someone else in addition to yourself?
          ix. How often has that occurred?
          x. What have you thought about doing to the other person?
          xi. What would be the outcome or benefit of this act toward this other person?
          xii. When does this thought occur?
          xiii. Recently, what specifically have you thought about doing to yourself?
          xiv. Have you taken any steps toward acquiring the means (gun, pills) of suicide? Do you presently have a weapon (gun) at home? What other equipment (bullets, rope, pills) is still in your home?
          xv. Have you thought when you would do this?
          xvi. Have you thought about where you would do this?
          xvii. Have you thought about what effect your death would have on your friends and others?
          xviii. You sound ambivalent or unsure about these plans. What are some of the reasons that have kept you from acting on them thus far?
          xix. More specifically, what are your feelings about religion, suicide, and God?

           xx. What are your thoughts about your responsibilities for your family and children if you kill yourself?
           xxi. What are your thoughts about other reasons for living and staying alive?
           xxii. What help would make it easier for you to cope with your current thoughts and plans?
           xxiii. Have you made any plans for your possessions or to communicate with people after your death such as a note or a will?
           xxiv. How does talking about this make you feel?

  3. Mood/emotional responses/coping
    a. Depression is a major risk factor for all age groups.
    b. Hopelessness is more predictive of suicide than depression.
    c. Individuals with personality disorders have an increased rate of suicide.
    d. Unrelieved anxiety disorder, particularly pain disorder
    e. Excessive guilt and self-blame
    f. Low self-esteem
    g. Chemical abuse

  4. Thoughts, beliefs, and perceptions
    a. Chaotic, disorganized, and/or irrational thinking
    b. Delusions of persecution
    c. Hallucinations, especially command hallucinations, telling the patient to commit suicide
    d. Poor judgment
    e. Poor impulse control

  5. Interpersonal relationships
    a. Recent loss of significant other(s) through death, divorce, separations
    b. Cumulative losses in a limited time frame
    c. Social isolation and withdrawal
    d. Recent psychotherapy termination/interruption of psychiatric treatment
    e. Availability of social support

  6. Physical illness
    a. Chronic, debilitating, terminal, or traumatic illness
    b. Chronic pain
    c. Recent, catastrophic loss of physical functions

B. Physical examination
  1. Level of treatment required
    a. First aid, emergency department care
    b. Hospital admission, routine care
    c. Critical care, aggressive technologic treatment

  2. Agent or method used
    a. Ingestion (overdose), cutting, stabbing
    b. Drowning, asphyxiation, self-strangulation
    c. Jumping, shooting

  3. Injury/Lesions/Toxicity
    a. Minimal
    b. Moderate
    c. Severe

4. Physical function recovery
   a. Good: complete recovery predicted
   b. Fair: recovery expected over time
   c. Poor: residual deficits expected
   d. Not reversible: no recovery expected
5. System assessment during critical care phase
   a. Cardiovascular system: Monitor for hemodynamic instability due to cardiovascular disruptions from overdose or direct traumatic injury.
   b. Respiratory system: Monitor respiratory function for possible aspiration, respiratory failure due to medication overdose, ingestion of toxic chemicals, or asphyxiation.
   c. Musculoskeletal system: Assess functional alterations due to traumatic injuries from motor vehicle crashes, jumping, stabbing, or gunshot wounds.
   d. Neurological: Assess central and peripheral nervous system function related to attempted suicide; monitor degree of impaired consciousness.
      i. No impairment demonstrated
      ii. Confusion
      iii. Stuporous
      iv. Comatose
C. Diagnostic parameters
   1. Comprehensive serum and urine toxicology screen: If the chosen method of suicide is medication overdose or toxic chemical ingestion, comprehensive serum/urine toxicology screens are necessary to obtain baseline data to plan medical/nursing care during the critical illness phase.
   2. *Hemoglobin/Hematocrit* is necessary to assess degree of hematologic stability, especially when the chosen method is cutting, stabbing, or jumping, which have produced significant overt/covert injuries and potential blood loss.
   3. Arterial blood gases: Monitor for acidoses pH less than 7.35, carboxyhemoglobin due to a carbon monoxide poisoning.
   4. Urinalysis: Myoglobinuria may exist due to muscle destruction (rhabdomyolysis) from toxic chemical ingestion or from remaining in a confined position after an overdose.

IV. Patient/family management

A. In planning comprehensive care in the patient who survives the suicide attempt, the nurse needs to use the following questions to direct care:
   1. Is the patient actively suicidal?
   2. What is the degree of lethality of the plan?
   3. Does the patient need to be in a protected environment? Does he or she need to be monitored closely until a protective environment is arranged?
   4. What is the level of commitment from the patient's support system?
B. Potential for self-directed violence related to suicidal ideation and poor impulse control
   1. Problem: self-harm, self-injury
   2. Intervention

a. Assess current suicide risk.

b. Seek consultation with medical psychiatry services to determine level of suicidality.

c. Implement appropriate level of observation/precaution; 1:1 if necessary (in accordance with hospital policy).

d. Notify all appropriate staff if patient is placed on suicide precautions.

e. Acknowledge feelings and explain precautions; inform patients that staff members will protect them until they are able to resist impulses.

f. Provide a safe physical and interpersonal environment based on level of suicide risk.

g. Do not promise absolute confidentiality about pertinent information that is important for the entire health team to know in planning and delivering care.

h. Document all patient/family contacts and planning; include assessment of risk and plan with specific restrictions, the method and frequency of observation, and staff responsibility for observation and escort if going out of unit for diagnostic procedures.

i. Arrange consultation and collaboration with psychiatric/mental health specialist and social worker to facilitate comprehensive psychosocial assessment and effective plan of care.

j. Transfer to psychiatric services when patient is medically stable.

3. Desired outcome

a. Patient remains safe.

b. Patient doesn't act on suicidal impulses while in hospital.

c. Patient/family verbalizes thoughts, feelings of suicide attempt.

C. Ineffective family coping: compromised due to completed suicide of patient

1. Problem: death of patient in critical care environment related to successful suicide

2. Intervention

a. Provide an opportunity for family to discuss the death of the patient.

b. Encourage consultation and use of psychiatric mental health specialist to assess and assist family in coping with loss and dealing with the impact of a successful suicide.

c. Discuss fears family members are experiencing.

d. Allow family members to express feelings (especially anger) toward the patient for abandoning them; allow family to discuss their feelings about not being able to prevent the suicide from occurring.

e. Refer to a survivors of suicide group such as the following:
   - Survivors of Suicide (SOS)
   - Loving Outreach to Survivors of Suicide (LOSS)
   - Striving to Reach Every Survivor of Suicide (STRESS)

V. Patient teaching and home health considerations

A. Patient survives suicide attempt

1. Confirm patient has been cleared by medical psychiatry services.

2. Assure that patient/family (if discharged from critical care unit) has outpatient referral appointments before leaving unit.

3. Ensure that both patient and family have written instructions concerning how to obtain emergency assistance if suicidal impulses return.
4. Review with patient/family indications of exacerbation of suicidality.
B. Patient dies from successful suicide
   1. Be available to family members and provide community support information after they return home.
   2. Encourage the survivor(s) to attend and participate in a support group.
   3. Review with survivors the importance of follow-up with mental health consultation to effectively manage psychologic trauma, shock, and grief.

Death/Dying

I. **Definition:** Death is an inevitable event every living being faces. Dying is a process, which can occur suddenly or over time and involves the dying person, family members, friends, colleagues, and the health care providers working with the patient.

   Death of the body as a whole is known as somatic death. When cessation of vital organs such as the heart, lung, and brain occurs, cellular death proceeds in a rapid though uneven manner. This downward spiral of function produces cellular death throughout the entire organism. The entire system does not fail simultaneously; instead, each organ ceases functioning at a different rate. This cessation of function can be specific for each individual.

   Understanding the complex physiologic interrelationships between cell death, somatic death, and the failure of vital organs is an integral but only initial step in developing nursing care for the dying patient and his or her family. Knowledge and attention to the underlying physiologic changes during the dying process can facilitate the health care provider's ability to alleviate pain, discomfort, and suffering, improving the overall quality of remaining life and minimizing the negative effects of the dying process on family members.

II. **Process of dying:** During the last hours of life, there are three important aspects of the dying process: the death watch, the death scene, and the final death. The death watch must be facilitated by the health care providers caring for the patient and family members. Physiologic control is achieved by aggressive pain control/management, sleep promotion, and relief of anxiety and restlessness while promoting overall comfort for the patient and family members. It is of primary concern to health care providers, family members, and friends that the patient not die in a tortured manner or alone. The death watch can last for hours, where the death scene is typically brief and terminates at the time of the patient's actual physiologic death and with the ritual of pronouncing death of the patient. Many times the family members are most intimately involved in this final aspect of the death process.

   There are several expected death patterns that describe when the patient is expected to die and in what type of predictable manner. Health care providers can assess when a patient will die and, therefore, can plan their nursing care in an appropriate manner. Death patterns can be delineated in the following five categories: (1) too sudden death, (2) fluctuating pattern, (3) certain death within a known time, (4) certain death within an unknown time, and (5) lingering.

III. Assessment

A. Pattern of patient's illness
   1. What are the medical diagnoses?
   2. When and how was the "bad news" given? How often and recent?
   3. Who delivered the "bad news" and how was it done?
   4. What does the patient and family understand about the illness?
   5. Is the patient still actively participating in decisions and treatment?
   6. Does the patient acknowledge physical limits and/or symptoms that are related to illness and treatment?

B. Stage of dying trajectory
   1. Acute phase: begins when the patient initially learns that death is a possibility
   2. Chronic living-dying phase: characterized by an increase in physical limitations, decreased functional status, and increase in dependence. This is a period of exacerbations and remissions; however, the general trajectory is a downward spiral.
   3. Terminal phase: characterized by generalized physical exhaustion. The patient is experiencing his last hospitalization.

C. Coping assessment
   1. Is the patient/family aware of the "terminal" diagnosis?
   2. How are the patient and family coping? What specific behaviors or defense mechanisms are being used by the patient and family?
   3. What degree of agitation or anger is present in the patient?
   4. What fears exist—unknown, loneliness, sorrow, loss of bodily function, loss of self-control, pain/suffering, loss of self-identity/self-worth, regression?
   5. How much control does the patient have over decisions in the remaining days?
   6. Is the patient/family requesting staff members to be in the room?
   7. Is the patient/family restricting visitors?

D. Pain assessment
   1. Degree of pain experienced
   2. What does the patient report reduces the pain? What increases the pain?
   3. What makes the patient comfortable?
   4. What is the patient's attitude toward the pain?

E. Spiritual and cultural assessment
   1. What hopes does the patient have?
   2. Who are the spiritual professionals important to the patient?
   3. What is the patient's and family's cultural view of death?
   4. What specific rituals are necessary or important?

F. Assessment of death preparations
   1. What are the "tasks" that the patient and family still need to accomplish?
   2. What preparations for dying has the patient made? (These include wills, funeral arrangements, living will, final messages.)
   3. Where does the patient want to die?

G. Assessment of past losses in life

H. Assessment of family coping
1. Is the family capable of carrying out the patient's wishes?
2. Does the family need additional support to make decisions when the patient is unable to do so?

IV. Patient/family management

A. Self-care deficit related to terminal phase of critical illness
1. Problem: increased dependence for physical care due to critical illness with active dying process
2. Interventions: physical care of the dying patient includes attention to the following aspects of nursing care
    a. Elimination: Keep the incontinent patient clean, dry, and odor-free, and assess for impaction; the nurse's attitude when dealing with the incontinent patient may communicate rejection or protective care.
    b. Hair: Cared-for hair has a great influence on self-image and self-esteem.
    c. Mucous membranes: The nose, mouth, and eyes need to be kept moist and clean; use of lubricants and mouthwashes is desirable.
    d. Nutrition and hydration: Small, frequent feedings of favorite foods are likely to be accepted; ice chips or favorite soft drinks need to be available constantly if the patient is capable of nutritional intake.
    e. Positioning: Frequent positioning is necessary to protect the patient from skin breakdown and to ensure that the airway is not partially or totally obstructed.
    f. Skin: Skin should be clean; lotion should be applied to provide moisture; and pressure areas should be protected from skin breakdown and decubitus formation. Massage therapy can be used for skin and muscle integrity, as well as a pain management and relaxation strategy.
3. Desired outcome: to provide physical care and maintain hygiene and comfort for the patient

B. Pain related to physiologic alterations due to terminal phase of critical illness
1. Problem: fear, procedural intolerance, emotional distress, anxiety
2. Intervention
    a. Use medications (both analgesics and antianxiety agents when appropriate) in *adequate* doses to provide pain relief.
    b. Consultation to clinical specialist in pain management to establish an effective regimen
    c. Utilize alternative measures such as hypnosis, guided imagery, massage, and acupunctural pressure therapy as adjuncts of pain medication. (At a late stage of dying, it is not appropriate to attempt imagery or hypnosis if the patient has not already used them.)
3. Desired outcome
    a. Patient and family report or acknowledge pain relief.
    b. Patient is able to participate in his or her care within restrictions of his physical condition.
    c. Absence of objective symptoms/signs of pain response
    d. Absence of or diminished level of agitation

C. Anxiety related to impending death due to helplessness, loss of control, and abandonment

 1. Problem: fear(s), anxiety, ineffective coping, increased sympathetic nervous system responses

 2. Interventions: emotional care of the dying patient and his or her family

   a. Spend time daily with patient, creating an accepting atmosphere.

   b. Listen rather than talk; allow for the expression of feelings.

   c. Allow and support the patient's own decision making in regard to planning time of care, visitors, and continued treatment.

   d. Use touch when the patient indicates through verbal or nonverbal behavior (crying, relating sad stories) that it is needed.

   e. Meet with family and significant others to answer questions, listen to feelings, provide information, and give support.

   f. Allow as much time as the patient needs with family and significant others.

   g. Make appropriate referrals, based on the patient's wishes, to social worker, psychiatric clinical specialist, lawyer, minister, priest, or rabbi.

   h. Aid the patient in completing unfinished business.

   i. If the patient is not able to be a decision maker, assist family members in making decisions.

   j. Use anxiolytic medication in conjunction with relaxation strategies to manage anxiety.

   k. Explain all tests and procedures to patient and family. Also include what the patient is expected to do during the process.

 3. Desired outcomes: Patient and family do the following

   a. Confront and express fears

   b. Express feelings

   c. Use support services offered to them

   d. Demonstrate a diminished level of death-related anxiety

   e. Complete preparations for death

D. Anticipatory grieving related to potential loss of significant other, death of self

 1. Problem: cognitive changes, behavioral changes, altered feelings, somatic symptoms

 2. Interventions

   a. Determine what is known or feared about potential loss.

   b. Encourage open discussion of fears and concerns.

   c. Identify and validate impact of previous experiences with loss.

   d. Avoid either reinforcing denial or causing a premature disruption of the denial process during the early stage of shock and disbelief.

   e. Instill hope for the abilities of patient and family to cope with loss.

   f. Identify the need for information of the patient and family.

   g. Provide family with ongoing, honest information concerning patient's clinical status and plan of care.

   h. Facilitate communication (when possible) between patient and significant others.

        i. Consult bereavement or mental health specialist and pastoral services to assist in supporting patient and family members.

        j. Encourage family members to maintain their own self-care.

        k. Identify any indications of dysfunctional grieving (suicidal ideation/ intent, pathologic denial, uncontrolled behavior such as violence).

3. Desired outcome

    a. Patient and family will express thoughts and feelings about the anticipated loss.

    b. Patient and family are able to make informed decisions related to the anticipated loss.

    c. Family members maintain constructive relationships.

    d. An "appropriate" death is achieved, which meets the following expectations:

        i. Conflict reduction

        ii. Reinforcement of significant relationships

        iii. Behavior is in alignment with patient's ideals and values.

        iv. Basic instincts and wishes are realized.

V. Interventions for health care provider staff to manage the impact of disenfranchised grief

A. Actively participate in staff meetings and support group meetings with mental health nurse specialist to explore nursing staff members' feelings about dying patients.

B. Clearly communicate, during report time and in team meetings, exactly what the patient and family know, with specific discussions about level of care decisions that have transpired.

C. Use ethics committee consultation for health care, patient, and/or family conflicts surrounding a difficult death event.

D. Use peer consultation to validate personal feelings of loss.

E. Use personal mental health consultation to assist in identification and management of disenfranchised grief.

VI. Patient and family teaching and home health considerations

A. Immediate "postloss" emotional care for family members

    1. Review care provided to patient.

    2. Determine if family members would like to see the patient before leaving the hospital.

    3. Consultation with spiritual leader, social worker, or mental health clinical specialist may be necessary if grief response is intense and family exhibits ineffective coping with loss.

    4. Provide referral to bereavement therapist.

    5. Arrange a mental health clinical specialist follow-up after 24 hours to determine level of coping.

    6. Provide referral to support group.

B. Patient leaving critical care unit to be cared for at home with high-technology–assisted nursing care

    1. Instruct patient and family on what to expect concerning illness trajectory.

2. Arrange a family member to "sleep over" in the critical care unit to facilitate family members' knowledge and skills in caring for patients.
3. Arrange referral and consultation to discharge planning team members to facilitate a smooth transition to the home care setting.
4. Encourage family members to participate in counseling if hospice or home care program has access to mental health specialist to explore impact of a family member dying at home.

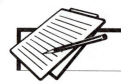

CHAPTER **3**

Trauma

Laurie Zone-Smith

I. Definition: Trauma is the physical injury caused by intentional and unintentional forces exerted on the body. Traumatic injuries kill nearly 150,000 Americans a year and leave 60 million injured and 300,000 permanently disabled. Trauma is the leading cause of death in persons 45 years old or younger and is ranked as the fourth major cause of death in all age groups [1]. *The trimodal death distribution* illustrates three peaks of death after injury [2].

A. Peak 1: 50% of deaths occur in the first few minutes after injury resulting from massive head or thoracic injuries, high spinal cord damage, large vessel transections (aortic), and exsanguination.

B. Peak 2: 30–35% of deaths occur 1–3 hours after injury resulting from hemothorax or pneumothorax; subdural or epidural hematoma; hypovolemic shock secondary to uncontrolled hemorrhage of the liver, spleen, femur; or pelvic fractures.

C. Peak 3: 10% of deaths occur days to weeks after injury as a result of sepsis, multisystem organ failure, and the secondary effects of trauma.

The trauma continuum of care begins at the event of injury and ends with full recovery, temporary or permanent disability, or death. Interventions by trained prehospital, medical, and nursing personnel can impact a trauma patient's outcome and potentially fatal complications.

II. Etiology. *Mechanism of injury:* Potential injuries and secondary complications can be predicted by knowing the mechanism of injury. The extent and nature of injury depend on the type of force applied and the body's response to the applied energy. Traumatic injuries are generally divided into blunt and penetrating assaults. Compression, crushing, shearing, acceleration, and deceleration forces can damage protective tissue, bones, organs, and muscle structures. Blunt trauma can be more life-threatening than penetrating trauma because of the potential for injuries to go unrecognized and undiagnosed. Burns are also considered traumatic injuries (see Chap. 10).

A. Blunt trauma patterns of injury: The cause of injury in penetrating trauma is the energy formed and transmitted by the penetrating instrument into the surrounding tissue. Organs commonly punctured include liver, small intestines, vascular structures, and spleen. Intestinal penetrating damage has significant mortality due to septic complications from fecal contamination. The injuries depend on the site of impact, the position of the assailant (angle of penetration), and type of instrument used.

1. Motor vehicle accidents: These accidents are the leading cause of death for Americans between the ages of 1 and 34 years [3].
   a. Head-on/rear-end collisions: Injuries of the aortic arch, liver, spleen, diaphragm, kidneys, and bowels causing tears and ruptures; lacerations to the face, chin, or mouth; anterior neck bruising; and injuries to the chest or abdomen with underlying cardiac contusion. Rear impact can result in hyperextension of the neck, commonly referred to as "whiplash."
   b. Lateral impact ("T-bone" impact): Impact on the driver's side will potentiate left-sided fractures and splenic injury. Impact on the passenger's side may cause right-sided injuries and liver involvement. May have contralateral injury of the head, neck and spine, pelvis, chest, abdomen.
   c. Rollover/ejection: High probability of multisystem injuries.
   d. Front-seat passenger/no safety belt: Injuries include fracture/dislocation of the ankle, knee, femur; posterior dislocation of the acetabulum; compression injuries of abdomen, chest, head, neck; and maxillofacial region.
   e. Limited use of safety devices: Shoulder harness alone can lead to bruising, severe lacerations, rib fractures, and neck injuries. Lap belt use only can cause facial, head, neck, chest, lumbar spine, and bladder injuries. A lap belt worn too high causes soft abdominal injury and thoracolumbar and spinal injuries.

2. Motorcycle and bicycle crashes: Head on, lateral impact, ejection, and laying the bike down commonly result in fractures to the skull, neck, ribs, or extremities; avulsions; abrasions; and "road rash." Head injury is the cause of 75% of motorcycle deaths. Head injuries are reduced with protective helmet use [4].

3. Pedestrian vs vehicle: Closed or open fractures of lower extremities including ankle, patella, tibia, fibula, femur, pelvis, head, thoracic, abdominal and spinal injuries

4. Falls or jumps: In general, in any fall greater than 15 feet, suspect internal injuries. Spinal and brain injury, bilateral skeletal fractures of the calcaneus (heel bone), lower extremities, long bones and pelvis; vertical shear and compression fractures. Axial loading (force applied upward or downward without bending) of cervical vertebral and lumbar spine may result in burst fractures, compression fractures, dislocations or disk extrusion, detachment of thoracic aorta and solid organs such as the liver or spleen, or Colles' fracture. Backward falls onto the occiput cause high-mortality skull fractures [5].

5. Aggravated assaults: Stomach perforation, diaphragmatic laceration and esophageal rupture, lacerated liver or spleen, or acute subdural hematoma.
6. Gunshot wound: Tissue cells move forward and laterally from the site, causing tissue compression and stretching in a process called *cavitation*. The result is tissue, bone, and organ destruction from burning, expanding gases. Bullet entry wounds may or may not have corresponding exit wounds. Usually, exit wounds are larger than entry wounds and have frayed edges. Each tissue wound and tract of the bullet trajectory should be considered carefully.
7. Impalement/stab wound: Impaled objects should only be explored and removed in the operating room. Diaphragmatic thoracic injuries (below the fourth intercostal space) may involve structures in the abdomen. One in four people sustaining penetrating abdominal injuries have associated chest injuries [6]. Extensive internal damage may result from weapon movement.

III. Nursing process. Bodily response to trauma: Each traumatized patient incurs varying disruptions in the hemodynamic, immunologic, and metabolic systems of the body. Improved survivability of trauma patients is accomplished by early and aggressive management of bleeding, airway complications, and infectious complications and by assurance of adequate nutritional intake.

A. Hemodynamic response: Trauma and injury are the most common causes of life-threatening hemorrhagic or hypotensive shock states. Hemorrhage (acute bleeding) may be obvious or occult. The extent of injury and sum of lost blood correlates with four stages of shock. Fluid replacement for all stages should include crystalloids.
1. Assessment
   a. Signs and symptoms (for a 70-kg person)
      i. Mild hemorrhage—up to 15% of blood volume (750 mL): slight hypotension due to low blood volume; tachycardia > 100 beats/minute to increase cardiac output; cool, pale skin; anxiety; dilated pupils; capillary refill (> 2 seconds); fluid shifts; sympathetic response; release of norepinephrine and epinephrine hormones, all in order to increase cardiac output. Responds to fluid resuscitation.
      ii. Moderate hemorrhage—up to 25% of blood volume (1250 mL): moderate hypotension (> 90 mm Hg systolic); hypoxia due to decrease in oxygen-carrying capacity; tachycardia (> 100 beats/minute); tachypnea; cool, pale skin; capillary refill poor; lethargy; weakness; decreased urine output (< 25 mL/hour); venous return decrease; "looks bad." Responds to fluid resuscitation.
      iii. Severe hemorrhage—up to 35% of blood volume (1800 mL): moderate to severe hypotension (60–90 mm Hg systolic); hypoxia; tachycardia (> 120 beats/min); cold; cyanosis; agitation; confusion; decreased urine output (< 15 mL/hour); shunting to

core organs (brain, heart, kidneys), metabolic dysfunction. Refractory to crystalloid fluid resuscitation. Likely to need blood transfusion and surgery to correct the underlying problem.

iv. Extreme hemorrhage—up to 50% of blood volume (2500 mL): profound hypotension (< 60 mm Hg systolic), severe hypoxia, bradycardia with decreased pulse pressures, skin cold and mottled, oliguria, unconscious; may result in irreversible cell and organ death. Exsanguination and circulatory failure lead to cardiac arrest [1].

b. Diagnostic tests

i. Serum

- *Trauma laboratory protocol:* Used for most patients with severe trauma. Includes complete blood count, chemistry, coagulation studies, arterial blood gases (ABG), toxicology screen, liver function tests (LFT), amylase, urine analysis, and blood tests for type and crossmatch.

- Complete blood count: Used as an indicator of the severity of blood loss, need for blood transfusion, and assessment of ongoing blood loss (based on progressively decreasing hemoglobin and hematocrit), and provides baseline values for white blood cells, red blood cells, and platelets.

- Chemistry: Provides data for assessment of electrolyte imbalances, particularly important in cases of hypovolemia and dehydration. Also helpful to evaluate renal function based on blood urea nitrogen (BUN) and creatinine values.

- Coagulation studies: Most commonly used are the prothrombin time and partial thromboplastin time. May be altered in cases of severe injury or when coagulopathy develops.

- ABG: Important for the assessment of respiratory dysfunction, hypoxemia, hypercarbia, and metabolic or respiratory acid–base imbalances.

- Toxicology: Useful for the assessment of alcohol intoxication and presence of illicit drugs, any of which may cause alterations in the patient's mental status.

- LFT: Frequently used as an early indicator of liver injury. Also helpful to assess for the presence of chronic liver disease.

- Amylase: Indicator of pancreatic injury. May also be elevated in cases of severe peritonitis.

ii. Urine

- Urine analysis: The presence of red blood cells in the urine may suggest renal or urogenital trauma. In addition, the urine can be used for toxicology screen and assessment of adequacy of renal function. Concentrated urine with high specific gravity is commonly seen with hypovolemia and dehydration.

iii. Other

- Plain radiographs: Commonly ordered x-rays in all patients with severe blunt trauma include: three-view cervical spine x-rays, anterior–posterior views of the chest and pelvis, and x-rays of any injured extremity. In penetrating trauma it is useful to mark the entry and exit sites (paper clips are good radiopaque markers) prior to obtaining x-rays, so that the piercing object trajectory and possible injuries can be assessed.

- Vascular contrast studies: The most frequently used is an aortogram to evaluate the presence of aortic or great vessel injuries in cases of enlarged mediastinum (by chest x-ray) or penetrating lower-neck and chest injuries.
- Computed axial tomography (CT) scan: Particularly helpful in the assessment of closed head injury (for head CT scan, intravenous contrast is not needed) or suspected spine injuries. Also used in the evaluation of blunt abdominal and pelvic trauma (in this case, oral and intravenous contrasts are very important to allow accurate assessment of visceral or retroperitoneal injuries).
- Ultrasound: Has been used on an experimental basis to evaluate abdominal trauma. This modality is more useful for the echocardiographic assessment of the heart and the pericardium (important in the management of myocardial contusion and pericardial tamponade). Doppler scans are also used in evaluating peripheral vessels.
- Gastrointestinal and urogenital contrast studies: These are essential for the assessment of suspected urethral or bladder injuries, as well as trauma involving the esophagus. Water soluble contrast (and not barium) should be used.
- Diagnostic peritoneal lavage (DPL): An invasive surgical procedure frequently used in the assessment of blunt abdominal trauma. The procedure involves the instillation of 1 liter of crystalloid solution in the peritoneal cavity. After 5–10 minutes the fluid is drained and analyzed for the presence of blood cells, bacteria, amylase, and foreign substances. The presence of 100,000 red blood cells/mm^3 or more and greater than 500 white blood cells/mm^3 is considered positive and operative intervention is indicated. If gross blood is found during the initial tap no further analysis is needed and the DPL is considered positive [1]. There is ongoing controversy regarding the use of DPL versus CT scanning in the assessment of blunt abdominal trauma.

2. Patient management
   a. Inadequate tissue perfusion related to actual fluid volume deficit caused by hemorrhage
      i. Problem: depleted blood volume; decreased cardiac output; decreased oxygen delivery with increased demand at the tissue level; cellular injury and death; multiple organ failure
      ii. Intervention
         - Resuscitative phase
         ○ Administer 100% oxygen; ventilatory support as needed.
         ○ Control bleeding (ie, direct pressure, pneumatic antishock garment; identify the source of hemorrhage.
         ○ Consider Trendelenburg position to increase venous return

○ Administer warmed fluid replacement through two large-bore IV catheters (14–16 g) with large-bore trauma tubing. Rapid bolus administration of 1–2 liters lactated Ringer's solution. General replacement rule: administer 3 mL of crystalloid solution for every 1 mL of blood loss, dependent on clinical picture.

○ Type and crossmatch for 4–6 U of packed red blood cells. In cases of severe hemorrhage and hypovolemia (> 35% loss of blood volume) significant impairment in venous return and cardiac output are present. Replacement of blood (type-specific or O-negative) in addition to crystalloid infusion is essential.

○ Monitor vital signs: a palpable radial pulse = a systolic blood pressure of 80 mm Hg or higher; a palpable femoral pulse = 70 mm Hg; and a palpable carotid pulse = 60 mm Hg.

○ Monitor urine output: urine output of at least 50 mL/hour indicates adequate resuscitation.

○ Recognize signs and symptoms of hemorrhagic shock: hypotension (< 90 mm Hg systolic); weak or thready fast pulse (≥ 120 beats/minute); decreased cardiac output; increased peripheral resistance; pale, cold, and clammy skin; level of consciousness dwindling (restless, anxious, combative to unconscious); delayed capillary refill greater than 2 seconds; shallow tachypnea; decreased urinary output; hypothermia; acidosis; complaints of thirst.

○ If pneumothorax or hemothorax is present, assist physician with chest tube placement. Connect chest tube to autotransfusion collection system and monitor for sudden increase or decrease in drainage; if blood not contaminated, autotransfuse within 4 hours; for continuous blood loss of greater than 200 mL/hour, consider thoracotomy for hemorrhage control.

○ Immediate surgical intervention for major trauma, including tube thoracostomy and emergency thoracotomy. Open thoracotomy cardiac massage can be life-saving with penetrating injury but rarely with blunt trauma.

▪ Critical care phase

○ Administer oxygen as needed; prepare to intubate and ventilate if necessary.

○ Monitor oxygen saturation, keep pulse oxygenation greater than 94%.

○ Adjust ventilator settings to keep end-tidal carbon dioxide tension less than 45 mm Hg.

○ Continue to administer crystalloids as needed to maintain systolic blood pressure greater than 90 mm Hg; heart rate less than 100 beats/minute; and cardiac output, pulmonary artery pressures, central venous pressure, and venous oxygen saturation normal. May need blood transfusion.

○ Monitor and document ABG results with every ventilator change or as needed (use pulse oximetry trend as a guide). Discuss needed changes with physician.

- ○ Consider administration of vasoactive drugs, but ensure that fluid repletion is completed before initiating (see Chap. 5).
- ○ Monitor and maintain urine output (UOP) greater than 50 mL/hour (must be greater than 1 mL/kg per hour for children). If myoglobin is present in urine from severe muscle or burn injury, maintain UOP greater than 100 mL/hour to avoid nephrotoxicity.
- ○ Assess pulses and skin temperature every hour.
- ○ Complete neurologic exams every 1–4 hours to assess cerebral perfusion.
- ○ Monitor chemistry lab work to assess renal function (BUN, creatinine) and LFT. Follow serial hemoglobin/hematocrit electrolyte imbalances.

   iii. Desired outcome
- Adequate oxygen perfusion of tissues and organs as evidenced by normal mentation, UOP greater than 50 mL/hour, normal renal and electrolyte lab values.
- Bleeding controlled with appropriate wound management or operative intervention. Remember that hemorrhage from solid organs (such as liver and spleen) can be self-limited if the extent of injury is not severe.
- Arterial pressure, cardiac output, venous oxygen saturation, and central venous pressure return to baseline.
- Vital signs return to normal range.
- Shock and fluid volume overload are avoided evidenced by clear lung fields and absence of edema.

 b. Anxiety related to acute decrease of health status and actual threat of death
   i. Problem: fear of dying, restlessness to combativeness, hopelessness, resistance to treatment.
   ii. Interventions
- Immediate nursing actions to reverse traumatic shock descent.
- Ensure patient has adequate pain medication coverage. Patients who use illicit drugs may require large doses of pain medications.
- Listen to the patient.
- Talk to the patient and family; explain interventions and provide information as appropriate.
- Maintain hopeful outlook.
- Allow family and patient private time.
- Encourage family members to remain close by as appropriate.
- Be prepared to repeat instructions many times.
- Administer antianxiety medications as needed.
- Accurately assess alcohol and illicit drug use prior to trauma.
- Alcohol withdrawal will cause severe anxiety and should be avoided with appropriate prophylactic treatment: lorazepam and oxazepam.

lorazepam, oxazepam
Action Depresses the CNS to decrease anxiety and agitation.
Administration Guidelines Lorazepam 2–6 mg orally daily in
  divided doses or 0.05 mg/kg intramuscularly or intravenously every
  4–6 hours; oxazepam: 15–30 mg orally three or four times daily.
Special Considerations Use cautiously in patients with
  myasthenia gravis or Parkinson's disease because drug may
  exacerbate symptoms; may cause lethargy.

- Consult psychologists, social workers, and clergy personnel as
  needed.
iii. Desired outcome
- Patient able to follow commands, verbalize feelings and complaints, and make appropriate health care and recovery decisions.
- Patient and family feel supported and cared for by the trauma
  team.
- Patient states pain and anxiety relieved.

B. Immunologic response: Early recognition of any form of infection in the
trauma patient is essential to avoid bacteremia, sepsis, and multisystem
organ failure. This will reduce morbidity and save lives. Increased bacterial
proliferation and colonization may activate acute inflammatory, chemical,
and cellular responses. Common sources of infection include wound and
extended pressure sites; respiratory and urinary tracts; and the gastrointestinal system, all of which can lead to bacteremia. Other potential sources
include bacterial translocation from the gastrointestinal tract; sinus infections; tooth, brain, abdominal/perirectal abscesses; organ and tissue infections of the heart lining, colon, pancreas, gallbladder, prostate, appendix, or
ears; and indwelling catheters and lines. See Table 3.1 for a list of common
infectious organisms in trauma.

1. Assessment
  a. Signs and symptoms
    i. Systemic infection: Suspect sepsis if there is a change in the
    clinical picture including chills followed by fever or hypothermia,
    tachycardia, tachypnea, oliguria, malaise, confusion, hemody-
    namic changes, and leukocytosis (increased leukocytes; white
    cells increase).
    ii. Localized infection: redness, tenderness, warmth, swelling, pu-
    rulent drainage from injury site, and dysfunction
  b. Diagnostic tests
    i. Serum
      - Serum: low platelet count; white blood cell count and differen-
        tial fluctuations and increases ($>10\%$) of bands (occurs with
        leukocytosis); electrolytes; glucose (hyperglycemia); lactate;
        must obtain blood cultures (for assessment of bacteremia and
        sepsis).

Table 3.1 Common Infectious Organisms in Trauma

Organism	Commonalities
Staphylococcus aureus Gram positive	Most common infectious agent; causative organism for necrotizing fasciitis
Group A beta hemolytic streptococci Gram positive	Most common in soft-tissue injuries
Streptococcus pneumoniae Gram positive	Concern for surgical patient; pneumococcal sepsis is potentially fatal for splenectomy patient
Clostridium perfringens (gas gangrene) Gram positive	Gas-forming soft-tissue infection; rapidly necrotizing; aggressive surgical debridement; surgical amputations to prevent spread
Escherichia coli Gram negative	Common in urinary tract infections, soft tissue, and bacteremia; normal flora for intestine; possible cause for peritonitis
Klebsiella Gram negative	"Barnyard" contaminations, soft tissue, bacteremia
Pseudomonas Gram negative	Nosocomial pneumonia, soft-tissue infections
Methicillin-resistant *S. aureus* (MRSA)	Virulent; usually in immunosuppressed patients; found in blood, sputum, and wounds; nosocomial pneumonia, strict reverse isolation

- ABG: acidosis
- Urinalysis culture and sensitivity
- BUN: increases; creatinine clearance: decreases
- Coagulation studies: disseminated intravascular coagulation may develop from sepsis
- Liver function tests and bilirubin: may be elevated in acalculous cholecystitis

ii. Cultures: always obtain prior to drug therapy or a change in antibiotic therapy. Document and specify drugs administered throughout the regimen; bedside bronchoscopy cultures.
- Aerobic and anaerobic cultures of the wound site and drainage sites [7].
- Blood cultures; total of two sets obtained from different sites and at times.
- Sputum; Gram stain and culture.
- Lumbar puncture.

iii. Radiographs
- Chest, abdominal, or sinus x-rays.
- Ultrasound or CT scan.

2. Patient management

   a. Potential for infection related to disruption of normal defense mechanisms.

      i. Problem: circulatory shock state, hypoxemia, pneumonias, sepsis and systemic inflammatory response syndrome.

     ii. Intervention

- Resuscitation phase
  - Use strict aseptic and sterile techniques during procedures.
  - Use universal precautions during the care of open wounds.
  - Exercise excellent hand-washing skills.
  - Institute infection control and isolation precautions (see Chap. 1).
  - Complete dressing changes on peripheral and central lines according to institutional policy.
  - Change intravenous catheter sites according to institutional policy.
  - Assess intravenous sites every shift for redness or signs of infection; discuss with physicians the need to change infected central lines; immediately discontinue any infected peripheral lines and start new intravenous lines in another site.
  - Discontinue all invasive devices as soon as possible.
  - If closed suction system used, change system every 24 hours; use closed suction if patient intubated longer than 48 hours.
  - After wound cultures are obtained, eliminate the possibility of infectious contamination with early treatments of irrigation, debridement, and surgical intervention if needed.
  - Administer intravenous antibiotics as prescribed.
- Critical care phase
  - Monitor for early signs of sepsis and systemic inflammatory response syndrome.
  - Document and trend quantity and quality of wound drainage.
  - Debride necrotic tissue with local wound care and frequent dressing changes.
  - Administer antibiotics judiciously to maintain adequate levels in blood; monitor drug incompatibilities closely.
  - Prevent pulmonary infections by repositioning patient and assisting in and out of bed frequently, completing chest physical therapy, using sterile suctioning techniques, and changing ventilatory tubing and closed suction per institutional policy.
  - Decrease exposure to nosocomial organisms by using basic infection control techniques (see Chap. 1)
  - Ensure adequate nutritional support: oral, enteral, or parenteral; obtain daily weights.
  - Maintain skin integrity: position and turn every 2 hours, provide a pressure relieving sleep surface, bathe patient using mild soap and warm water, protect skin from urine and fecal exposure.

- ○ Transfer to intermediate care unit as soon as possible to decrease frequency of nosocomial exposures found in the intensive care unit.
  - iii. Desired outcome
    - Absence of signs and symptoms of infection.
    - Blood, urine, sputum, and wound cultures are negative.
    - Prevention of nosocomial infection
- b. Altered tissue perfusion related to hyperdynamic state of septic shock and sepsis
  - i. Problem: catabolic metabolism; ineffective wound healing; diminished cerebral, coronary, and organ blood flow.
  - ii. Intervention:
    - Attempt to identify source of infection; obtain urine, serum, sputum, and wound cultures.
    - Provide pulmonary support: oxygen, ventilation and positive end-expiratory pressure, constant repositioning with head of bed up as necessary
    - Correct fluid volume deficits with crystalloids. Administer fluids (lactated Ringer's solution or normal saline) to maintain systolic blood pressure greater than 90 mm Hg and UOP greater than 50 mL/hour.
    - Transfuse colloids (blood products) according to hemoglobin, hematocrit results in order to improve oxygen-carrying capacity.
    - Administer vasopressors, but only after fluid volume has been replaced, to maintain adequate blood pressure.
    - Steroid use to decrease capillary leak is controversial and is not recommended in the trauma patient at present
    - Monitor arterial pressure, central venous pressure, pulmonary artery pressures, and ABGs; if changes occur, discuss plan of care with physician.
    - Monitor BUN and creatinine to assess renal functioning and recognize need for dialysis.
    - Monitor LFT to determine hepatic functioning.
    - Assess orientation and mental functioning to determine cerebral perfusion.
    - Provide adequate nutritional support: calculate to account for increased caloric requirements caused by the hyperdynamic state.
    - Monitor and document intake and output.
  - iii. Desired outcome
    - Fluid volume overload is prevented as evidenced by normal central venous and pulmonary artery pressures.
    - Oxygenation of blood is adequate as evidenced by pulse oxygenation greater than 94% and normal ABG.
    - Organ perfusion is adequate as evidenced by normal mentation, adequate urine output, palpable pulses, warm dry skin, normal LFT.

c. Hyperthermia related to inflammatory process, hypermetabolic state, or circulating pyrogens
  i. Problem: increased oxygen consumption and increased metabolic requirements
  ii. Intervention
  - Identify infectious source and organism by obtaining urine, serum, sputum, and wound cultures.
  - Document and trend core temperatures every hour for ineffective thermoregulation.
  - Monitor heart rate; fever is often associated with tachycardia.
  - If febrile administer antipyretic drug therapy, as ordered.
  - After patient has reached maximum temperature assist with cooling techniques: cool room, maximize airflow, provide cool water bath, provide dry clothing.
  - Assist with surgical drainage of exudative lesions and abscesses.
  - Minimize invasive therapies, discontinue invasive lines and tubes as soon as possible.
  - Administer systemic antibiotics based on suspected pathogens, culture results and the organism's antibiotic sensitivity, as ordered.
  - Monitor caloric intake to ensure that nutrition meets increased metabolic demands (see Chap. 4).
  iii. Desired outcome
  - Restoration to normal core body temperature (37°C)
  - Caloric intake sufficient to meet demands
  - Heart rate returns to baseline.

C. Metabolic response: Injured and critically ill patients experience varying stress levels that can trigger the breakdown of carbohydrates, protein, and fat (catabolic state). Increased stress and energy demands due to injury and decreased intake of life-sustaining nutrients necessitate a nutritional assessment and replenishment within 48–72 hours postinjury. Hypermetabolic states increase oxygen demand and consumption as well as basal energy needs. If nutrients are not readily available, there will be a delay in wound healing, compromise of immune response, and loss of energy reserves and muscle mass. The key to prevention of metabolic deficiencies is early nutritional support with adequate protein and calories.
  1. Assessment
    a. Signs and symptoms
      i. Edema
      ii. Weight loss, fat loss, and muscle wasting
      iii. Fatigues easily
      iv. Pulmonary insufficiency and inability to wean
      v. Opportunistic infections
    b. Diagnostic tests
      i. Serum
      - Blood volume deficiencies of sodium, potassium, serum albumin, transferrin, prealbumin, low total lymphocyte count, creatinine, glucose, magnesium, phosphorus, and trace elements.

        ii. Urine
- Urinalysis: measure nitrogen levels and glycosuria.

2. Patient management

    a. Alterations in nutrition, less than body requirements, related to increased metabolic demand

        i. Problem: insulin resistance, protein depletion, malnutrition, impaired wound healing, increased infection and organ dysfunction, negative nitrogen balance (urine nitrogen loss due to increased protein catabolism)

       ii. Interventions
- Nutritional assessment and early supportive strategies are required to replenish stores of carbohydrates, proteins, and fats with oral intake, tube feedings (enteral), or sterile intravenous (parenteral) administration.
- Early consultation with dietician.
- Calculate caloric requirements and monitor daily weights. Must estimate Basal Energy Expenditure and multiply by 1.5 to obtain caloric requirement during recovery from severe injury.
- Maintain accurate calorie counts.
- Obtain a 24-hour urine sample once a week to monitor for creatinine clearance and nitrogen balance.
- When initiating parenteral nutrition obtain finger-stick blood sugars frequently.
- Administer insulin, potassium, multivitamins, trace minerals, and other nutritional adjuncts as needed.
- Monitor input and output frequently.
- If oral nutritional supplements ordered, space administration so that patient is hungry at meal time. Add flavors to enteral formulas (such as strawberry or chocolate syrup).
- If patient can eat, encourage family members to bring in favorite foods to stimulate caloric intake.
- Monitor for diarrhea (see Chap. 4).

     iii. Desired outcome
- Patient consumes minimal daily requirements and vitamins. Must ensure adequate intake of proteins, carbohydrates, and fats on a diet plan.
- Adequate wound healing
- Fluid and electrolyte balance normal
- Positive nitrogen balance
- Weight gain
- Return to normal basal metabolism needs: 1500–1800 calories day (6300–7560 J/day) or 1 calorie/kg per hour (4.2 J/kg per hour).
- Return to normal diet as soon as possible.
- Return of appetite

IV. Severity categories of trauma. Penetrating injuries causing transections or severe lacerations to heavily vascularized areas or vital organs are life-threatening injuries. Multisystem injuries have varying degrees of shock. Burns vary depending upon intensity of heat and amount of time of body surface contact with the heat source. Blood loss and hypotension vary depending upon the time to definitive intervention (direct pressure, adequate fluid replacement, and surgical procedure).

A. Life-threatening: injuries incompatible with life involve massive crushing injuries to vital structures in chest, abdomen, pelvis, head, or neck.
  1. Injuries
     a. Disruptions of oxygen exchange or lung processes: airway obstruction or respiratory insufficiency; open or tension pneumothorax, massive hemothorax, flail chest and pulmonary contusion; tracheal disruption; and airway inhalation injury.
     b. Disruptions of circulatory status or organ processes: great vessel or arterial disruptions such as aortic transection or rupture, intimal disruption, or pericardial tamponade.
     c. Disruptions of neurologic status: loss of sympathetic tone, unconsciousness, high cord injuries, intracerebral hemorrhage, brain stem compression, or hemispheric damage.
     d. Disruptions of bone continuity or vascular processes: orthopedic injuries such as pelvic crush and extremity amputations.
  2. Complications
     a. Apnea or hypoxia = anoxia; may be immediately fatal.
     b. Severe hypotension, severe shock, or exsanguination.
     c. Ischemia (muscle, tissue, and brain).
     d. *Adult* respiratory distress syndrome.
     e. Aspiration or nosocomial pneumonia.
     f. Sepsis and systemic inflammatory response syndrome.
     g. Coagulopathies (frequently due to hypothermia).
     h. Brain death.
     i. Cardiac arrest.
B. Potentially life-threatening
  1. Injuries
     a. Disruptions of oxygen exchange or lung processes: respiratory insufficiency; pneumothorax, pulmonary contusions with or without flail segment, tracheobronchial disruption and traumatic diaphragmatic rupture
     b. Disruptions of circulatory status or organ systems: hemodynamic compromise possibly due to cardiac contusion, abdominal organ injuries (liver and spleen most common), esophageal disruption, or eviscerations
     c. Disruptions of neurologic status: altered level of consciousness, brain anoxia, cerebral edema, increased intracranial pressure, paralysis, or loss of sensation possibly due to head or spinal trauma or degloving injury

      d. Disruptions of bone continuity or vascular processes: arterial or intimal disruption, open or closed multiple fractures or dislocations, flail chest, first rib fracture with possible underlying subclavian artery injury, blunt chest or abdominal trauma, crushed pelvis, two or more proximal long-bone fractures, maxillofacial trauma, or traumatic amputations

  2. Complications

      a. Hypotension or occult bleeding.

      b. Severe medical problems induced by the traumatic event (ie, myocardial infarction).

      c. Brain death.

      d. Septicemia.

      e. Nerve injury (phrenic, laryngeal, vagus, brachial plexus).

      f. Vascular problems: deep vein thrombosis, arteriovenous fistula, pseudoaneurysm.

      g. Pulmonary or fat emboli.

      h. Disseminated intravascular coagulation.

      i. Loss of a limb

C. Non–life-threatening: Some dramatic injuries may look extremely severe and seem to warrant immediate intervention; however, they may not be life-threatening (such as orbital blow-out fractures). Always address basic and advanced life support needs before proceeding.

  1. Injuries

      a. Disruptions of lung processes: lung contusion or simple hemothorax or pneumothorax

      b. Disruptions of bone continuity or vascular compromise: orthopedic injury, digital amputations, simple fractures, surface trauma, or peripheral vascular injury

      c. Disruptions of mental health: psychologic or emotional problems induced by traumatic accident

  2. Complications

      a. Volkmann's contractures (contractures resulting from injury to the blood supply to that area).

      b. Compartment syndrome (damage caused by ischemia secondary to increased compartment pressure).

      c. Inappropriate behavior threatening injury to themselves or someone else.

V. Specific extremity injuries

A. Fractures

  1. Definition: Normal bone continuity is disrupted and usually involves a zone of injury including adjacent soft-tissue structures. Fractures are described according to the three following classifications:

      a. Anatomic site: epiphyseal (head of a long bone), metaphyseal (wider shaft, growth zone), diaphyseal (shaft of the long bone), or intra-articular (joint). A diaphyseal fracture can be further described as distal, medial, or proximal third of the shaft.

      b. Type of displacement: closed (simple), open (comminuted), complete, incomplete, compression, displaced, greenstick (twisting), impacting, or overriding

      c. Plane of fracture: linear, longitudinal, oblique, spiral, or transverse

  2. Etiology: The mechanism of injury and the extent and duration of an energy source impacting the specific body region forecast injuries to surface tissue and bone.

  3. Nursing process

      a. Assessment: Important data include prehospital extrication time, immobilization techniques, resuscitative stabilization measures, and mechanism of injury comorbidities (motor vehicle accidents [most common], ejection from a vehicle, falls, crush/compression injuries, violent assaults, industrial). Examine any photographs accompanying chart.

         i. Signs and symptoms

- Primary survey (airway, breathing, circulation, disability [neurologic status], and exposure/environmental control [prevent hypothermia]) is executed first [1].
- Estimate blood loss
○ Secondary-survey orthopedic assessment (Table 3.2).
○ Fractures and associated injuries (Table 3.3).

         ii. Diagnostic tests

- Radiographs of all fractures should include anterior–posterior and lateral views in order to evaluate multiple angles of the injury and determine extent of disruption. Oblique and comparison views of the unaffected extremity, and films of joints above and below the injury, may also be necessary.
- Arteriogram/angiography: Used when vascular involvement is suspected.
- Magnetic resonance imagery: identifies soft-tissue injury, disk involvement of spinal injuries, ligamentous injuries

Table 3.2 Secondary-Survey Orthopedic Assessment

Limb adduction/abduction	Point tenderness, quality, and location
Edema	Pulses quality and equality distal to injury
Color	Sharp and dull sensation
Ecchymosis	Proprioception
Capillary refill	Movement prior to injury
Temperature	Muscle spasms over the injury
Pain	Motor dysfunction
Compare shape with opposite extremity	Deformity
Inability to bear weight	Crepitus
Shortening or rotation of a limb	Breaks in skin, lacerations, and abrasions
Estimated blood loss resulting in hypo-volemic shock	

Table 3.3 Fractures and Associated Injuries

Fracture Site	Associated Injuries
Femur	Tibia/fibula, hip, acetabulum, femoral neck, pelvic ring disruption, patella, ligaments
Abdomen	Pelvis, ribs, lumbar spine
Calcaneous	Low vertebral burst
Knee	Femur, tibia/fibula, posterior hip (dislocation), popliteal artery disruption, ligaments
Long bones	Joints above and below fracture site

- CT scans and myelograms identify fractures undetected by plain films, document amount of dislocation, confirm amount of comminution and stability of the fracture.
- Urethrogram/cystogram identify disruption of urethral system by bony displacement secondary to impact.
- Serum
  ○ Trauma laboratory protocol (see Hemodynamic response, p. 38)
  ○ Hemoglobin and hematocrit for blood loss
  ○ Chemistries for fluid balance; monitor for a decrease of serum calcium, magnesium, and phosphate.
  ○ Type and crossmatch to prepare for possible transfusion.
  ○ Coagulation studies for hemorrhage potential
  ○ Urinalysis for toxicology screen and myoglobin; adequate output = 0.5–1.0 mL/kg per hour urine output for an adult
  ○ ABG or pulse oximetry measurements preferred
  b. Patient management
    i. Impaired physical mobility related to immobilization devices and pain.
      - Problem: Interferes with ability to perform activities of daily living, potentiates the development of deep vein thrombosis, constipation/ileus, pressure ulcers, fluid and electrolyte abnormalities, foot drop, and pneumonia
      - Intervention: resuscitation phase
      ○ Early intervention in prehospital and emergency department (first 24 hours). Urgent surgical intervention by orthopedic surgeon can reduce the extent of extremity disability.
      ○ Immediate immobilization and reduction/realignment of bony injury within 8 hours. Immobilize joints above and below injury. Consider use of a pneumatic antishock garment (PASG) to temporarily immobilize pelvis or femur fractures and tamponade pelvic hemorrhage. However, the clinician must monitor hidden external bleeding under the PASG. The PASG should not be used in patients with congestive heart failure or pregnant patients.
      ○ Apply insulated ice, splint, and elevate extremity above level of heart to reduce swelling and pain.

- ○ Continue reevaluation of circulatory and neurovascular status of injured extremity. Assess pulses (palpable and Doppler) and skin temperature. Observe for compartment syndrome. The presence of a pulseless extremity, pallor of the skin, paresthesia, and pain are highly suggestive of compartment syndrome.
- ○ Assist with fasciotomy if indicated.
- ○ Monitor for external bleeding.
- ○ Assist in temporary fracture reduction measures.
- ○ Provide pain and anxiety relief with short-acting, IV analgesics and anxiolytics after neurologic examination and determination of associated injuries. Ensure that pain medications have been administered before fracture reduction (see Morphine).
- ▪ Intervention: critical care phase
- ○ Ensure that pulses are present distal to immobilization site.
- ○ Avoid manipulation of injury.
- ○ Apply sterile dressing and complete dressing changes to wounds and immobilization pin sites as ordered.
- ○ Pulmonary management: Encourage patient to get out of bed as soon as possible. Instruct or assist patient to turn, cough, and complete deep-breathing exercises or spirometry every 2 hours and as needed.
- ○ Consult physical therapy and occupational therapy as soon as possible.
- ○ Review allowable positioning in and out of bed with patient. Use padding to pressure points. Maintain clean, dry skin surfaces.

---

morphine
Action Decreases pain.
Administration Guidelines 2–10 mg intravenously every 1–2 hours.
Special Considerations Monitor respiratory rate and blood pressure when administering large doses.

midazolam
Action Depresses the central nervous system to decrease anxiety.
Administration Guidelines 1–4 mg intravenously during procedures.
Special Considerations Monitor respiratory rate and blood pressure frequently; have airway management equipment immediately available.

lorazepam
Action Depresses central nervous system to decrease anxiety.
Administration Guidelines 2–6 mg orally daily in divided doses or 0.05 mg/kg intramuscularly or intravenously every 4–6 hours.
Special Considerations Use cautiously in patients with myasthenia gravis or Parkinson's disease because drug may exacerbate symptoms or may cause lethargy.

- Fracture realignment management: appropriately utilize and maintain traction devices, sterile cleansing of pin sites, circulatory and neurovascular limb reassessment.
- Initiate rehabilitative exercises early. Encourage patient to participate actively in passive range of motion exercises, including plantar flexion and dorsiflexion of feet. Consider using foot splints to prevent foot drop.
- Instruct patient to assess pain on a scale of 0–10 and document every 2 hours or after any pain-relieving interventions; provide pain relief as appropriate.
- Provide distraction such as movies, music, games, and reading materials.
- Desired outcome
- Skin integrity disruption prevented.
- Further damage prevented.
- Patient reports pain relieved.
- Restore mobility to optimal level, healing of fracture without malunion.
- Patient verbalizes understanding and assists with care procedures, adaptive devices, and exercises.

ii. Potential for infection related to contaminants of open fractures and soft-tissue injury.
- Problem: Nosocomial infection, slowed healing process, sepsis, tetanus, gas gangrene, and osteomyelitis.
- Intervention (resuscitative phase)
- Obtain aerobic and anaerobic wound cultures prior to irrigation.
- Use wet saline dressing on exposed tissue. Avoid iodine-based solutions due to tissue irritation and delayed wound healing.
- Provide irrigation and contaminant debridement with copious amounts of saline. This procedure may be done in the operating room.
- Use sterile technique diligently to avoid further contamination.
- Administer appropriate broad-spectrum antibiotics to cover suspected organisms. Be sure to administer on time to maintain adequate levels in blood.
- Administer tetanus toxoid immunization or booster to prevent tetanus.

---

tetanus toxoid

Action Stimulates antibody production to provide passive immunity against tetanus infection.

Administration Guidelines 0.5 ml intramuscularly only; booster given every 10 years.

Special Considerations Do not give to patients with acute respiratory infection, convulsive disorders, immunosuppression, or active tetanus infection.

- Intervention (critical care phase)
- ○ Monitor for signs of infection: erythema, edema, pain, wound drainage, fever, chills, changes in vital signs.
- ○ Administer antibiotics as ordered; give on time to maintain adequate levels in blood.
- ○ Use sterile technique during dressing changes and pin-site care; wash hands before and after each patient contact.
- ○ Maintain skin integrity especially at skin/device contact.
- ○ Observe for signs of osteomyelitis, common to open fractures and marked contamination: low-grade fever, swelling, tenderness, pain at site, and purulent drainage.
- ○ Observe for signs and symptoms of gas gangrene: pain, swelling, color changes in the zone of injury, purulent drainage, hemorrhagic bullae (blisters), tachycardia, fever, altered sensorium.
- ○ Provide adequate hydration and nutrition
- ○ Apply antimicrobial topical agents as ordered.
- ○ Instruct patient how to maintain clean wound sites.
- ○ Instruct patient to inform nurse if new pain at site occurs.
- Desired outcome
- ○ Absence of infection evidenced by normothermia, white blood cell counts less than 15,000 mm^3, negative wound cultures, absence of foul-smelling drainage
- ○ Resolution of infection and identified organism treated with antibiotics in timely manner
- ○ Good skin color and temperature
- ○ Absence of swelling
- ○ Patient demonstrates aseptic wound self-care.

iii. Potential for impaired gas exchange related to pulmonary occlusion caused by pulmonary embolus/fat embolus from fat globule release secondary to manipulation of fracture or from prolonged immobility.
- Problem: acute hypoxia from pulmonary artery occlusion.
- Interventions
- ○ Monitor for signs of respiratory distress (dyspnea, tachypnea); provide ventilatory support as needed; assist with intubation as needed.
- ○ Obtain vital signs every 4 hours; obtain temperature every hour if fever develops.
- ○ Assess for petechiae on chest, axillae, and conjunctivae. Notify physician if present.
- ○ Monitor ABG data and arterial oxygen saturation (by pulse oximetry); maintain arterial oxygen saturation greater than 94%; make needed ventilatory changes.
- ○ Assess breath sound every 4 hours to ensure adequate gas exchange in all lobes.
- ○ Monitor for thrombocytopenia (platelet level < 150,000–250,000/mm^3).

- ◦ Assess neurologic status every hour due to the potential for cerebral ischemia.
- ◦ Limit movement of fracture to avoid mobilization of fat.
- ▪ Desired outcome
- ◦ Normal gas exchange evidenced by normal respirations, arterial oxygen tension greater than 80 mm Hg, arterial carbon dioxide less than 45 mm Hg, arterial oxygen saturation greater than 94%, arterial blood pH 7.35–7.45.
- ◦ Restlessness secondary to dyspnea is diminished.

B. Traumatic amputations

1. Definition: Severed parts can be life-threatening, but bleeding is usually well managed with direct pressure to wound or stump. Amputations are classified as traumatic, partial, complete, incomplete, or surgical. Descriptive types include the following:

   a. Cut or guillotine: well-defined wound edges and localized damage to soft tissue, vessels, and nerves

   b. Crush wound: diffuse soft-tissue damage involving arterial intima

   c. Avulsive amputation: tearing or stretching of tissue with nerve and vasculature torn away from injury site; degloving (shearing) injury.

2. Etiology

   a. Most common cause of upper-extremity amputation is motor vehicle accidents, then farming accidents, industry-related crush injuries, and violent assaults.

   b. Other mechanisms include saws, knives, hatchets, and lawn mowers.

   c. Common sites of amputations include digits (fingers and toes); hand; forearm; arm; ear; nose; penis; transmetatarsal; and below, through, and above the knee.

3. Nursing process

   a. Assessment

      i. Signs and symptoms

      - ▪ Decreased systolic blood pressure (<90 mm Hg) if extensive bleeding at injury causes hypovolemia.
      - ▪ Decreased UOP (<30 mL/hour) from hypovolemia.
      - ▪ Increased heart rate from hypovolemia.
      - ▪ Diminished mentation related to decreased cerebral perfusion.

      ii. Diagnostic tests

      - ▪ X-rays of both the stump and amputated part to determine presence of foreign body.
      - ▪ Trauma laboratory protocol: same as mentioned under Hemodynamic response, p. 39.

   b. Patient management

      i. Actual fluid volume deficit related to blood loss

      - ▪ Problem: Possible tissue or organ destruction from decreased perfusion.
      - ▪ Intervention (resuscitation phase)
      - ◦ Address life-threatening injuries first, by primary and secondary assessment.

- ○ Determine mechanism of injury to consider possible contamination at stump site.
- ○ Control hemorrhage with direct pressure and saline-moistened dressings; elevate and immobilize stump; avoid use of tourniquet, since circulation can be compromised further.
- ○ Monitor hemoglobin and hematocrit; administer blood products if necessary.
- ○ Frequent checks of vital signs and neurologic status.
- ○ Estimate actual blood loss as outlined in Hemodynamic response, p. 38.
- ○ Administer warmed intravenous fluid and blood products.
- ○ Fluid replacement with two large-bore intravenous catheters in unaffected limb with lactated Ringer's solution.
- ○ Administer oxygen by face mask.
- ○ Insert a Foley catheter to monitor hourly UOP. Maintain at least 50 mL/hour during resuscitation phase.
- ○ Provide stump, amputated part, and reimplantation care (Table 3.4).
- ▪ Intervention: critical care phase
- ○ Monitor central venous pressure, pulmonary artery wedge pressure, and other hemodynamic data.
- ○ Monitor intake and output measurements
- ○ Consult psychiatry to address body image concerns, sensory changes

Table 3.4 Stump, Amputated Part, and Reimplantation Care

Stump
1. Control active bleeding by direct pressure and elevation
2. Splint as necessary
3. Irrigate profusely with saline and dress with damp sterile dressings with protective wrapping

Amputated Part
1. Irrigate and remove contaminants by rinsing with saline and pat dry
2. Wrap in saline moistened gauze, sterile dressing
3. Place part in resealable plastic bag and place in larger bag containing ice and water
4. Never use dry ice
5. *Do not freeze or soak part*
6. Hypothermia will enhance viability up to 18 hours as opposed to 4–6 hours at room temperature
7. Assure part is labeled with patient's name; accompanies patient everywhere and to the operating room

Reimplantation
1. Parts can be used as graft material to the stump if the amputated part is not able to be reimplanted
2. Common parts reimplanted include thumb, digits at metacarpal level, wrist, forearm, any amputation in children
3. Contraindications to reimplantation: severe crush with vascular damage, multiple level amputations, severe contamination, thrombosed vessels in amputated part

○ Use aseptic technique when completing dressing changes; assess site carefully for signs of infection (redness, swelling, pain, or purulent drainage)
- Desired outcome
○ Vital signs within normal limits.
○ Lab data reflect adequate hemoglobin and hematocrit levels.
○ Further bleeding prevented

ii. Potential for infection of stump.
- Problem: Localized infection causes pain and has potential for systemic infection.
- Intervention
○ Debride and irrigate wound thoroughly; remove all necrotic tissue; may require operating room.
○ Prevent edema by using nonrigid sterile dressing application; consult physical therapy and occupational therapy to select appropriate stump wrapping.
○ Administer tetanus immunization and antibiotics as ordered
○ Use strict hand-washing and sterile technique
○ Immediately consult orthopedic surgeon.
○ Support partial amputation by immobilizing the area.
- Desired outcome
○ Absence of infection
○ Wound healing

iii. Impaired physical mobility related to pain and contractures
- Problem: Loss of limb, dysfunctional ambulation, altered balance, coordination deficit, contractures, alteration in sensory function.
- Intervention
○ Provide prescribed skin care of stump.
○ Consult physical therapy early.
○ Encourage and assist with isometric exercises of involved extremity with repetition. Above-the-knee amputation: avoid hip flexion and abduction; do not elevate stump on pillows.
○ Reposition patient and stump frequently
○ Stump wrapping with *elastic fabric bandage*; always wrap distal to proximal to prevent swelling; and shrink and shape stump for prosthetics.
○ Encourage range-of-motion exercises to increase muscle strength and flexibility.
○ Provide sufficient pain control with analgesics to ensure compliance with exercises
○ Instruct family in physical therapy assistant role and patient's needs for functional activities.
- Desired outcome
○ Absence of contractures
○ Optimal range of motion
○ Pain controlled

iv. Disturbance in body image and self-concept related to disfigurement
- Problem: Loss of limb or part, powerlessness, anger, fear, depression, unwillingness to accept loss or view stump
- Intervention
  ◦ Consider psychologic consultation.
  ◦ Discuss with the patient feelings of loss and the normal grief cycle. Provide a supportive environment to assist in grieving process.
  ◦ Allow patient to make as many choices as possible (food, routine, naps) to gain a sense of control.
  ◦ Discuss plan of care related to prosthesis fitting.
  ◦ Encourage patient to participate in plan of care and decision making.
- Desired outcome
  ◦ Patient exemplifies adequate coping mechanisms.
  ◦ Patient is actively involved in rehabilitative phase.

C. Compartment syndrome
1. Definition: A complication of orthopedic trauma when a nerve, tendon, vessel, or muscle is constricted within a closed space that is surrounded by membranes that do not stretch. May also result from acute arterial occlusion. Restricted circulation due to microvasculature changes causes ischemia of nerve and muscle (Volkmann's ischemic contracture).
2. Etiology: Compartment syndrome is a function of time and pressure. Increased duration of stressor and pressure produce symptoms. Internal pressure is from bleeding or edema, external pressure from restrictive devices such as casts, or prolonged inflation of the PASG. Injuries at risk of developing compartment syndrome include closed fractures accompanied by tissue contusion and bone displacement, compression/crush injuries, open fractures, arterial injuries from gunshot wounds, and burns.
3. Nursing process
   a. Assessment
      i. Signs and symptoms: Presence of all of the following denotes very advanced ischemia from compartment syndrome.
         - Pain: related to muscle ischemia.
         - Pallor: skin color changes related to lack of blood supply to the area.
         - Pulses: may be diminished or absent related to arterial inflow compression.
         - Paresthesia of the affected area due to sensory nerve ischemia.
         - Paralysis: due to ischemia of motor nerves.
      ii. Diagnostic tests
         - Serum: myoglobin may be present if muscle necrosis has occurred.
         - Urine: myoglobin present if muscle necrosis has occurred.
         - Other: intracompartmental pressure measurements with monitoring device to measure the intracompartmental pressure at the injury site.

- ○ Pressure less than 20 mm Hg: normal
- ○ Pressure 20–30 mm Hg: limited tissue perfusion
- ○ Pressure 30–60 mm Hg: ischemic damage and immediate need for pressure reduction. Arterial blood flow is not usually obstructed by compartment pressures of 30–60 mm Hg. Distal pulses may still be palpated.

b. Patient management
   i. Potential for decreased tissue perfusion and neurovascular compromise related to increased compartment pressure
     ▪ Problem: pain, edema, paresthesia, myoglobinuria, necrosis.
     ▪ Interventions
     ○ Ascertain time of injury and time since onset of symptoms; damage can occur within the first few hours after injury, may present on admission to emergency room.
     ○ Identify site and mechanism of injury.
     ○ Suspect associated injuries: soft-tissue contusions, hematomas, fractures or dislocations.
     ○ Assess and monitor for pain, pallor, pulses, paresthesia, and paralysis ("the five Ps").
     ○ Investigate pain complaints of throbbing disproportional pain at injury site unrelieved by analgesic drugs and increased in response to passive stretch of the muscle.
     ○ Examine firmness or tenseness of compartments by comparing with uninjured extremity.
     ○ Observe pallor and capillary refill delay distal to the compartment.
     ○ Identify paresthesia or loss of sensation. These are late signs indicating pressure on the nerves and may manifest as numbness and tingling. Examine with two-point discrimination, sharp and dull touch.
     ○ Assess for limited or weak motor ability of extremity because of pain from pressure.
     ○ Assess pulses distal to injury. Check pulses with palpable and Doppler method every 1–2 hours; if diminished, late sign and irreversible, presence of pulses does not rule out compartment syndrome. The mechanism of injury and accompanying signs and symptoms are the keys to detection.
     ○ Maintain the extremity at heart level to decrease swelling, yet maintain perfusion.
     ○ Release constrictive devices such as casts or tight dressings
     ○ Monitor and record trends in patient's pain patterns and effects of medication.
     ○ Trend compartment pressures and notify physician of rising pressures indicating compartment syndrome; measure circumference of extremity.
     ○ Prepare patient for operating room when surgical decompression of the compartment's fascial sheath by fasciotomy is required.

- Intervention (postfasciotomy)
  - Assess neurovascular status hourly, patterns of response to interventions, and continued limb assessment (crucial to prevent further disability). Fasciotomy should immediately return pulse.
  - Monitor for skin infection, assuring sterility of fasciotomy sites and wet-to-wet (open tissue) or wet-to-dry sterile saline dressings as appropriate.
  - Monitor for bleeding.
  - Monitor clinical signs of increasing compartment pressure due to immobilization, persistent edema, or venous leaking.
  - Assist with compartment syndrome measurements.
  - Expect delayed primary or secondary skin closure with grafts after swelling has receded.
- Desired outcome
  - Increased arterial blood flow and improved venous return to injured area
  - Intracompartmental pressure less than 20 mm Hg.
  - Prevention of neuromuscular deterioration and irreversible sequelae
  - Absence of signs of infection to fasciotomy sites
  - Skin graft heals properly

ii. Impaired physical mobility related to pain, pressure, and fasciotomy incisions
- Problem: Decreased extremity function, weak motor responses, and fear of pain
- Intervention
  - Early intervention to relieve pressure and subsequent destruction to microvasculature
  - Initiate range-of-motion exercises early.
  - Identify pressure points and pad appropriately to avoid pressure sores.
  - Ensure sufficient pain control to improve compliance with exercises.
- Desired outcome
  - Full range of motion of injured extremity
  - Functional ability to complete activities of daily living
  - Prevention of contractures
  - Patient participates in rehabilitative phase.

VI. Discharge planning for the trauma patient

A. Patient, caretaker, and family have been provided and understand all written discharge instructions.
  1. All questions answered.
  2. Understanding of appropriate locations to return to for continued health care needs.
  3. Knowledge of names and telephone numbers of personnel to call for answers to questions.

B. Home health care agency and rehabilitation arrangements are complete prior to discharge.
   1. Home environment conducive to recovery, especially for elderly and challenged populations.
   2. Home assessment for running water, electricity, cleanliness, and caretaker support.
   3. Nutritional requirements met and healthy foods identified.
C. Patient and caretaker understand and demonstrate wound care.
   1. Infection prevention techniques.
   2. Hand-washing technique.
   3. Understanding of signs and symptoms of infection.
   4. Understanding of sterile versus nonsterile environment.
   5. Recognition of signs and symptoms of wound infection.
D. Patient and caretaker understand causes and treatment of pain.
   1. Distinction of pain types: acute pain (compression, tearing, cramping, edema) and chronic pain (phantom limb pain, incorrect joining of bone fractures).
   2. Knowledge of medication appropriate for types of pain.
   3. Mobility and range-of-motion exercises encouraged as appropriate.
   4. Proper use of crutches or mechanical equipment.
E. Patient and family offered support group.
   1. Counseling for body image changes or abuse (victims and their abusers).
   2. Substance abuse counseling.
   3. Spiritual support groups.
   4. Financial counseling.
   5. Legal guidance (living wills, power of attorney, organ donation).
   6. Psychological counseling for anxiety, depression, suicidal tendencies.
   7. Return to work as soon as possible encouraged.
F. Prescriptions filled and instructions explained.
   1. Medication side effects and contraindications.
   2. Dosage, route, and regularity of administration.
G. Trauma-prevention education and behavior modification.
   1. Stress management for patient and caretaker.
   2. Seatbelt, child safety seat, and helmet use.
   3. Pedestrian and bicycle traffic safety.
   4. Education about guns and knives, and violence avoidance strategies.
   5. Education about drinking, driving, and drugs, avoidance strategies.
H. Follow-up appointments are made and explained to family.
   1. Determine how patient will return to clinic.
   2. Facilitate arrangements to assure return to clinic.

References

1. American College of Surgeons Committee on Trauma. *Advanced Trauma Life Support Instructor Manual* (5th ed). Chicago: American College of Surgeons, 1993. Pp. 11, 21.
2. Trunkey D. The value of trauma centers. *Am Coll Surg Bull* 67:5, 1982.

3. National Safety Council. *Accident Facts* (1987 ed). NSC: Chicago, 1987.

4. Creel JH. In JE Campbell (ed), *Basic Trauma Life Support Advanced Prehospital Care* (2nd ed). Englewood Cliffs, NJ: Prentice-Hall, 1988. P. 13.

5. Young HA, Schmidek HH. Complications accompanying occipital skull fractures. *J Trauma* 22:914, 1982.

6. Vanore ML. Module 2. In EW Bayley, SA Turcke (eds), *A Comprehensive Curriculum for Trauma Nursing*. Boston: Jones and Bartlett, 1992. P. 19.

7. Lyerly HK. *The Handbook of Surgical Intensive Care: Practices of the Surgery Residents at the Duke University Medical Center*. Chicago: Year Book, 1989: Chap. 16.

CHAPTER **4**

Nutrition

Nancy Evans

I. Definition: Hospitalized patients are at high risk for the development of malnutrition. Some suggest that as many as 50% of hospitalized patients have documented moderate to severe protein-calorie malnutrition. Protein-calorie malnutrition is associated with increased morbidity and mortality. As the most common form of malnutrition in the hospital setting, it is characterized by decreased levels of visceral and somatic proteins as well as depleted fat stores and muscle wasting.

A. Marasmus: Inadequate calorie intake results in decreased fat stores and depleted muscle mass; most common in the moderately stressed patient

B. Kwashiorkor: Inadequate supply of amino acids to support protein synthesis; results in decreased levels of plasma proteins, anemia, impaired immune response and edema

C. Mixed kwashiorkor/marasmus (protein-calorie malnutrition): Characterized by skeletal muscle wasting, decreased fat stores, and depleted visceral proteins; deficits in energy and protein are most common in severely stressed patients who are catabolic

II. Etiology: The response to critical illness and injury is characterized by two distinct phases: ebb phase and flow phase.

A. Ebb phase: Goal is to maintain bloodflow and oxygenation of vital organs; short duration; characteristics include the following:
1. Decreased cardiac output
2. Decreased core temperature
3. Decreased oxygen consumption
4. Increased levels of catecholamines, glucagon
5. Decreased insulin
6. Increased serum glucose level
7. Hepatic glucose production normal

B. Flow phase: Goal is to provide fuel for organ function and tissue repair; peak elevations occur 5–10 days after injury; characteristics include the following:
1. Increased cardiac output
2. Increased core temperature

3. Increased oxygen consumption
4. Increased levels of catecholamines, glucagon
5. Normal or increased insulin
6. Serum glucose normal or increased
7. Hepatic glucose production markedly elevated
8. Hypermetabolism and hypercatabolism
    a. Flow phase is mediated by counterregulatory hormones (cortisol, glucagon, catecholamines, growth hormone) and cytokines (interleukin-1, tumor necrosis factor, interferon).
    b. Alterations in substrate metabolism occur during flow phase.
        i. Carbohydrate metabolism
            - Increased hepatic glucose production
            - Increased glucose consumption by wounds, cells of the reticuloendothelial system, inflammatory tissue
            - The increased glucose production is not reduced with exogenous glucose administration.
            - Insulin resistance results in hyperglycemia.
        ii. Fat metabolism
            - Breakdown of fat from adipose tissue stores
            - Increased levels of free fatty acids
            - Fatty acids oxidized for fuel or recycled back to peripheral tissue
        iii. Protein metabolism
            - Accelerated breakdown of skeletal muscle
            - Liver utilizes amino acids from skeletal muscle catabolism to synthesize acute-phase–reactant proteins, which support immune function and wound healing.
            - Increased catabolism of skeletal muscle results in negative nitrogen balance.

III. Nursing assessment

A. Assessment: within 24 hours of the patient being stabilized
B. Signs and symptoms
    1. General appearance
        a. Depletion of muscle and fat stores
            i. Temporal wasting
            ii. Obvious tissue wasting around bony prominences such as ribs, iliac crest, scapula
        b. Edema—severe hypoalbuminemia disrupts oncotic pressure and may cause fluid to leak from vascular space into surrounding tissues.
        c. Skin texture—dryness or scales can be secondary to essential fatty acid deficiency.
        d. Skin turgor—indication of hydration status.
        e. Teeth, mouth, and gums—poor condition, bleeding may indicate vitamin deficiency.
        f. Condition of hair and nails—hair loss is associated with zinc deficiency.

2. Muscle strength
   a. Decreased ability to assist in turning or transferring from bed to chair
   b. Reduced hand-grasping strength
3. Cardiac
   a. Hemodynamic assessment—blood pressure, central venous pressure, pulmonary artery pressure (PAP), pulmonary artery wedge pressure (PAWP), cardiac output
      i. Assess for indications of overhydration or underhydration.
      ii. Decreased blood pressure, decreased cardiac output may preclude enteral feeding, because inadequate bloodflow to the intestine will not support digestion and could cause intestinal ischemia.
   b. Identify need for fluid restrictions
4. Respiratory
   a. Respiratory rate, tidal volume, vital capacity, minute ventilation
      i. Decreased diaphragm muscle mass will increase tidal volume, decrease vital capacity, increase respiratory rate and minute ventilation.
      ii. Overfeeding nonprotein calories will increase CO_2 production.
   b. Delayed progress in weaning from mechanical ventilation
5. Renal
   a. Urine output—assess quantity and quality of urine output
      i. Decreased urine output
      ii. Fluid overload
      iii. Decreased creatinine clearance
   b. Electrolytes, blood urea nitrogen, creatinine
      i. Accumulation of urea in blood: This will rise in the hypercatabolic patient as skeletal muscle is mobilized. It also rises during protein administration without dialysis.
      ii. Increased potassium, magnesium, and phosphorus
      iii. Increased creatinine indicates worsening renal function.
   c. Type and frequency of dialytic therapy
      i. Dialysis is a catabolic therapy and contributes to protein depletion.
      ii. Continuous arteriovenous hemofiltration dialysis or peritoneal dialysis is a significant source of nonprotein calories.
6. Gastrointestinal
   a. Quantify output from any tubes accessing the GI tract
      i. Fluid/electrolyte depletion can occur with excessive losses from the GI tract.
   b. Measure abdominal distention.
   c. Stool output—quantify amount, describe consistency
      i. Excessive stool or fistula losses contain significant amount of measurable nitrogen.
   d. Auscultation of bowel sounds—least useful information, and absence of bowel sounds does not mean GI tract is nonfunctional.
C. Anthropometric data
   1. Admission weight and height
      a. Evaluate degree of weight loss; greater than 10% is significant.

   2. Calculate ideal body weight (IBW)
      a. Men: IBW = 106 lb for first 5 ft; 6 lb for each additional in.
      b. Women: IBW = 100 lb for first 5 ft; 5 lb for each additional in.
      c. Calculate % IBW (Table 4.1) [1]
         ▪ Severe malnutrition less than 70% of IBW
         ▪ Moderate malnutrition 70–80% of IBW
         ▪ Mild malnutrition 80–90% of IBW
      d. Skin fold measures are less reliable during acute periods of stress.
D. Metabolic assessment
   1. Visceral protein status—catabolic illness results in depletion of albumin, prealbumin, and transferrin because of a decreased production of these proteins to support increased synthesis of acute-phase–reactant proteins.
      a. Albumin—long half-life (21 days) limits its usefulness as a marker of nutritional deficit; however, it is a good indicator of the severity of critical illness. Fluid status will affect serum measures: Overhydration results in decreased albumin, underhydration results in elevated values.
      b. Prealbumin—a shorter half-life (2 days) makes this a more reliable measure of protein repletion. Renal impairment will falsely elevate serum levels because excretion is decreased. Serum measures are decreased with liver failure.
      c. Transferrin—half-life is approximately 8–10 days. Levels appear low when iron stores are low such as with massive hemorrhage.
   2. Measures of immune function—total lymphocyte count and skin antigen testing
      a. Less reliable measure of nutritional status in the critically ill because impaired immunocompetence results from stress, trauma, and many chronic diseases
   3. Energy expenditure—total energy expenditure is usually increased in proportion to the severity of injury and stress.

Table 4.1 Calculations Used to Determine Protein and Energy Needs

Calculation of Ideal Body Weight

$$\% \text{ ideal body weight} = \frac{\text{current body weight}}{\text{ideal body weight}} \times 100$$

Harris-Benedict Equation—estimates basal metabolic rate (BMR)
BMR (Male) = 66.47 + 13.7 (kg weight) + 5 (cm height) − 6.7 (age)
BMR (Female) = 655 + 9.6 (kg weight) + 1.85 (cm height) − 4.68 (age)
    BMR multiplied by 1.3 to 1.5 = basal energy expenditure

Nitrogen Balance
Calculated using a 24-hour urine collection for urine urea nitrogen (UUN)

$$\text{Nitrogen balance} = \frac{\text{g protein intake}}{6.25} - [\text{UUN} + 4]$$

Data from Ackerman, M. H., Evans, N. J., and Ecklund, M. M. Systemic inflammatory response syndrome, sepsis, and nutritional support. *Crit. Care Nurs. Clin. N. Am.* 6:321, 1994.

    a. Estimating metabolic rate: Harris-Benedict equation (BMR)

      i. Equation predicts basal metabolic rate (see Table 4.1).

      ii. Equation underestimates needs during critical illness and over-estimates energy needs in patients who are in barbiturate coma.

      iii. Predictive equations are typically multiplied by stress factors to define the total daily nonprotein calorie prescription.

    b. Measuring resting energy expenditure (REE): indirect calorimetry

      i. Measures oxygen consumption and CO_2 production

      ii. Requires a portable metabolic cart

      iii. Most accurate way to determine energy expenditure; greater than 120% reflects hypermetabolism

4. Nitrogen balance

    a. Nitrogen balance = nitrogen intake − nitrogen output.

    b. Collect 24-hour urine for urine urea nitrogen and creatinine.

    c. Negative nitrogen balance is characteristic of acute illness.

5. Serum chemistry measures: Electrolytes—serum levels fluctuate rapidly during periods of acute illness.

    a. Potassium, magnesium, phosphorus—serum levels drop in response to aggressive refeeding because potassium, magnesium, and phosphorus ions are driven into the cell to support anabolism.

    b. Blood urea nitrogen and creatinine—increases may reflect hydration status and signal worsening renal function.

    c. Serum glucose—hyperglycemia (> 200 mg/dL) characteristic feature during severe stress

    d. Serum triglyceride—hypertriglyceridemia may reflect decrease clearance of lipid.

    e. Hemoglobin/hematocrit—chronic anemia is common with protein-calorie malnutrition.

IV. Patient management

A. Alteration in nutritional/metabolic status related to hypermetabolism and hypercatabolism caused by the response to severe stress/acute illness.

    1. Problem: weight loss, negative nitrogen balance, delayed wound healing

    2. Intervention

      a. Nutritional support is indicated if patient will be taking nothing orally for more than 5 days.

      b. Determine energy needs

        i. Caloric needs are based on the goals for fat stores/body weight.

          ▪ Weight gain: (resting energy expenditure [REE] $\times$ 1.5)—not recommended during critical illness

          ▪ Weight maintenance: (REE $\times$ 1.2)

          ▪ Weight loss: (REE $\times$ 0.8–1.0)—no less than 800 nonprotein kcal/d

        ii. Estimated needs during critical illness

          ▪ Weight maintenance = 35–40 kcal/kg body weight per day.

          ▪ Use ideal body weight if patient is morbidly obese.

    c. Determine protein needs.
       i. Protein repletion is usually required for highly catabolic patients.
      ii. 2.0 g/kg body weight per day
      iii. Measure nitrogen balance weekly.
  3. Desired outcome
    a. Meet goals for fat stores and body weight.
    b. Reduce net negative nitrogen balance.
      i. Difficult to achieve positive nitrogen balance during periods of extreme catabolism
    c. Decrease morbidity and mortality
B. Nutritional deficit related to inability to use GI tract during period of hypercatabolism and hypermetabolism secondary to severe hemodynamic instability (reduced bloodflow to intestine); disruption of the continuity of the GI tract because of obstruction, fistula, or ileus; decreased absorption caused by GI bleeding, acute pancreatitis, or intractable diarrhea.
  1. Problem: potential weight loss, negative nitrogen balance, delayed wound healing, increased morbidity and mortality
  2. Intervention: total parenteral nutrition (TPN)
    a. Energy supply—dextrose (1 g = 3.4 kcal)
      i. Provide 60–70% of total nonprotein calorie needs.
      ii. Do not exceed 7 g dextrose/kg body weight per day.
      iii. Minimal requirement is 200 g/d (700 kcal).
      iv. Dextrose solutions available in concentrations ranging from 5% to 70%
    b. Energy supply—lipid (1 g = 9 kcal)
      i. Provide 30–40% of total nonprotein caloric needs.
      ii. Do not exceed 2.5 g fat/kg body weight per day.
      iii. Lipid solutions available in 10% or 20% concentrations
    c. Protein supply
      i. Standard amino acid formulas contain a mix of essential and nonessential amino acids.
      ii. Amino acid solutions available in concentrations ranging from 8.5% to 14%
    d. Electrolytes
      i. Add electrolytes to total parenteral nutrition (TPN) regimen daily for maintenance
        • Sodium—70–100 mEq/d
        • Potassium—70–100 mEq/d
        • Chloride—80–120 mEq/d
        • Magnesium—15–20 mEq/d
        • Phosphorus—20–30 mmol/d
        • Calcium—10–20 mEq/d
        • Acetate—0–60 mEq/d
        • Daily adjustments based on daily laboratory values
    e. Vitamins
      i. Add daily parenteral vitamin supplement to TPN

        ii. 1 mg vitamin K added to TPN for maintenance

        iii. 10 mg vitamin K IM × 3 days for repletion if there are clotting abnormalities

        iv. Additional thiamine, folate, vitamin B_{12} with alcohol abuse

    f. Trace elements

        i. Add daily parenteral trace element mix to TPN.

        ii. Standard solution contains zinc, copper, manganese, chromium, and selenium.

        iii. Additional zinc required during acute catabolic stress

        iv. Reduce copper and manganese in the setting of biliary obstruction and liver failure.

    g. Administration techniques

        i. Delivery requires central vascular access because of increased osmolarity of the TPN solutions.

- May use existing lines that have been properly maintained
- Femoral catheters can be used.
- Proximal ports of hemodynamic monitoring lines can be used.
- Initiate TPN at goal: no rationale to slowly tapering solutions.
- Check blood glucose every 6 hours for 48 hours and then, if stable, daily.
- Monitor serum magnesium, calcium, potassium daily for 3 days, then every 3 days.
- Discontinuation of TPN: No rationale supporting the need to slowly taper down TPN solutions before discontinuing

    h. Prevent potential complications of TPN

        i. Metabolic complications: (1) hyperglycemia: monitor blood glucose and adjust glucose calories accordingly, add short-acting insulin to TPN to keep sugar less than 200 mg/dL, increase amount of nonprotein calories provided as fat; (2) hypertriglyceridemia: monitor baseline serum triglycerides, reduce lipid calories if triglycerides are greater than 500 mg/dL, monitor postinfusion triglyceride level to assess clearance; (3) hypercapnia: avoid overfeeding to prevent increased carbohydrate production; (4) hepatic dysfunction: avoid overfeeding, expect mild transient elevations in transaminase and alkaline phosphatase that peak within 10–15 days of starting TPN, monitor liver function tests weekly.

  3. Desired outcome

    a. Goals for weight/fat stores met

    b. Reduced net negative nitrogen balance

    c. Increased visceral protein levels (prealbumin, albumin, transferrin)

    d. Serum electrolyte levels within normal limits

C. Nutritional deficit related to inability to eat and meet requirements during periods of hypermetabolism and hypercatabolism secondary to upper GI tract obstruction, ileus, fistula; pancreatitis; risk of aspiration; decreased pharyngeal reflexes or depressed mental status

  1. Problem: potential for weight loss, negative nitrogen balance, delayed wound healing, and increased morbidity and mortality

2. Intervention: initiate enteral feeding

    a. Determine where in the GI tract to feed: stomach or small intestine.

        i. Gastric ileus common in severe head injury, after extensive abdominal surgery, and during severe sepsis

        ii. Delayed gastric emptying can occur from pharmacologic intervention or is associated with chronic illness such as diabetes.

        iii. Postpyloric enteral feeding will reduce the risk of feeding-related aspiration.

    b. Select enteral access device (Table 4.2)

        i. Determine if enteral feeding will be short-term (<1 month) or long-term (>1 month).

        ii. Permanent enteral access is indicated if forced feeding is necessary greater than 1 month.

    c. Select enteral formula

        i. Standard polymeric formula—contains 1 kcal/mL and is 70–80% free water. Most contain approximately 40 g of protein per liter and are indicated for moderately stressed patients.

        ii. Calorically dense formula—contains 1.5–2.0 kcal/mL and is 60–70% free water. Use in fluid-restricted patients.

Table 4.2 Selection of Enteral Feeding Tubes

Type of Tube	Tube Tip Location	Advantages	Disadvantages
Nasoenteric tube	Stomach or proximal small intestine	Easy insertion Small bore designed for short-term use (<1 month)	Tip migration common High-risk of clogging Poor cosmetic appearance
Gastrostomy tube	Stomach	Avoid complication of nasal intubation Designed for long-term use (>1 month) Large diameter minimizes clogging	Open surgical procedure Does not eliminate risk of aspiration
Percutaneous endoscopic gastrostomy (PEG)	Stomach	Not an open surgical procedure Reduced anesthesia risk Ease of delivery	Does not eliminate risk of aspiration Procedure constraints— morbid obesity, ascites, esophageal obstruction
Jejunostomy tube	Jejunum	Maximal reduction of aspiration risk Early postop feeding	Open surgical procedure Anesthesia risk Requires pump for delivery

       iii. High-protein formula—contains greater than 50–60 g of protein per liter and is indicated for highly catabolic patients.

       iv. Predigested formula—limited application but may be of use in pancreatitis or malabsorption syndromes

       v. Enteral formulas contain vitamins, trace elements.

  d. Administration techniques

       i. Intermittent feeding: Enteral feeding is administered via gravity drip every 4–6 hours. This delivery method is only for intragastric feeding. Each feeding should infuse over 30–60 minutes. Each intermittent feeding should not exceed 480 mL. Introduce feeding at 120 mL every 4 hours and advance as tolerated to goal regimen.

- Monitor tolerance to feeding regimen
  - Check gastric residuals before each feeding: Hold if residual is greater than 150 mL.
  - Assess for nausea vomiting or bloating—may indicate gastric motility is slowed

       ii. Continuous feeding can be delivered into the stomach or small intestine. Start feeding at a rate of 30–50 mL/h and advance in increments of 30 mL until hourly rate reaches goal. Feedings into the small intestine must be continuous via a pump to prevent diarrhea.

- Monitor tolerance to regimen
  - Check gastric residuals every 4 hours.
  - Monitor abdominal girth—hold feedings for increased abdominal distention.
  - Monitor for nausea and vomiting—may indicate tube tip has migrated from small intestine to stomach.
  - Monitor for diarrhea: Rule out infectious causes, dilute hypertonic medications that are delivered via the feeding tube with water, and treat with routine administration of antidiarrheals.

  e. Prevent complications of enteral feeding

       i. Overhydration: select enteral formulas that are calorically dense that contain less free water.

       ii. Dehydration: dilute enteral formulas with water to meet calculated daily fluid requirements.

       iii. Aspiration: keep head of bed elevated 30–45 degrees, use coloring agent to detect feeding in tracheal aspirate, use pH testing or glucose testing on tracheal aspirate to detect presence of feeding, administer enteral feeding post pylorically, use only small-bore nasoenteric tubes.

       iv. Diarrhea: exclude and/or treat other causes of diarrhea; consider fiber formula for severe diarrhea caused by a malabsorption syndrome; consider an elemental or peptide-based formula.

       v. Administer loperamide

       vi. Feeding tube blockage; avoid medication administration if possible; if no other route available, use liquid medications or thoroughly crushed pills; flush tube every 3–4 hours with warm water during continuous feeding and before and after each intermittent feeding.

Ioperamide

Action Slow intestinal transit time.

Administration Guidelines 2 mg PO every 4–6 hours; compatible with enteral formula.

Special Considerations No central nervous system side effects.

---

3. Desired outcome
   a. Meet goals for weight/fat stores.
   b. Reduce net negative nitrogen balance.
   c. Reduce morbidity and mortality.
   d. Minimize complications of enteral feeding.
D. Alterations in fluid and electrolyte status related to impairment of organ function (renal, liver, cardiac, respiratory) complicating delivery of nutritional goals.
   1. Problem: Deteriorating organ function impairs clearance/tolerance of calories, protein, fluid and electrolytes resulting in fluid overload, abnormal serum electrolytes, increased BUN, increased CO_2 production.
   2. Intervention: Adjust nutrient prescription to account for worsening organ function.
      a. Renal
         i. Protein prescription: Decrease total amount of standard amino acids (1.4 g/kg per weight) if dialysis is ineffective or contraindicated.
         ii. Keep blood urea nitrogen (BUN) less than 100 g/dL.
         iii. Specialized renal formulas (essential amino acids) are only indicated in patients who cannot be dialyzed. The efficacy of these specialized formulas is controversial.
         iv. Maximally concentrate all nutrient solutions.
         v. Restrict/delete magnesium, potassium, and phosphorus.
         vi. Provide additional acetate.
         vii. Calculate caloric contribution of dialytic therapies such as CAVHD and peritoneal dialysis.
      b. Hepatic
         i. Protein prescription: Slowly introduce standard amino acid solutions (0.8–1 g/kg per weight) and advance as tolerated, monitoring for worsening encephalopathy.
         ii. Restrict hepatic formulas (branched-chain amino acid formula) for patients with worsening encephalopathy who are unresponsive to medical therapy.
         iii. Provide at least 150–200 g of glucose/d.
         iv. Restrict fluid and sodium.
         v. Supplement vitamin K 1 mg daily, monitor clotting studies.
         vi. Delete copper and manganese.
      c. Respiratory
         i. Avoid overfeeding patients (> 150% of measured energy expenditure).
         ii. Select a 50:50 mix of glucose and fat to meet daily nonprotein calorie requirements.

Table 4.3 Suggested Guidelines for Monitoring Patients During Nutritional Support

Parameter	Frequency
Nursing Assessment	
Intake/Output	Hourly to every 8 hours
Parenteral or enteral infusion rate	Every 4 hours
Weight	Daily
Temperature	Every 8 hours
Nutritional Measures	
Albumin, prealbumin, transferrin	Weekly
PT, PTT	Weekly
Serum triglyceride	Preinfusion, postinfusion, then weekly
Resting energy expenditure	Weekly
24-hour urine—calculate nitrogen balance	Weekly
Fluid/Electrolyte status	
Serum electrolytes	Daily
Magnesium, calcium, phosphorus	Daily × 3 days, then every 3 days
Liver function tests	Preinfusion, then weekly
Glucose	Every 6 hours × 24 hours, then daily

     d. Cardiac
         i. Maximally concentrate all enteral and parenteral solutions.
         ii. Restrict sodium as indicated.
         iii. Supply potassium, particularly in patients receiving digitalis.
         iv. Additional potassium and magnesium during aggressive diuresis.
         v. Do not use the GI tract if the patient is on multiple vasopressor agents.
     e. Monitoring. Daily monitoring parameters for the patient receiving nutritional support are outlined in Table 4.3.
   3. Desired outcomes
     a. Fluid balance
     b. Serum electrolytes within normal levels
     c. Minimize metabolic complications: hepatic encephalopathy, uremia, increased CO_2 retention, hyperglycemia

Reference

1. Ackerman, M.H., Evans, N.J., and Ecklund, M.M. Systemic inflammatory response syndrome, sepsis, and nutritional support. *Crit. Care Nurs. Clin. N. Am.* 6:321, 1994.

Disorders in Patients in Critical Care

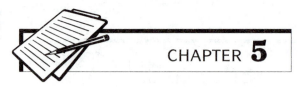

CHAPTER **5**

Cardiovascular Disorders

Jennifer Hebra

Coronary Artery Disease/Angina

I. Definition: The process of atherosclerosis causes thick, nonflexible plaque to adhere to the walls of arterial lumens. Over time, as these plaques increase in size, they cause obstruction of blood flow through the lumen. Plaques tend to build in areas of turbulent flows and in vessel bifurcations. This progressive narrowing of the coronary arterial lumens by atherosclerosis is known as coronary artery disease (CAD). CAD can be linked directly to several cardiac disorders including angina pectoris, myocardial infarction, congestive heart failure, and cardiogenic shock.

A. Angina is chest pain resulting from inadequate oxygen supply for the oxygen demanded by the myocardium. This oxygen supply is limited because of the occlusive nature of the atherosclerotic lesions in CAD. The classic or exertional angina is created by an increase in the myocardial oxygen demand. Demand requirements are enhanced by increases in heart rate (HR), systolic blood pressure (SBP), myocardial wall tension, and contractility. Prinzmetal's, or variant, angina results from a decrease in oxygen supply, while the demand remains constant. In addition to atherosclerotic occlusion, angina may also be caused by coronary vasoconstriction or vasospasm. These two concepts can work in tandem to result in mixed angina, a combination of vasospasm and increased demand. Angina can also be caused by hypertension, cardiac dysrhythmias, aortic stenosis and regurgitation, anemia, and hyperthyroidism.

B. Stable angina is chest pain, usually following exertion and lasting approximately 1–5 minutes, relieved by rest or nitroglycerin, and remaining unchanged over several months; ST-segment depression may be noted on the electrocardiogram (ECG) during episodes of chest pain.

C. Unstable angina is the first episode of chest pain, pain at rest, postinfarction pain, or stable angina that has changes in frequency, timing, or duration and lasts about 10 minutes despite rest or use of sublingual nitroglycerin.

D. Silent ischemia is the presence of objective data to support ischemic myocardium (ie, ECG or other studies) in an asymptomatic patient.

II. Etiology: The clinical etiology of atherosclerosis is the occlusive nature of the plaque formation. As the plaque continues to build, the vessel becomes stenotic, and thrombus may form over the plaque itself or over an area of plaque separation from the intima (innermost layer). Eventually, this may cause complete occlusion. The complete occlusion of a coronary artery may result in myocardial ischemia or infarction.

III. Nursing process

A. Assessment
   1. Signs and symptoms
      a. Chest pain
         i. Pressure or heaviness
         ii. Substernal, posterior thorax, intrascapular area, left shoulder and down the left arm, often involving the third and fourth fingers, and/or jaw
         iii. Patient often uses fist to describe the sensation
         iv. Patient sometimes mentions burning or itching
      b. Cardiac dysrhythmias: high risk of occurring when the patient is experiencing chest pain due to discrepancy in oxygen supply and demand
         i. Potentially lethal ventricular dysrhythmias and atrioventricular blocks
      c. Associated symptoms
         i. Nausea, vomiting, diaphoresis, dyspnea, cool and clammy skin, increased HR, increased blood pressure: All result from sympathetic nervous system stimulation.
         ii. Symptoms typically subside when the angina resolves.
   2. Diagnostic tests
      a. Serum: *Serum enzymes* may be elevated if acute myocardial infarction (AMI) (see section "Acute Myocardial Infarction" later in this chapter).
      b. Urine: no specific changes
      c. Other
         i. *Continuous monitoring* detects premature ventricular contractions (PVCs), ventricular tachycardia (VT), and ventricular fibrillation (VF) from the irritability and instability of the injured area; atrioventricular (AV) blocks especially if ischemia involves right coronary artery (RCA), because the RCA supplies the AV node in most patients.
         ii. *Twelve-lead ECG* ST-segment elevation or depression in leads corresponding with myocardial area suffering ischemia. ST-segment changes are thought to result from alterations in repolarization of the ischemic cells.
         iii. *Holter monitoring* records cardiac rhythm over time. Patients keep a diary to compare ECG changes with patient activity.
         iv. *Exercise ECGs* detect ECG changes associated with exertion.
         v. *Radionuclide imaging* enhances exercise testing by improving sensitivity and specitivity.
         vi. *Cardiac catheterization* (or coronary arteriography) determines the presence or extension of CAD and provides information to support medical or surgical interventions. Significant coronary artery occlusion is greater than 70% obstruction of the vessel.

B. Patient management: must differentiate diagnosis from AMI. See section "Acute Myocardial Infarction" for appropriate interventions.

   1. Potential for myocardial injury related to the discrepancy between myocardial oxygen supply and demand

      a. Problem: Myocardial muscle injury or infarction may result in cardiac dysfunction and chest pain.

      b. Interventions

         i. Maintain hemodynamic stability.

- Monitor blood pressure (BP) and HR every 1–2 hours, with drug titrations, with complaints of chest pain, and as needed.

        ii. Pharmacologic therapy (Table 5.1) [1, 2].

- Oxygen: 2–4 liters via nasal cannula to enhance oxygen delivery
- Nitrates (nitroglycerin, nitroprusside) dilate vascular and selected smooth muscles, both venous and arterial. Decreases venous return, thereby decreasing preload, which alleviates wall tension. This results in reduced myocardial oxygen demand.
- Beta-adrenergic blocking agents (labetolol, propranolol) block the effects of catecholamines. Negative inotropic (contractility) and chronotropic (HR) effects decrease contractility, rate, and oxygen demand; effects are enhanced by concomitant use with nitrates.
- Calcium channel blockers (verapamil, nifedipine, diltiazem) inhibit the movement of calcium across myocardial and vascular smooth muscle cells decreasing myocardial contractility and conductivity and vasodilating the coronary arteries, collateral vessels, and the peripheral arterial system, thereby decreasing myocardial oxygen demand and BP and increasing oxygen supply.

      iii. For all medication administration

- Titrate until pain relieved
- Maintain BP greater than 90 mm Hg systolic
- When discontinuing IV vasoactive medications, always aspirate drug from IV tubing before flushing.
- Monitor side effects of nausea, vomiting, hypotension, bradycardia, dysrhythmias, dizziness, palpations, dyspnea.

      iv. Intervene rapidly to reverse oxygenation discrepancy.

      v. Continuously monitor the ECG leads that have documented ST-segment changes when the patient experiences angina.

      vi. Monitor ECG for dysrhythmias and possible T-wave inversion.

      vii. Instruct patient to recognize and to report to nurse immediately if pain or discomfort recurs.

      viii. Obtain a 12-lead ECG immediately if patient experiences chest pain or changes in the ST segment are noted.

      ix. Maintain patent IV.

      x. Assess efficacy of pharmacologic therapy.

      xi. Modify activity levels to decrease oxygen demand.

- Provide adequate rest periods.
- Plan appropriate visiting goals with the patient and family.
- Avoid large meals.
- Avoid extreme weather temperatures.

Table 5.1 Cardioactive Medications

Drug Class and Drug Name	Action	Administration Guidelines	Special Concerns
Vasodilators and antihypertensives Nitroglycerin Nitroprusside Diazoxide Isosorbide dinitrate	Vasodilation of the systemic arteries, collateral coronary arteries, systemic veins, and relaxation of smooth muscles in epicardial vessels Nitroglycerin $\rightarrow \downarrow$ Pain in ischemia $\rightarrow \downarrow$ Venous return $\rightarrow \downarrow$ Preload and O_2 consumption Nitroprusside $\rightarrow \downarrow$ Preload and afterload $\rightarrow \downarrow$ Myocardial O_2 consumption $\rightarrow \uparrow$ Cardiac output	Nitroglycerin 0.4 mg SL q5min × 3 doses IV: must be mixed in a glass bottle; mix 50 mg/250 mL D5W (200 µg/mL); begin infusion at 5 µg/min up to 10–200 µg/min; titrate to response. Topical: 1½–2 in. of 15 mg per in. ointment Nitroprusside IV: mix 50 mg/250 mL D5W (250 µg/mL); begin infusion at 0.5–10 µg/kg/min; continuous IV infusion Diazoxide IV: 1–3 mg/kg (max 150 mg) IV push; may repeat q5–15 min for HTN crisis Isosorbide dinitrate 2.5–10 mg SL or 10–40 mg PO qid or sustained release 40 mg q6–12h	Monitor BP and HR q1h and after each titration Continuously monitor PAP and CVP; obtain CO, PAWP, and SVR q1–4h or with titrations Monitor urine output and maintain >30 mL/h to assess renal perfusion Maintain patient in recumbent position during all titrations; especially when administering diazoxide May cause hyperglycemia and sodium and water retention Nitroglycerin must be weaned off Nitroprusside is photosensitive and requires protection from light; also monitor for cyanide toxicity Monitor patient for headache, dizziness, nausea and vomiting, palpitations, and abdominal cramping All IV vasodilators should be aspirated from line before flushing
Beta-blockers Labetalol Propranolol	Block beta-adrenergic receptor sites resulting in: $\rightarrow \downarrow$ HR $\rightarrow \downarrow$ Myocardial contractility Slowed AV conduction $\rightarrow \downarrow$ BP $\rightarrow \downarrow$ Myocardial oxygen demand	Labetalol IV: 20 mg IV injection over 3–5 min, may repeat with 40–80 mg in 10 min to maximum of 300 mg PO: 100–400 mg 2 ×/d	Continuously monitor for HR and dysrhythmias Check BP q5min during administration and 2 × afterward Patient must remain recumbent for 30 min after IV injections

Table 5.1 *Continued*

Drug Class and Drug Name	Action	Administration Guidelines	Special Concerns
Beta-blockers (*cont.*)	↓ Dysrhythmias by decreasing circulating catecholamine effects	**Propranolol** IV: 1–3 mg IV no faster than 1 mg/min, repeat dose after 2 min once only, to a total dose of 0.1 mg/kg PO: 10–20 mg, 3–4×/d	Notify physician if BP drops more than 20 mm Hg or if SBP <100 mm Hg Assess for rales and wheezing frequently; may cause bronchospasms, report to physician promptly Avoid use in bradycardia, hypotension, CHF, pulmonary edema, COPD
Calcium channel blockers Diltiazem Nifedipine Verapamil	Influx of calcium into muscle cells dictates the resting tone and activation of muscle contraction; calcium channel blockers relax vascular smooth muscle and cause peripheral vasodilation, thus decreasing BP, force of contraction, and delay AV nodal conduction; used to control BP and angina; decreases refractoriness of the AV node and terminates AV nodal reentry dysrhythmias	**Diltiazem** IV: 0.25 mg/kg IV over 2 min (20 mg avg), if response not adequate after 15 min, 0.35 mg/kg over 2 min, then start infusion of 150 mg/150 mg NS (1 mg/mL) at 10–15 mg/h PO: 60–120 mg 2×/d **Nifedipine** PO: 10–20 mg 3×/d, may be punctured and administered SL **Verapamil** IV: 2.5–5 mg IV over 2–3 min, may repeat after 30 min with 5–10 mg to a maximum dose of 20 mg PO: 80 mg 3×/d	Monitor BP q5min during all IV injections and q5min 2× Monitor BP q1h with diltiazem infusion Monitor for 2nd- and 3rd-degree heart blocks; atropine may assist in improving HR Assess for signs and symptoms of CHF and peripheral edema Notify physician if SBP drops more than 20 mm Hg or to <100 mm Hg Ensure resuscitation equipment is available, especially with verapamil injection; rapid ventricular rate or severe hypotension may be seen Patient should remain recumbent at least 1 hour after IV injections Avoid verapamil and diltiazem in AV block, Wolff-Parkinson-White syndrome, severe cardiac failure, and sinus nodal dysfunction

Inotropes
Digoxin
Dopamine
Dobutamine
Amrinone

Increase the force of contraction, while there is an increase in myocardial oxygen demand, this is usually balanced by a decrease in chamber size, thereby reducing wall tension

Digoxin
↑ Contractility
↓ Heart rate

Dopamine
Precursor to norepinephrine; stimulation of alpha, beta, and dopaminergic receptors; depends on infusion rate
↑ Heart rate

Dobutamine
↑ Stroke volume
↑ Cardiac output
↑ BP
↑ Heart rate

Amrinone
Vasodilates by relaxing vascular smooth muscle

Digoxin
IV: 0.25–0.50 mg q4–6h to total 1.0 mg, then 0.125–0.5 mg daily
PO: 0.5–0.75 mg followed by 0.25–0.5 mg q6–8h to total 1.0–1.5 mg then 0.125–0.5 mg daily

Dopamine
IV: mix 400/250 mL D5W (1.6 mg/mL)
Infuse at renal dose (dopaminergic): 0.5–3.0 μg/kg/min; inotropic dose (beta): 3–10 μg/kg/min; alpha: 10–20 μg/kg/min

Dobutamine
IV: 500 mg/250 mL (2 mg/mL); infuse at 2.5–4.0 μg/kg/min

Amrinone
IV: 0.75 mg/kg; IV push: over 2–3 min; if in peripheral line dilute with NS to avoid irritation, then mix 400 mg/250 mL NS (1.6 mg/mL), start infusion at 5 μg/kg/min

Monitor for digoxin toxicity (nausea, vomiting, visual disturbances, dysrhythmias), especially if acidotic or electrolytes imbalanced
Monitor potassium level B/C hypokalemia; increases incidence of digoxin toxicity
Carefully monitor HR, BP, dysrhythmias (VT, SVT) and urine output during infusions
Assess IV site frequently to detect infiltrations
Correct hypovolemia before administration
Dopamine and dobutamine inactivated by alkaline solutions
Amrinone will precipitate with furosemide; do not mix with dextrose solutions

Table 5.1 *Continued*

Drug Class and Drug Name	Action	Administration Guidelines	Special Concerns
Beta-adrenergic stimulators Isoproterenol	Stimulate beta receptor sites to increase cardiac contractility and HR **Isoproterenol** Pure beta-adrenergic stimulator ↑ Cardiac output ↑ ↑ ↑ Myocardial oxygen consumption Vasodilator, therefore ↓ BP	IV: mix 2 mg/250 mL D5W (8 µg/mL); infuse at 2–10 µg/min; titrate for HR response; *never* give IV push	Monitor BP q1h, prn, and with each dosage change Continuously monitor HR Reduce dose if HR >110; greatly increases myocardial oxygen demand Due to ↑ in myocardial oxygen demand, may extend myocardial ischemia
Anticoagulant agents Heparin	Anticoagulates by preventing the conversion of prothrombin to thrombin and the conversion of fibrinogen to fibrin	IV injection: 10,000 U initially, then 5000–10,000 U q4–6h IV infusion: 5000–10,000 U IV as a loading dose, then mix 25,000 U/500 mL D5W (50 U/mL) and start infusion at 500–1500 U/h; titrate to keep APTT 1.5–2 times control value SQ: 10,000–20,000 U initially, then 8000–20,000 U q8–12h	Monitor frequently for bleeding (petechiae, bruising) and thrombocytopenia (platelet count <150,000/mm³) Have protamine sulfate and heparin antagonist immediately available in case of heparin overdose Monitor APTT 1 hour after each change in IV infusion rate and q4h until dose stabilized; check results before each injection
Angiotensin-converting enzyme inhibitors Captopril Enalapril	Inhibit ACE from converting inactive angiotensin I to active angiotensin II in the plasma and lungs (angiotensin II has pressor effects and stimulates the secretion of aldosterone); thus, ACE inhibitors decrease peripheral vascular resistance and salt and water retention	**Captopril** PO: 12.5–25 mg 2–3 ×/d **Enalapril** PO: 10–40 mg/d in 1–2 divided doses IV: 1.25 mg q6h over 5 min; if patient also receiving diuretics, 0.625 mg IV over 5 min	IV enalapril: monitor BP q15min 2×, then q30min 2×, then q2h; hypotension may not be seen for 4 hours after dose Check for orthostatic hypotension before getting out of bed Monitor fluid status daily (input and output)

Drug	Mechanism	Dosage	Nursing Considerations
Diuretics Bumetanide Ethacrynic acid Furosemide	Diuretic; inhibits tubular reabsorption of sodium and chloride, resulting in high-volume urine excretion Furosemide ↑ Venous capacity; therefore, ↓ preload	**Bumetanide** PO: 0.5–2.0 mg/d IV: 0.5–1.0 mg, repeat in 2–3 h until desired response, maximum 10 mg **Ethacrynic acid** PO: 50–100 mg/d IV: 0.5–1.0 mg/kg over 1–2 min, may be repeated with dose of 50 mg; reconstitute in D5W or NS; do not use if cloudy **Furosemide** PO: 20–80 mg per dose; do not exceed 600 mg/d IV: 20–40 mg dose IV over 1–3 min; increase dose by 20 mg q2–3h until desired response	Monitor sodium, chloride, and potassium levels daily or more frequently, depending on dosing Monitor fluid balance (input and output) carefully Obtain urine output q1h Replace IV doses with oral doses as soon as possible Obtain orthostatic BP before getting out of bed
NSAIDs Ibuprofen	Blocks the synthesis and release of prostaglandins, thus decreasing pain and capillary leakage	**Ibuprofen** PO: 400–800 mg 3–4 ×/d; do not exceed 3200 mg/d	If possible, administer drug with food or antacid Assess patient for GI symptoms of nausea, vomiting, or anorexia; may try lower dosages at more frequent intervals

Table 5.1 *Continued*

Drug Class and Drug Name	Action	Administration Guidelines	Special Concerns
Class Ia antiarrhythmic Quinidine	Class Ia antidysrhythmic that prolongs the action potential; prolongs the refractory period; may terminate atrial fibrillation and flutter and suppresses SVT and ventricular dysrhythmias; may prevent VT and VF	200–300 mg PO q6–8h IM: administration very painful, larger dose required IV: rarely given and can cause cardiovascular collapse	Must monitor QT intervals, notify physician if QT_c ($QT_c = QT/\sqrt{RR}$) increases Prolongs AV nodal conduction; do not give in conduction disorders Absolutely contraindicated in torsades de pointes: it will potentiate rhythm and progress to VF (secondary to prolonged QT) GI side effects: diarrhea and abdominal cramping
Catecholamines Epinephrine Norepinephrine	Stimulate alpha and beta receptors within the sympathetic nervous system	Epinephrine IV: cardiac arrest: 0.5–1.0 mg IV push (1:10,000) Continuous infusion: 2 mg/250 mL D5W (8 µg/mL); infuse 1–8 µg/min Norepinephrine Continuous infusion: 4 mg/250 mL D5W (16 µg/mL) and infuse at 2–10 µg/min Dilute in D5W only	Check BP before, immediately after, 5 and 15 minutes after and at least q1h after dose or initiation of administration or with titrations Continuously monitor for ventricular dysrhythmias (PVCs, VT, and VF) Do not mix with alkaline solutions May see transient increase in WBC count Assess IV access frequently to avoid extravasation (necrosis and sloughing of surrounding tissue may occur)

QT_c, rate-corrected QT interval; other abbreviations as defined in text.
Adapted from Malseed, R. T. *Pharmacology Drug Therapy and Nursing Considerations* (3rd ed.). Philadelphia: J. B. Lippincott, 1990; and Underhill, S. L. et al. (eds.). *Cardiovascular Medications for Cardiac Nursing*. Philadelphia: J. B. Lippincott, 1990.

- Create an activity plan with the patient and family and closely monitor patient's tolerance to the activity level (ie, increases in HR, BP, respiratory rate).
- Meet comfort and privacy needs

xii. Increase coronary artery lumen size—percutaneous transluminal coronary angioplasty (PTCA): Inflate a balloon-tipped catheter inside the affected coronary artery to press the plaque against the lumen wall, thus increasing lumen size (see Appendix A).

c. Desired outcomes

  i. Absence of symptoms of myocardial oxygen discrepancy such as pain, increased HR, decreased BP, ST-segment changes, T-wave inversion, or dysrhythmias noted on ECG

  ii. AMI avoided

  iii. Verbalizes relief of pain

  iv. No complications resulting from PTCA

2. Potential for hemodynamic instability with ischemic episodes related to decreased myocardial tissue perfusion

a. Problem: Increase in HR and decrease in BP results in increased oxygen demand, decreased tissue perfusion, and transient left-sided heart dysfunction.

b. Intervention

  i. Monitor BP and HR every 1–2 hours, after each drug administration or titration, with all episodes of pain, and as needed.

  ii. Reevaluate need for any negative inotropic drugs (ie, beta-adrenergic blockers) because of possible heart failure.

  iii. Monitor closely for dysrhythmias (ie, PVCs, VT, and VF), since they may worsen cardiac function.

c. Desired outcome

  i. BP and HR remain normal.

  ii. Patient avoids left-sided heart dysfunction or failure.

  iii. Patient remains in normal sinus rhythm without ectopy.

3. Differentiate angina from AMI

a. Problem: Treatment options differ for AMI.

b. Intervention

  i. Obtain complete pain description

---

angina
- Should last less than 20 minutes
- Should be relieved by nitroglycerin alone, without additional analgesics
- Usually does not involve sense of impending doom

AMI
- Should have ECG changes consistent with ischemia or necrosis (see section "Acute Myocardial Infarction" for typical ischemic changes)
- AMI will have elevated cardiac enzymes
- Often has sense of impending doom

        c. Desired outcome
          i. Patient receives treatment based on the appropriate differentiation of angina from AMI
  C. Discharge planning
    1. Patient discharged with knowledge about modifiable risk factors and methods to reduce the following risks:
      a. Reduce fat intake
      b. Reduce cholesterol intake
      c. Smoking cessation
      d. Diabetes control
    2. Able to identify activities that precipitate an anginal event and verbalizes action necessary to avert or treat
    3. Sublingual nitroglycerin, one tablet (0.4 mg) every 5 minutes three times or one tablet prophylactically before events known to cause chest pain
    4. Verbalizes symptoms that require seeking health care intervention
    5. States knowledge of correct discharge instructions including medications, activity level, self-assessment of HR, and follow-up requirements

Acute Myocardial Infarction

  I. **Definition:** Necrosis of cardiac cells most often as a result of decreased blood supply to the myocardium from atherosclerosis. Mortality from an AMI is greatest within 2 hours of the onset of pain and can be reduced by prompt intensive care hospitalization and the control of dysrhythmias.

  II. **Etiology:** Coronary arteries with reduced lumen size as a result of plaque formation are vulnerable to the sudden cessation of blood flow due to thrombosis, platelet aggregation, or spasm. This sudden disruption in perfusion, most often from the formation of thrombus, ranging from minutes to hours, can cause irreversible damage to the myocardium distal to the affected coronary artery. Thrombus formation is thought to result from plaque rupture, bleeding into the plaque, or erosion of the intimal layer area over the lesion.

  III. **Nursing process**

  A. Assessment
    1. Signs and symptoms
      a. Chest pain that lasts greater than 20 minutes, is not relieved by nitroglycerin alone, creates high anxiety, and may involve a sense of impending doom (see description of chest pain on pp. 77, in "Coronary Artery Disease/Angina")
      b. Hypotension related to decreased cardiac output (CO) from left ventricular dysfunction (see Cardiogenic Shock, p. 96)
      c. Hypertension related to reflexive sympathetic nervous system stimulation, vasoconstriction to combat low CO, and pain
      d. Tachycardia in response to decreased stroke volume and pain
      e. Bradycardia may result from conduction abnormalities caused by myocardial ischemia (ie, heart blocks).

   f. Dysrhythmias—injury irritability or increased wall tension enhance
      dysrhythmia probability; continuously monitor for VT, VF, atrial fibril-
      lation and flutter, and AV blocks
   g. Cool, clammy extremities and diaphoresis due to cardiogenic shock
   h. Third or fourth heart sound (S_3 or S_4) on auscultation from heart
      failure or decreased ventricular compliance, respectively
   i. Heart murmurs and rubs may be auscultated as a result of turbulent
      blood flow and abnormal heart muscle movement; a pericardial rub is
      most often heard on the fourth day after myocardial infarction (MI).
   j. Jugular venous distention (JVD) secondary to decreased systolic emp-
      tying from ventricular dysfunction
   k. Complications that should be anticipated include cardiogenic shock,
      congestive heart failure (CHF), dysrhythmias, pulmonary emboli, rup-
      tures of the septum and papillary muscle, and aneurysm.
2. Diagnostic parameters
   a. Serum
      i. Enzymes: Enzyme elevations that reflect damage specifically to
         the myocardium include creatine kinase MB isoenzyme (CK-MB)
         and lactate dehydrogenase (LDH) isoenzymes. Although CK-MB
         is indicative of myocardial necrosis, it may not be as a result of MI.
         If the LDH_2/LDH_3 ratio is greater than 1, the diagnosis of MI is
         supported (Table 5.2).
   b. Urine. No specific changes
   c. Other
      i. The electrocardiogram may show ST-segment elevation or
         peaked or inverted T waves, especially in the cardiac monitoring
         leads that are sensitive to the area of the infarct. Although Q waves
         demonstrate septal activation and are normal in some leads (I,
         aVL, and V_6), they are not normal in all leads. Abnormal Q waves
         appear when extensive myocardial ischemia results in conduc-
         tion delays under the sensing electrode. A Q-wave infarct refers to
         MIs that increase the depth or duration of normal Q waves or
         when new Q waves appear that were not previously apparent.
         Usually, pathologic Q waves develop within 2–9 hours of infarct or
         in patients with a long history of ischemia. ECG changes may
         appear for reasons other than myocardial ischemia and must be
         differentiated from pericarditis, cardiomyopathy, pulmonary em-
         boli, and chronic obstructive pulmonary disease. Table 5.3 [2, 3]

Table 5.2 Timetable of Enzyme Elevations that Reflect Myocardial Damage

Enzyme	Elevation Onset	Elevation Peak	Return to Normal
CK-MB	4–6 h	12–20 h	36–48 h
LDH_2 and LDH_3	Both increase in 12 h	24–48 h	3–4 d

Abbreviations as defined in text.

Table 5.3 Probable Coronary Arteries Responsible for Myocardial
Infarctions and Corresponding Leads that Are Most
Likely to Demonstrate Ischemic Changes

Infarction	Coronary Artery Involved and Comments	Leads that May Show Ischemic Changes
Anterior wall	Usually LAD; septal involvement is common	V_1–V_4; if chest lead already used for continuous dysrhythmia monitoring, also use III or aVF
Inferior wall	RCA (most people) or LCA	II, III, and aVF
Lateral wall	LCA	I, III, aVL, aVF, V_5, and V_6
Posterior wall	RCA (most people) or LCA	V_1 and V_2: reciprocal changes of tall R waves and ST-segment depression; possibly II, III, and aVF if also inferior involvement

LAD, left anterior descending coronary artery; LCA, left circumflex artery; other abbreviation as defined in text.
Adapted from Underhill, S. L., et al. (eds.). *Cardiovascular Medications for Cardiac Nursing.*
Philadelphia: J. B. Lippincott, 1990; and Stillwell, S. *Quick Critical Care Reference.* St. Louis:
C. V. Mosby, 1990.

is a list of MI sites, the probable coronary artery responsible, and
the leads most likely to demonstrate these changes.

ii. Two-dimensional echocardiography provides images that define
the cardiac structures and allows for visualization of wall motion
abnormalities. Blood flow in the heart can be distinguished, and
valvular dysfunction may be seen.

IV. Patient management

A. Pain related to decreased myocardial tissue perfusion
   1. Problem: Pain increases myocardial oxygen consumption and circulating
      catecholamines, which increases myocardial workload.
   2. Interventions
      a. Oxygen: 2–4 liters via nasal cannula; some patients in respiratory distress
         may require a face mask; obtain an arterial blood gas only if patient is in
         distress, because of the possibility of administering thrombolytics; be
         prepared to assist in intubation and mechanical ventilation if hypoxia
         persists (arterial oxygen saturation < 90% and arterial carbon dioxide
         tension ($Paco_2$) > 45–50 mm Hg) with 100% oxygen therapy
      b. Sublingual nitroglycerin—0.4 mg every 5 minutes, up to three doses.
         If hypotension occurs, elevate extremities and administer an IV saline
         infusion.
      c. Administer morphine sulfate.
      d. Monitor BP and pulse every 5 minutes during the administration of
         analgesics.

---

morphine sulfate
Action Causes venodilation, which reduces preload and decreases afterload.
Administration Guidelines 1–4 mg IV and repeated every 5–10 minutes until pain is controlled or side effects occur.
Special Considerations Look for nausea, vomiting, hypotension, dizziness, and respiratory depression.

---

  e. Frequently assess pain relief using an objective pain scale and document.
  f. Administer beta-adrenergic blockers such as labetalol or propranolol to decrease myocardial oxygen demand, thereby decreasing pain (see Table 5.1).
  3. Desired outcome: Pain is relieved as evidenced by patient confirmation using objective pain scale.
B. Minimize myocardial cell injury related to decreased myocardial tissue perfusion from coronary artery occlusion.
  1. Problem: Continued occlusion increases infarct size and leads to worsening cardiac muscle function, possible cardiogenic shock, and death.
  2. Intervention
    a. Obtain pertinent data to determine that an infarct has or is occurring: Obtain ECG immediately; obtain lab values, including cardiac enzymes at the prescribed times; avoid IM injections that may alter enzyme results; assess chest pain for frequency, duration, and severity.
    b. Administer beta-adrenergic blocking agents (labetalol, propranolol): reduce HR, BP, and myocardial contractility, which results in decreased oxygen demand. (See Table 5.1 for a list of drugs and administration guidelines.)
    c. Nitroglycerin has been shown to limit infarct size when administration is started early and hypotension does not occur.
    d. Heparin therapy may decrease mortality, but bleeding complications should limit use to patients with large anterior MIs, those at risk for developing cardiac wall thrombi, or those at risk for a recurrent MI.

---

heparin
Action Inhibits the clotting of blood by preventing conversion of prothrombin to thrombin and fibrinogen to fibrin.
Administration Guidelines 5000 USP (United States Pharmacopeia) units IV, followed by 1000 USP units per hour continuous infusion; titrate to maintain partial thromboplastin time (PTT) at 1½ to 2 times normal value.
Special Considerations Monitor PTT with each dose adjustment until value normalizes, then every 8 hours to every day; monitor for bleeding from skin and mucous membranes and presence of hematuria or hemoptysis.

---

e. Consider reperfusion of the myocardium.

   i. Thrombolytic agents induce clot lysis and restore perfusion of the myocardium; Table 5.4 [1] provides descriptions of thrombolytic agents.
   - Start at least two IV catheters before administration of thrombolytics.
   - If arterial blood-gas analysis is absolutely required, use radial site for puncture, since pressure can be applied easily.
   - Initiate therapy within 4–6 hours of the onset of chest pain.
   - Heparin administered concomitantly to maintain the activated partial thromboplastin time (aPTT) at two times the control value speeds the rate of coronary reperfusion
   - Aspirin 325 mg PO may decrease mortality when administered with streptokinase.

   ii. Thrombolytic therapy is indicated for patients with the following:
   - Ischemic symptoms persisting longer than 30 minutes
   - New ST-segment elevation of at least 0.1 mV in at least two leads reflecting changes of the inferior, anterior, or lateral wall or ST-segment depression reflecting posterior damage; see Table 5.3 for the ECG leads most likely to display ST-segment changes.

   iii. Thrombolytic therapy is contraindicated for patients with the following:
   - Documented bleeding disorder
   - Recent history of GI or genitourinary bleeding
   - Documented BP greater than 200/120 mm Hg
   - History of a cerebrovascular accident, head trauma, or surgery
   - Prolonged cardiopulmonary resuscitation
   - Pregnancy
   - Suspected aortic dissection, diabetic hemorrhagic retinopathy, or presenting with a serious illness

f. PTCA: See Appendix A for a description of this treatment modality.

g. Coronary artery bypass graft: See Appendix A for a description of this treatment modality.

h. Maintain patent IV access for the administration of analgesics and antidysrhythmic agents.

i. See sections "Congestive Heart Failure/Pulmonary Edema" and "Cardiogenic Shock" for the assessment and management (including hemodynamic monitoring) of these complications.

j. See the American Heart Association advanced cardiac life support (ACLS) algorithms in Appendix C for the treatment of cardiac arrest.

k. Continuously monitor the ECG in the leads most appropriate to detect reocclusions of the involved arteries [4,5]. See Table 5.3 for appropriate monitoring leads.

l. Administer antidysrhythmic medications as quickly as they are needed based on ACLS guidelines (see Appendix C).

Table 5.4 Thrombolytic Therapy

Drug Name	Action	Administration Guidelines	Special Concerns (All Agents)
All thrombolytic agents	Convert plasminogen to plasmin degrading fibrin clots, plasma proteins, and fibrinogen	See specific agents, below	Most effective if therapy initiated within 4–6 h of *onset of symptoms*; the sooner therapy started, the more likely infarct area will be limited
Urokinase (generalized lysis)	Uses enzymes from human kidneys to activate plasminogen directly Half-life: 20 min	IV: reconstitute 250,000 IU vial with 5.2 mL of sterile water until dissolved, then mix in 500 mL D5W or NS (500 U/mL); give 4400 U/kg over 10 min; then administer 4400 U/kg per hour for 12 h	Monitor ECG rhythm continuously; be aware ventricular ectopy is common Have emergency equipment immediately available (see Advanced Cardiac Life Support guidelines in Appendix C)
Streptokinase (generalized lysis)	Uses beta-hemolytic streptococci to link with plasminogen to ultimately form plasmin Half-life: 23 min	IV: 250,000 U initially, then 100,000 U/h for 24 h or 1,500,000 U in single IV infusion over 1 h. Check streptokinase resistance levels before initiating therapy, do not give if >1,000,000 U	Assess patient for signs and symptoms of bleeding; hematuria, bleeding from IV sites, etc. Discontinue therapy if serious bleeding occurs Secure IV access (at least two) before initiating therapy
Alteplase (tissue plasminogen activator) (clot specific)	Uses tissue culture by recombinant DNA methods to bind with fibrin to convert plasminogen to plasmin with limited systemic effects Half-life: <10 min	IV: total 100 mg by administering 60 mg 1st h (6–10-mg bolus 1st 1–2 min), then 20 mg over 2nd h, then 20 mg over 3rd h; reconstitute with sterile water only	Avoid arterial punctures for 48 h; if required, use radial artery and hold direct pressure for an uninterrupted 30 min Monitor for allergic reaction (wheezing, decreased BP)

Abbreviations as defined in text.
Adapted from Malseed, R. T. *Pharmacology Drug Therapy and Nursing Considerations* (3rd ed.). Philadelphia: J. B. Lippincott, 1990.

    m. Anticipate the development of life-threatening dysrhythmias by avoiding hypoxia, acidosis, electrolyte imbalances, left ventricular failure, hypotension, and recurrent ischemia.

    n. Initiate transvenous or transcutaneous pacing as indicated for asystole, second-degree type II or third-degree heart block, symptomatic bradycardia refractory to atropine administration, new left bundle branch block, and a new right bundle branch block when left anterior or posterior hemiblock exists. (See Appendix A for the care of a patient with a pacemaker.)

    o. Institute an activity plan with the agreement of the patient and family to limit stress and myocardial workload.

    p. Provide sedation as required to assist with myocardial oxygen perfusion.

    q. Avoid large meals, caffeine, and beverages that are too hot or cold.

    r. Provide stool softeners as needed to prevent straining.

  3. Desired outcome

    a. Adequate myocardial tissue perfusion is attained as evidenced by absence of ST-segment elevation, dysrhythmias, and pain.

    b. Complications of an AMI are avoided as evidenced by patient progressing through recovery phase without event.

C. Discharge planning

  1. Ensure that patient has knowledge base about avoidable risk factors and how to control them.

  2. Review patient's plan for a cardiac rehabilitation program.

  3. Review information about follow-up appointment with patient and family.

  4. Ensure patient has knowledge of medications and treatments and has an understanding of the importance of adherence to medication and therapy regimens.

Congestive Heart Failure/Pulmonary Edema

  I. Definition: Congestive heart failure (CHF) is the inability of the cardiac muscle to contract with sufficient force and effectiveness to maintain adequate cardiac output and tissue perfusion despite adequate venous return.

  II. Etiology: CHF may result from complications of AMI, sequelae of cardiomyopathy, or undue stress on the heart by fluid overload, anemia, or thyrotoxicosis. Incomplete systolic emptying of blood returning from the systemic vessels causes volume accumulation and edema formation. CHF can affect the right or left ventricle depending on the location of muscle dysfunction.

  III. Nursing process

  A. Assessment

    1. Signs and symptoms

      a. Relative to both left- and right-sided failure

        i. Tachycardia: an attempt to increase CO

     ii. Decreased CO, cardiac index (CI): pump failure and incomplete systolic emptying impede forward blood flow

     iii. Increased systemic vascular resistance (SVR): constriction reflexive from decrease in CO

     iv. Increased right atrial pressure (RAP), pulmonary artery pressure (PAP), and pulmonary artery wedge pressure (PAWP): due to incomplete systolic emptying and backflow of blood

     v. Possible hypotension: pump failure

  b. Left-sided heart failure (pulmonary edema)

     i. Wet cough and frothy sputum: Backflow of blood into the pulmonary and systemic vasculature increases the pressure causing interstitial leak to occur.

     ii. Interstitial leak interferes with gas exchange of oxygen and carbon dioxide possibly resulting in the following:

       • Dyspnea, nocturnal dyspnea, orthopnea, carbon dioxide retention acidosis, anxiety, crackles or wheezing, cyanosis, pallor, or oxygen saturation by pulse oximetry less than 94%

     iii. Elevated PAP, PAWP, SVR: reflects left ventricular failure and incomplete systolic emptying

     iv. S_3: rapid ventricular filling

     v. S_4: atrial contraction forcing blood into a distended ventricle

  c. Right-sided heart failure. Backflow of blood into the systemic circulation causes the following:

     i. Jugular vein distention

     ii. Peripheral, possibly pitting edema

     iii. Systemic fluid retention; ascites

     iv. Right pleural effusion

     v. Nausea, vomiting, loss of appetite; abdominal pain

  d. Decreased urinary output: less than 30 mL/h secondary to renal venous congestion with decreased glomerular filtration rate

  e. Hepatomegaly: secondary to venous congestion

2. Diagnostic tests

  a. Serum

     i. Secondary to pulmonary congestion

       • Arterial blood gas analysis

        ◦ Arterial oxygen tension (PaO_2) less than 80 mm Hg: Fluid in alveoli decreases gas exchange.

        ◦ $PaCO_2$ less than 35 mm Hg: Increased respiratory rate (RR) lowers carbon dioxide level.

        ◦ pH greater than 7.45: result of decreased carbon dioxide levels and resulting alkalosis

     ii. Secondary to systemic venous congestion

       • Sodium less than 140 mEq/L if diluted from edema

       • Potassium less than 3.5 mEq/L from uncontrolled diuretic medication use

       • Potassium greater than 5.0 mEq/L if renal failure present

     iii. Elevated liver enzymes secondary to liver dysfunction

- Serum glutamic oxaloacetic transaminase (SGOT) greater than 40 U/L
- Serum glutamate pyruvate transaminase (SGPT) greater than 35 U/L
- LDH greater than 250 U/L
- Alkaline phosphatase (ALP) greater than 35 U/L
- Bilirubin: direct greater than 0.2 mg/dL and total greater than 1.0 mg/dL

b. Urine: no specific changes

c. Other

   i. ECG may show various dysrhythmias, most frequently atrial flutter and fibrillation; the fluid that accumulates in the heart chambers causes the myocardium to stretch; increased wall tension enhances myocardial irritability and increases dysrhythmia probability.

  ii. X-ray may demonstrate cardiomegaly, pleural effusion, pulmonary congestion, and enlarged liver.

B. Patient management

  1. Decreased CO and tissue/organ perfusion related to impaired myocardial function and pulmonary and systemic fluid accumulation

   a. Problem: poor tissue/organ perfusion and cellular injury and possible death

   b. Intervention

    i. Administer medications in collaboration with physicians to include the following (see Table 5.1):

- Vasodilators: morphine to decrease venous return and myocardial oxygen consumption. Nitrates increase venous capacity, thus reducing venous blood return, which decreases central venous pressure (CVP), RAP, pulmonary artery pressures (PAP), and PAWP (preload). Nitroprusside dilates arterial vessels, thus reducing SVR and myocardial workload.
- Inotropes to enhance myocardial contractility and ventricular ejection of blood volume (digitalis, dopamine, dobutamine, and amrinone)
- Diuretics to reduce actual circulating blood volume (furosemide, bumetanide, and ethacrynic acid)
- Angiotensin-converting–enzyme (ACE) inhibitors decrease preload and afterload while increasing cardiac output by preventing angiotensin I from converting to angiotensin II (captopril and enalapril)

   ii. Monitor and report changes in CVP, PAP, PAWP, SVR, and CO every hour, as needed, or with every drug titration. (See Appendix H for normal values and formulas for calculation.)

  iii. Monitor BP closely for hypotension, notify physician, and titrate drugs to keep SBP greater than 90 mm Hg.

  iv. Continuously monitor mixed venous oxygen saturation ($S\bar{v}o_2$) if available and attempt to maintain between 70% and 80%.

    v. Limit fluid intake to support reducing circulating volume, carefully monitor and document intake and output hourly.

   vi. Maintain urine output greater than 30 mL/h.

  vii. Weigh patient every day; 1 kg = 1 liter of fluid.

 viii. Limit patient activity to conserve myocardial oxygen utilization.

   ix. Assess physical symptoms of fluid retention every 4 hours: pedal (pitting) edema, jugular vein distention, S_3.

    x. Continuously monitor for cardiac dysrhythmias and treat according to ACLS guidelines (see Appendix C).

   xi. Maintain patent IV/central lines for medication administration.

  xii. Monitor digitalis levels to maintain in therapeutic range; assess for digitalis toxicity even if level is within normal range, especially in the presence of electrolyte imbalances and acidosis.

 xiii. Maintain serum potassium greater than 4.5 mEq/L, especially if administering digitalis and diuretics.

 xiv. May administer heparin 5000 U SC to prevent thrombus formation, if patient is undergoing bed rest.

  xv. Monitor and control chest pain (ischemia secondary to inadequate myocardial perfusion)

c. Desired outcome

    i. Patient maintains adequate CO and tissue perfusion as evidenced by HR, BP, CVP, PAP, PAWP, SVR, CO, and $S\bar{v}o_2$ within normal range.

   ii. Jugular venous distention (JVD) diminished

  iii. Lung fields clear

  iv. Appropriate mentation

   v. Urine output greater than 30 mL/h

2. Alteration in gas exchange related to interstitial fluid leak in the pulmonary vasculature interfering with alveolar–capillary exchange of oxygen and carbon dioxide

  a. Problem: Decreased tissue oxygenation may cause cellular injury and possible death.

  b. Intervention

    i. Administer oxygen 2–4 liters per nasal cannula to maintain Pao_2 greater than 80 mm Hg to support perfusion efforts; be prepared to provide mechanical ventilation if necessary.

   ii. Monitor arterial O_2 saturation by pulse oximetry; attempt to maintain greater than 94%.

  iii. Continuously monitor $S\bar{v}o_2$ and attempt to maintain between 70% and 80%.

  iv. Monitor CVP, PAP, PAWP, SVR, CO, and PVR; document values and report changes in trends to physician.

   v. Calculate and monitor alveolar–arterial O_2 tension gradient (see Appendix H); report findings to physician.

  vi. Obtain arterial blood gases as needed to monitor adequate oxygenation; collaborate with physicians for changes needed in oxygen therapy.

       vii. Assess breath sounds every 2 hours for crackles, rhonchi, or wheezing.

      viii. Assist patient to a position that maximizes chest expansion.

      ix. Encourage patient to cough frequently to expel sputum.

      x. If intubated, suction as needed to control frothy secretions.

      xi. Prevent pneumonia and atelectasis by encouraging patient to cough and deep breath or use incentive spirometer every hour while awake.

   c. Desired outcome:

      i. Arterial blood gas results within normal limits; respiratory rate (RR) 12–20 breaths/minute; absence of adventitious breath sounds; adequate tissue perfusion

      ii. No dysrhythmias

      iii. Hemodynamic parameters within normal limits

C. Discharge planning

   1. Ensure patient understands low sodium diet, rational for pharmacologic treatment, anxiety control, symptoms that require medical attention, and risk factor modification.

   2. Ensure patient is aware of need for frequent rest periods and activity limitations.

   3. Review considerations in section "Acute Myocardial Infarction." See Discharge planning, pp. 86, 92.

Cardiogenic Shock

  I. Definition: All forms of shock are characterized by decreased tissue perfusion. Cardiogenic shock is caused by a dysfunction of the myocardium, usually as a result of an MI that involves greater than 40% of the heart muscle. Cardiogenic shock can also result from cardiac surgery, cardiac tamponade, cardiomyopathy, CHF, massive pulmonary emboli, ventricular septal defects, papillary muscle rupture, valvular disorders, or any cardiac dysfunction that interferes with stroke volume.

  II. Etiology: CO decreases as a result of ventricular dysfunction, causing a decrease in blood pressure. As a compensatory mechanism, epinephrine and norepinephrine are released in order to improve contractility and HR. If the cardiac function cannot be improved adequately by compensatory mechanisms to meet the metabolic needs of the body, cell injury occurs. As the cycle continues and more cells are destroyed, multisystem organ failure eventually transpires.

  III. Nursing process

  A. Assessment

   1. Signs and symptoms

    a. Signs congruent with an AMI (see Signs and symptoms in "Acute Myocardial Infarction," p. 86)

    b. Hypotension: Systolic blood pressure (SBP) less than 90 mm Hg and mean arterial blood pressure (MAP) less than 65 mm Hg secondary to decreased cardiac function that results in decreased CO

c. Tachycardia: Increased HR is a compensatory mechanism to improve CO.

d. Skin cold, clammy, pale and weak thready pulses from decreased peripheral perfusion

e. Tachypnea: RR greater than 20 breaths/minute due to pulmonary congestion and anxiety

f. Pulmonary congestion: Pressure from failing left ventricle leads to decreased ventricular emptying and thus pulmonary backflow.

g. Peripheral edema: As the ventricles fail, systemic congestion results.

h. Increased filling pressures: pulmonary artery systolic pressure (PAS) >30 mm Hg, pulmonary artery diastolic pressure (PAD) >15 mm Hg, PAWP >18 mm Hg, due to incomplete systolic emptying

i. Decreased CI: <2 L/min per m^2, due to left ventricular failure

j. Increased SVR: greater than 1400 dyn, due to compensatory vasoconstriction

k. Mixed venous oxygenation decreased: S$\overline{v}$o$_2$ less than 70% secondary to decrease in supply from failing ventricle

l. Neurologic deficits: Possible confusion, lethargy from decreased cerebral perfusion

m. Urine output less than 30 mL/h from decreased renal perfusion and a compensatory mechanism to conserve volume

2. Diagnostic tests
   a. Serum
      i. Blood urea nitrogen (BUN) and creatinine (Cr) may be elevated from renal impairment.
      ii. Cardiac enzymes may be elevated if myocardial ischemia has occurred.
      iii. Arterial blood gases may demonstrate acidosis or hypoxemia from poor tissue perfusion.
      iv. Blood glucose elevated from glycogenolysis from sympathetic nervous system stimulation
      v. Hyperkalemia: Potassium greater than 5.0 mEq/L secondary to decreased renal perfusion
      vi. Lactate levels may be increased if anaerobic metabolism has occurred.
   b. Urine: No specific changes
   c. Other. Chest radiography: The heart may be enlarged, and pulmonary congestion may be present due to inadequate systolic emptying.

B. Patient management
   1. Decreased tissue perfusion related to left ventricular failure and the inability to provide an adequate cardiac output to meet tissue demands
      a. Problem: Poor tissue perfusion leads to cellular and organ injury and possible death.
      b. Intervention
         i. Monitor BP and HR every 1–2 hours, with drug titrations and prn.

      ii. Continuously monitor PAP, S$\bar{v}o_2$, and CVP; be sure to correlate findings with pharmacologic interventions.

      iii. Obtain PAWP, SVR, and CO every 4 hours and collaborate with physician if treatment changes are required.

      iv. Assess pulses and capillary refill every hour to monitor peripheral perfusion.

      v. Avoid Trendelenburg's position for hypotension because worsening of heart function from further fluid overload may result.

      vi. Monitor urine output every hour to assess fluid status; keep output greater than 30 mL/h.

      vii. Perform neurologic exam hourly to assess cerebral perfusion.

      viii. Pharmacologic therapy (see Table 5.1)

- Positive inotropes should be administered to increase CO by improving contractility of the functioning myocardium (dopamine, dobutamine, amrinone).
- Vasopressors will support BP to enhance tissue perfusion (epinephrine, norepinephrine).
- Diuretics are administered to decrease fluid overload (furosemide, ethacrynic acid).
- Morphine given IV will increase venous capacity and decrease volume return to the heart, thus decreasing overload.

      ix. For all medication administration, do the following:

- Titrate carefully, obtaining vital signs 5–10 minutes after each change.
- Maintain BP greater than 90 mm Hg systolic.
- Monitor side effects of nausea, vomiting, hypotension, bradycardia, dysrhythmias, dizziness, palpations, dyspnea.

      x. Notify physician and prepare to correct acidosis and electrolyte imbalances as they occur.

      xi. Continuously monitor the ECG for dysrhythmias that may be life-threatening; be prepared to intervene immediately per ACLS guidelines if needed (see Appendix C).

      xii. Maintain patent IV.

      xiii. PTCA may be used to reperfuse the myocardium if necrosis has not yet occurred (see Appendix A).

      xiv. An intra-aortic balloon pump (IABP) reduces afterload and improves coronary blood flow and renal perfusion; IABP will increase BP, CO, and cerebral and coronary artery perfusion (see Appendix A)

      xv. Ventricular assist devices (VADs) decrease the workload of the ventricles by supporting the heart's pumping action (see Appendix A).

c. Desired outcomes

      i. Hemodynamic stability is achieved as evidenced by normal arterial blood gases; BP, heart rate (HR), PAP, CI, and SVR; clear mentation, urine output greater than 30 mL/h; palpable pulses, skin warm and dry; and brisk capillary refill.

      ii. No complications resulting from PTCA, IABP, or VAD

2. Alteration in gas exchanges at the cellular level related to greatly diminished cardiac output

   a. Problem: Cellular functioning will be impaired if anaerobic metabolism occurs, leading to cell injury and death.

   b. Intervention

      i. Maximize oxygenation by administering oxygen at 2–4 liters per nasal cannula to maintain PaO_2 greater than 80 mm Hg; oxygen mask, nonrebreather, or intubation and mechanical ventilation may be required.

         ▪ Assist with intubation by providing supplies and comforting patient through procedure.

         ▪ Collaborate with physician and respiratory therapist to determine ventilator settings.

      ii. Monitor arterial blood gas results.

      iii. Keep oxygen saturation by pulse oximetry greater than 94%.

      iv. Auscultate lung fields every 2 hours and as needed to assess fluid status.

      v. Assist patient to a comfortable position to maximize chest expansion; however, do not raise head of bed above 30 degrees to prevent decreasing preload dramatically.

      vi. Continuously monitor $S\bar{v}O_2$; attempt to keep between 70% and 80%.

      vii. Modify activity levels to decrease oxygen demand.

         ▪ Provide adequate rest periods.

         ▪ Plan appropriate visiting goals with the patient and family.

         ▪ Create an activity plan with the patient and family and closely monitor patient's tolerance to the activity level (ie, increases in HR, BP, RRs).

         ▪ Meet comfort and privacy needs.

   c. Desired outcomes

      i. RR 12–20 breaths/minute

      ii. Arterial blood gas results remain within normal limits.

      iii. Normal mentation

      iv. Absence of adventitious breath sounds

      v. Oxygen saturation by pulse oximetry greater than 96%

      vi. PaO_2 greater than 80 mm Hg

C. Discharge planning

   1. Patient has knowledge of medications and therapy regimens and understands the importance of adhering to treatment.

   2. Patient and family are aware of the limitations of activity to preserve myocardial functioning and avoid overexertion.

   3. Patient and family know how to contact an appropriate health care professional in the event of an emergency.

Hypertensive Crisis

  I. Definition: Hypertensive crisis is defined as a sudden rise in blood pressure with a resulting diastolic pressure of greater than 120–140 mm Hg. This situation most commonly occurs in patients with poorly controlled hypertension and individuals who suddenly discontinue taking hypertensive medications. Hypertensive crisis is an emergency and must be treated urgently to thwart irreversible damage to various end organs. Injury is most commonly associated with kidneys, brain, and myocardium and may result in death. Emergency intervention is especially critical if the hypertension is associated with aortic dissection, encephalopathy, pulmonary congestion, chest pain or ECG changes, intracranial bleeding, eclampsia, or pheochromocytoma (catecholamine-producing tumor of chromaffin tissue usually located in the adrenal medulla).

II. Etiology: Hypertension is an increase in peripheral resistance due to vessel narrowing or vasoconstriction. Crisis events are most often associated with primary hypertension (also called essential hypertension) and are of unknown etiology. Secondary hypertension results from other pathologic conditions including pheochromocytomas, aldosterone-producing tumors, Cushing's disease, and renal–vascular hypertension; some congenital disorders; pregnancy; and selected medications (ie, steroids).

III. Nursing process

A. Assessment

    1. Signs and symptoms

        a. Hypertension: sudden increase in diastolic BP to greater than 120–140 mm Hg; bounding pulses

        b. Headache: related to intense vasodilation in the brain

        c. Nausea: an autonomic response that results from the stimulation of the medullary vomiting center

        d. Retinopathy: changes to the retina by vasoconstriction of the arterioles and veins in an attempt to respond to the increased BP; papilledema, fluid transudation, exudates, and hemorrhage may be seen

        e. Encephalopathy: Excessive intra-arterial pressure causes vasospasm, decreased cerebral blood flow, and increased capillary permeability resulting in edema; symptoms include irritability, confusion, lethargy, seizures, and coma.

        f. Renal dysfunction: possible renal failure—oliguria or anuria; edema from increased vascular pressure

        g. Associated complications: Monitor for signs and symptoms of CHF, AMI, and aortic dissection.

    2. Diagnostic tests

        a. Serum

            i. BUN and Cr: elevated due to renal damage from increased pressure

            ii. Red blood cell (RBC) count: may be decreased due to hematuria

        b. Urine

            i. Specific gravity: may be decreased if renal impairment results in glomerulonephritis; renal impairment decreases ability to concentrate urine.

            ii. Proteinuria: Renal impairment leads to protein spillage.

c. Other
    i. Chest radiography: may demonstrate signs of pulmonary congestion or enlarged cardiac silhouette due to left ventricular hypertrophy

B. Patient management

  1. Potential for (organ) injury related to extreme hypertension

    a. Problem: Cellular injury and possible death occurs in organs due to hypertension; severe complications if not controlled immediately.

    b. Intervention

      i. Continuously monitor blood pressure and document every hour or with any changes.

- Assist with the insertion of an arterial line; describe procedure to patient, support infection control measures.
- Notify physicians with sudden changes in pressure; if decreased too rapidly, reflexive organ damage may occur from hypoperfusion.

      ii. Pharmacology: see Table 5.1

- Nitroprusside: vasodilates rapidly by acting on the vascular smooth muscles of the arteries
- Diazoxide: also very powerful vasodilator by directly relaxing the resistance vessels
- Beta-adrenergic blockers: inhibit sympathetic nervous system activity resulting in decreased HR and systemic vascular resistance; these include labetalol, propranolol
- Calcium channel blockers: block calcium channel entry resulting in peripheral and coronary arterial vasodilation; includes verapamil, nifedipine, diltiazem
  ◦ Monitor drug response closely, titrate as needed to maintain adequate HR and BP

     iii. Continuously monitor for dysrhythmias and ST-segment changes that may indicate myocardial ischemia.

     iv. Monitor urine output every hour to assess renal functioning.

     v. Monitor respiratory status frequently; assess for signs of pulmonary edema: crackles, frothy sputum, restlessness.

     vi. Obtain and evaluate arterial blood gases as needed to assess pulmonary status.

     vii. Assess neurologic status frequently; neurologic exam at least every 4 hours; assess patient for headaches

    viii. Provide pain medications as needed and appropriate

     ix. Assist physician staff with the accurate diagnosis and treatment of the underlying cause of secondary hypertension; once patient becomes stable and hypertension is controlled, patient may require surgical intervention; support patient and family if surgery (ie, tumor resection or renal–vascular repair) is required.

    c. Desired outcome

      i. BP will return to patient's baseline or to less than 140/90 mm Hg.

     ii. Normal mentation

    iii. Urine output greater than or equal to 30 mL/h

      iv. BUN less than 20 mg/dL, and Cr less than 1.5 mg/dL
      v. Pulses equal without bounding on palpation
      vi. Patient states headache pain improved

C. Discharge planning

1. Patient learning will occur in the areas of medication regimen, risk factor reduction, stress management, and symptom recognition.
2. The nurse should stress that uncontrolled hypertension and medication dose infrequency may lead to crisis.
3. Ensure patient has a follow-up appointment.
4. Educate patient and family in obtaining BP daily and to document the results in a diary.

Cardiac Tamponade

I. Definition: Cardiac tamponade results from fluid accumulation in the pericardial space. It may also be seen when fluid accumulates in the anterior mediastinal space in patients who have had a pericardiotomy during open heart surgery. Fluid may accumulate with very little change in pericardial pressure at first. However, because the pericardium's stretch is limited, a small additional increment in fluid volume will cause an abrupt increase in intracardiac pressures that drastically restricts ventricular filling capabilities. Secondary to the inability of the heart to fill with blood, the CO dramatically decreases or ceases, resulting in cardiogenic shock.

II. Etiology: Bleeding into the pericardium may occur secondary to blunt or penetrating trauma (ie, gunshot wound, vehicular collision, stabbing, etc), cardiac surgery or catheterization, thrombolytic or anticoagulation therapy, discontinuation of epicardial pacing wires, or myocardial infarction with myocardial wall disruption. Fluid accumulation may also result from acute pericarditis or the presence of a metastatic tumor. The drastic increase in intracardiac pressures disrupt systolic emptying bringing the stroke volume (SV) (volume ejected with each heartbeat) close to zero. With no SV, there is minimal CO and significant decrease in tissue perfusion.

III. Nursing process

A. Assessment

1. Signs and symptoms
   a. Beck's triad: (1) muffled heart sounds: The fluid-filled pericardium muffles the auscultation of valve closure sounds. (2) Distended neck veins: Decrease or absence of ventricular emptying creates a backflow of blood to the systemic circulation, thereby distending the neck veins (possibly not as apparent in the acute trauma patient). (3) Hypotension: The decreased SV diminishes the cardiac output; when the CO is insufficient, BP falls, and shock develops.
   b. Paradoxical pulse is a drop in BP by at least 15 mm Hg during inspiration caused by the increased pressure in the thorax and on the great vessels; this increased pressure further impedes the filling capacity of the ventricles.

    c. Cardiac pressure equalization: The CVP, PAWP, PAS, and PAD become almost equal (usually > 20 mm Hg), because the increased pressure on all cardiac chambers causes global ventricular impairment and failure.

    d. SVR increases as vasoconstriction occurs as an attempt to compensate for diminished CO.

    e. Hypotension is a late sign related to very diminished CO.

    f. Pulsus alternans: Alternating strong and weak pulses result from the failing left ventricle.

    g. Sinus tachycardia: As the baroreceptors sense a low CO, the sinus node attempts to increase HR to supplement low SV (CO = SV × HR).

    h. Sudden cessation of mediastinal chest tube output following open heart surgery: If fairly high output of drainage from the mediastinal chest tubes suddenly stops, immediately notify physician and suspect impending tamponade.

  2. Diagnostic tests

    a. Serum

      i. No finding specific to tamponade

    b. Urine

      i. No specific changes

    c. Other

      i. X-ray shows possible widening of the mediastinum from the fluid accumulation, dilated inferior superior vena cava from the backflow pressure.

      ii. Echocardiogram may demonstrate dilated inferior and superior vena cava from backflow pressure.

B. Patient management

  1. Decrease in CO related to restricted ventricular filling caused by pericardial fluid accumulation

    a. Problem: Decreased tissue perfusion may lead to cell injury, cell death, or organ dysfunction.

    b. Intervention

      i. Continuously monitor for all signs and symptoms of cardiac tamponade after cardiac surgery; most frequently occurs in first 24 hours after bypass and then again in 10–14 days; if suspected, intervene immediately and notify physician; physician may open chest to avoid cardiac arrest.

        ▪ Have wire cutters immediately available.

        ▪ Set up sterile suction equipment to evacuate the anterior mediastinal space.

        ▪ Prepare patient for emergency return to the operating room.

      ii. Assist physician with pericardiocentesis: drainage of the pericardium through needle aspiration; surgical exploration may be warranted.

        ▪ Monitor patient for dysrhythmias, chest pain (myocardial laceration), hemothorax or pneumothorax (punctured lung or bleeding into the pleural space; signs include decreased breath sounds and dyspnea).

      iii. Administer fluids to expand intravascular volume; lactated Ringer's solution, colloid solutions, and blood products are commonly used; very rapid infusion may be necessary

      iv. Administer nitroprusside to decrease afterload (see Table 5.1).

      v. Administer positive inotropic agents to enhance cardiac contractility and effectiveness (see Table 5.1).

      vi. Be prepared for emergency intubation/mechanical ventilation if needed.

      vii. If patient on mechanical ventilation, consider decreasing positive end-expiratory pressure (PEEP); PEEP increases thoracic pressure and may decrease venous return.

      viii. Maintain at least two patent large-gauge IVs.

      ix. Monitor BP, HR at least every 15 minutes; be alert for pulsus paradoxus.

      x. Monitor cardiac pressures (PAP, CVP, SBP, DBP) for equalization.

      xi. Monitor SVR and pulse pressure to evaluate response to therapy.

      xii. Assess patient for Beck's triad (see earlier).

      xiii. Obtain urine output hourly; less than 30 mL/h may demonstrate decreasing CO.

      xiv. Assess neurologic status frequently to determine cerebral perfusion.

      xv. Monitor skin temperature and color and capillary refill to assess perfusion.

   c. Desired outcome

      i. Normal cardiac output as evidenced by: HR within 20 beats of baseline, BP within 20 mm Hg of baseline, at least greater than 90 mm Hg systolic, normal mentation, urine output greater than 30 mL/h, skin warm with brisk capillary refill, SVR, PAWP, CVP, and PAP within normal limits, and normal sinus rhythm

      ii. Absence of Beck's triad; clear auscultation of heart sounds, no jugular venous distention

C. Discharge planning

  1. Ensure patient and family have clear understanding of medication regimen.

  2. Review with patient and family the activity limitations set by health care team/cardiac rehabilitation.

  3. Cardiac tamponade is usually a complication of an underlying pathologic condition; review the discharge instructions needed for the primary diagnosis.

Infectious Processes

Endocarditis

I. Definition: Acute endocarditis is an infection of the endocardial (innermost) lining or the valves of the heart. The infecting organisms are usually bacteria, fungi, rickettsiae, or yeasts. Endocarditis occurs more often in men than women and is associated with prosthetic heart valves, congenital heart disease, stenotic or insufficient valves, IV drug use, and invasive procedures such as cardiac surgery or dental work. *Staphylococcus* and *Streptococcus* are the two bacterias and *Candida albicans* is the fungus that most commonly cause endocarditis.

II. **Etiology:** The infectious process involves inflammation of the endocardium and possibly the growth of vegetations (lesions) on the leaflets of the affected valve or valves. The mitral and aortic valves are most often affected. A circulating microorganism adheres to the valve surface secondary to numerous complex processes. After colonization occurs, the vegetative process begins. This vegetation interferes with the normal functioning of the heart and its ability to circulate blood volume. CHF and infarctions of end organs are serious complications seen with endocarditis.

III. **Nursing process**

A. Assessment
   1. Signs and symptoms
      a. Acute infection: may see fever, anorexia, tachycardia, fatigue, and diaphoresis associated with the primary offending organism
      b. Murmur: Various murmurs may be auscultated and are associated with either stenosis or insufficiency of the particular valve involved. (See "Valvular Disorders," p. 110, for description of murmur.)
      c. Embolism: Fragments of the vegetation can break off and travel with the blood flow causing the following various sequelae:
         i. Pulmonary infarct: fragments from the right heart; chest pain and hemoptysis
         ii. Cerebral: left heart fragments; paralysis, meningitis, sudden blindness, and change in level of consciousness
         iii. Skin and mucous membranes: related to the microemboli that travel to the skin; classic findings include the following:
            - Osler's nodes—tender, painful reddened papules on the finger pads and the soles of the feet
            - Janeway's lesions—small, nontender, red-blue spots found on palms and the soles of the feet
            - Roth's spots—small white spots near the optic disc in the retina usually surrounded by areas of hemorrhage
            - Splinter hemorrhage—linear hemorrhage under the nailbeds
   2. Diagnostic tests
      a. Serum
         i. Blood cultures may be positive and may isolate the offending organism.
         ii. Blood count: white blood cell (WBC) count and sedimentation rate increased secondary to infective process; anemia due to microemboli and hemorrhage.
      b. Urine
         i. Hematuria due to microemboli hemorrhage in the kidneys
      c. Other
         i. Chest radiography: CHF is a complication often seen with endocarditis; x-ray findings are consistent with CHF: cardiomegaly, pleural effusion, and pulmonary congestion.

      ii. Echocardiography can establish a diagnosis of endocarditis, but a negative test does not rule out the diagnosis; vegetations may be visualized on the valves, and hemodynamic information can assist in the management of the patient.

B. Patient management

  1. Endocardial and valvular infection related to the adherence of microorganisms to the inner layer of the heart allowing for colonization and vegetation formation

    a. Problem: Vegetative lesions cause valvular stenosis or insufficiency and may break off causing embolic complications.

    b. Intervention

       i. Obtain blood culture adhering to strict aseptic technique to prevent contamination; several sets may be necessary.

      ii. Monitor temperature and HR as response to fever; if patient's tachycardia is incongruent with temperature, suspect heart failure.

    iii. Administer antipyretics to combat fever discomfort if febrile.

     iv. Administer organism-sensitive antibiotics closely adhering to schedule to maintain consistent levels in blood, usually required for 4–6 weeks; maintain patent IV.

      v. Assist with and encourage mouth care to prevent thrush due to antibiotic use; consider nystatin administration.

---

nystatin

Action Antifungal antibiotic.

Administration Guidelines 5 mL swished in mouth, then swallowed four times per day, or if a pastille, allow to dissolve in mouth (do not chew or swallow) four to five times per day.

Special considerations Large doses may cause adverse GI reactions.

---

      vi. If PA catheter in place obtain CO, PAP, and PAWP and calculate SVR and CI every 4 hours to assess for signs of septic shock (high CO and low SVR).

    vii. Maintain aseptic techniques with all invasive procedures

   viii. Provide routine IV catheter care: change every 72 hours or per institutional protocol.

     ix. Provide urine catheter care at least daily to defend against invading organisms; wash with soap and water, do not allow urine to backflow into the bladder during transfers, assess urine for cloudiness and odor, and support catheter bag to prevent urethral trauma.

    c. Desired outcome

       i. Offending organism is identified and antibiotic-sensitive antibiotics are administered in a timely manner.

      ii. WBC returns to normal range.

    iii. Temperature and HR are within normal range.

     iv. SVR, PAP, PAWP, and CO are within normal limits.

2. Decrease in cardiac output related to dysfunction of infected valves
  a. Problem: Decreased CO leads to decreased tissue perfusion, cellular injury, and possibly cellular death.
  b. Intervention
    i. Monitor vital signs every 1–2 hours and as needed.
    ii. Assess peripheral pulses every hour and capillary refill every 4 hours along with skin temperature.
    iii. Assess heart sounds every 4 hours to monitor presence or change in murmurs; S_3 and S_4 may indicate heart failure.
    iv. Monitor for other signs of congestive heart failure (ie, pulmonary crackles, shortness of breath, murmurs, and tachycardia). (See "Congestive Heart Failure/Pulmonary Edema," p. 94, for interventions.)
    v. Continuously monitor PA and central venous pressures and document every hour.
    vi. Obtain CO, and calculate SVR and CI every 4 hours or as needed; notify physician of changes in trends.
    vii. Administer positive inotropic drugs as needed to enhance CO; see Table 5.1 for description of dopamine, dobutamine, amrinone, and digoxin.
    viii. Continuously monitor $S\bar{v}o_2$ and document every hour; make further assessments if alteration in trend occurs; plan patient activities with patient and family to decrease oxygen demands.
    ix. Document urine output every hour, and notify physician if less than 30 mL/h.
    x. Monitor pulse oximetry and blood gases to assess oxygenation; administer oxygen via nasal cannula or mask to meet demands.
    xi. Monitor level of consciousness and neurologic response every hour.
    xii. Prepare patient and family for valvular replacement surgery if indicated; a 6-week regimen of antibiotics is usually completed before patient is ideal candidate; emergency surgery may be required depending on degree of heart failure.
  c. Desired outcome
    i. Patient will maintain adequate cardiac output and tissue perfusion as evidenced by HR and BP within normal limits; CO, PAP, PAWP, SVR, CI, and $S\bar{v}o_2$ within normal range; adequate mentation, and urine output of greater than 30 mL/h.

C. Discharge planning
  1. Ensure patient and family know when and where to go for follow-up appointment.
  2. Ensure that patient and family have knowledge of medication dose, route, regimen, and importance of adhering to the administration schedule.
  3. Instruct patient to notify dentist and other health care professionals of endocarditis before any procedures are done so that prophylactic antibiotics may be administered.
  4. Instruct patient to notify health care provider of any signs of infection or heart failure.

Pericarditis

I. Definition: The pericardium is a membrane that surrounds the heart and portions of the vena cava, aorta, and pulmonary arteries and veins. The normal pericardium provides protection for the heart from inflammation and disease of nearby structures and reduces the friction caused by cardiac contractile movements. Acute pericarditis is defined as inflammation of the pericardium that may be related to a viral infection, respiratory infection, neoplasm, trauma, or myocardial infarction or may be of idiopathic origin. Gram-negative organisms may also be at fault, but usually only in the immunosuppressed or debilitated patient. Pericarditis often involves effusion of fluid into the pericardial space.

II. Etiology: Inflammation of the pericardium causes leukocytes to accumulate in the membrane sac and possibly the superficial layer of the epicardium or the connecting pleurae. In addition to the fluid accumulation, vascularity of the pericardium may increase, and fibrin deposits may form. If progression of the inflammation and fluid accumulation is rapid or of substantial volume, it may interfere with SV and CO due to direct pressure exerted on the chambers.

III. Nursing process

A. Assessment

1. Signs and symptoms

   a. *Chest pain* may be described as dull, sharp, or aching; difficult to differentiate from ischemic pain, however, pericarditis is suspected if the pain correlates with movements such as position changes or respiratory excursion; the pain is associated with the pleural involvement by inflammation or effusion.

   b. *Dyspnea* related to pain on chest expansion or from direct pressure of the enlarged pericardium on the bronchial structures.

   c. *Friction rub* will be auscultated and best heard with the diaphragm of the stethoscope from the fourth or fifth intercostal space, close to the left sternum; intensity may increase on inspiration; a friction thrill may be palpated; caused by the rubbing together of the fibrous pericardium and the epicardial surface of the heart or from the outer pericardium and adjacent structures.

   d. *Fever* may be present if purulent effusion exists.

   e. *Pulsus paradoxus* (SBP decreased by at least 15 mm Hg on inspiration) may be present due to the compression of the great vessels on inspiration caused by the stretching of the inflamed and stiff pericardium.

   f. *Cardiac tamponade* is a serious threat if the pericardial fluid is of significant volume or accumulates rapidly. (See "Cardiac Tamponade" p. 101.)

2. Diagnostic tests

   a. Serum

      i. *Blood cultures* may be positive if pericarditis is a result of infection.

      ii. *Cardiac enzymes* may show small elevations in CK-MB if epicardial damage has occurred.

   b. Urine

      i. No significant changes

   c. Other

      i. Chest radiography may demonstrate cardiac silhouette enlargement if significant effusion is present.

      ii. ECG changes caused by alterations in repolarization from inflammation or injury to the epicardium; possible changes may include ST-segment elevations in leads I, II, aVL, aVF, and V_3–V_6 with ST-segment depression in leads aVR and V_1 [6].

B. Patient management

  1. Pain related to the inflammatory process of pericarditis

   a. Problem: interferes with daily activities, causes stress and anxiety

   b. Intervention

      i. Administer nonsteroidal anti-inflammatory drugs (NSAIDs) to decrease the inflammation and to decrease pain. These may include aspirin, ibuprofen, or others (see Table 5.1 for administration guidelines).

      ii. Administer steroids as needed if nonsteroidal anti-inflammatory drugs (NSAIDs) prove ineffective; prednisone is the agent of choice.

---

prednisone

Action Decreases inflammation.

Administration Guidelines 2.5–15 mg PO two, three, or four times daily; should be individualized and may also be given IV; must be tapered, never discontinue abruptly, since withdrawal could be life-threatening.

Special Considerations If pericarditis is thought to be viral or bacterial, be sure to cover adequately with anti-infective agents, because prednisone increases susceptibility.

---

      iii. Assist patient to find a comfortable position that alleviates pain.

      iv. Assist patient and family in limiting activities to decrease pain; possibly limit visits and enforce bed rest.

      v. Treat underlying cause of inflammation with appropriate antibiotic therapy; administer on tight schedule to maintain adequate levels in blood.

      vi. Utilize objective pain scale to assess patient's pain; document interventions and response to interventions.

      vii. Prepare patient and family for possible surgery: pericardiectomy (removal of part or all of the pericardium); interventions include preoperative education, surgical preparation, and postoperative management involving dysrhythmia, pain, fluid, and cardiac function management.

    c. Desired outcome

        i. Patient states pain has been relieved.

        ii. Objective pain scale verifies pain has been relieved.

        iii. Physical evidence correlates with pain relief: ability to rest quietly, decreased anxiety, absence of facial grimacing or physical discomfort.

2. Potential for alteration in CO due to pressure on the cardiac structures from pericardial effusion

    a. Problem: Decreased CO results in decreased tissue perfusion, cellular injury and possible death, and altered mentation.

    b. Intervention

        i. Continuously monitor ECG signals for changes in the ST segments described earlier and for atrial and ventricular dysrhythmias caused by pressure on the myocardium; atrial fibrillation is common.

        ii. Continuously monitor pulmonary artery catheter readings for equilibrium in cardiac pressures that may indicate cardiac tamponade. (See "Cardiac Tamponade," p. 101.)

        iii. Continuously monitor $S\bar{v}O_2$ and report changes in trends.

        iv. Measure PAWP and CO and calculate SVR every 4 hours.

        v. Assess pulses every 4 hours.

        vi. Assess patient frequently for neck vein distention, especially on inspiration, which may signal cardiac tamponade.

        vii. Assist physician and support patient if pericardiocentesis is necessary to remove excess fluid accumulation; needle aspiration is used to drain fluid; ensure aseptic technique is followed closely.

    c. Desired outcome

        i. Patient will maintain CO within normal range.

        ii. Patient will avoid cardiac tamponade.

        iii. Adequate perfusion will be maintained as evidenced by normal mentation, palpable pulses, warm skin, and absence of dysrhythmias.

3. Ineffective breathing pattern related to pain on chest expansion

    a. Problem: Pain will cause guarding and decreased depth in breathing, thus increasing risk for decreased tissue oxygenation and the development of pneumonia.

    b. Intervention

        i. Administer pain medications and NSAIDs as ordered, and frequently assess efficacy of interventions.

        ii. Assist patient in optimal position to decrease pain on inspiration. (Sitting upright often decreases discomfort.)

        iii. Assess respiratory depth patterns for ineffective patterns.

        iv. Monitor pulse oxygenation frequently, and maintain above 94%.

        v. Obtain arterial blood gases if respiratory status deteriorates.

        vi. Provide supplemental oxygen via nasal cannula or mask if needed to maintain adequate oxygenation.

        vii. Assist patient in completing incentive spirometry exercises every hour while awake.

        viii. Assess lung fields every 4 hours for decreased breath sounds or crackles in the bases.

        ix. Provide a pillow to splint chest during coughing and spirometry exercises.

    c. Desired outcome

        i. Oxygen saturation by pulse oximetry remains greater than 94%.

        ii. Arterial blood gases are within normal limits.

        iii. Chest expansion is adequate to provide oxygenation as evidenced by normal mentation and adequate tissue oxygenation.

        iv. Patient avoids pneumonia complications.

        v. Only vesicular (normal) breath sounds are heard.

C. Discharge planning

    1. Ensure patient and family have the knowledge required to take medications correctly and at the appropriate times.

    2. Instruct patient to report signs of infection (ie, fever, pain) to health care provider immediately.

    3. Instruct patient to limit activity and to take frequent rest periods throughout the day to promote the further decrease in inflammation.

Valvular Disorders

  I. Definition: Valvular heart disease in the acute care setting primarily consists of valvular regurgitation or stenosis. Regurgitation refers to the backflow of blood through an incomplete valve closure and causes distention of the heart chamber that precedes the damaged valve. This is primarily due to damage to or near the valve, rheumatic heart disease, trauma, or infection. Stenosis is defined as impedance to forward blood flow through a stiff or incompetent valve. This may be caused by calcification or fibrosis of the valve leaflets.

  II. Etiology: Acute valvular dysfunction most commonly involves the mitral or aortic valves. Table 5.5 [7] lists the valvular dysfunctions and the etiologies, signs and symptoms, and treatments that are specific to the pathologic dysfunction of the valve.

  III. Nursing process

    A. Assessment (see Table 5.5)

    B. Patient management

      1. Alteration in CO related to valvular dysfunction and poor left ventricular function (also see treatment for congestive heart failure)

        a. Problem: decreased tissue perfusion and cellular injury

        b. Intervention

          i. See interventions specific to valve dysfunction in Table 5.5.

          ii. Control ventricular response to atrial fibrillation with quinidine and digoxin (see Table 5.1 for administration guidelines).

          iii. If the onset of atrial fibrillation with rapid ventricular response has been recent, cardioversion may be considered; use with caution due to emboli formation from blood stasis; 4–6 weeks of anticoagulation therapy may be required if time period for atrial fibrillation is unknown.

Table 5.5 Most Common Valvular Disorders: Etiology, Signs and Symptoms, and Valve-Specific Treatment

Valvular Disorder and Etiology	Assessment: Signs and Symptoms	Valve-Specific Treatment
Mitral valve regurgitation Etiology: incomplete closure of the mitral valve allowing backflow of blood into the left atrium caused by Rheumatic heart disease Congenital anomaly Ischemic papillary muscle rupture Endocarditis Mitral valve prolapse Ruptured chordae tendineae	Atrial fibrillation Backflow of blood to the atria stretches and thins the atrial walls; wall tension causes atrial fibrillation High left atrial pressure 12–20 mm Hg due to backflow of blood PAP elevated due to backflow of blood from left ventricle PAWP: giant V waves indicate severe regurgitation to a noncompliant left atrium Pulmonary edema if onset of regurgitation is acute, as seen in chordae rupture secondary to MI or trauma; large increase in left atrial pressure causes pulmonary congestion Heart sounds: split S_2 and a pansystolic, blowing murmur heard at the apex and radiating toward the axilla due to incomplete valve closure and turbulent blood flow Sinus tachycardia: decreased stroke volume is ejected into aorta because excess volume is unloaded back into the atria; HR increases to maintain forward CO Chest radiography: if chronic regurgitation, may show increased heart size due to hypertrophy Cardiac catheterization used to determine left ventricular size and contractility, intracardiac pressures, and severity of regurgitation; poorly tolerated in the acute mitral valve regurgitation; poorly functioning left ventricle may contraindicate surgery	IABP may be used to decrease afterload which will encourage forward blood flow (see Appendix A) Surgery Valve repair or replacement: repair is preferred to retain the chordae function. See Appendix A for the care of the postoperative cardiac surgical patient
Mitral stenosis Etiology: Stiff or incompetent mitral valve impedes the forward flow of blood caused by rheumatic heart disease and causes fibrosis of the chordae tendineae and/or papillary muscles, calcification of the valve leaflets, and fusion of the valve openings	Dyspnea occurs with exertion; progresses to dyspnea with minimal exertion, periods of orthopnea or pulmonary edema; forward blood flow impeded resulting in back pressure in the pulmonary vasculature Hemoptysis frothy pink sputum: pulmonary vein rupture/pulmonary infarction Ortner's syndrome (hoarseness): compression by enlarged left atrium or dilated pulmonary artery on the left recurrent laryngeal nerve	Administer dobutamine and isosorbide to decrease pulmonary congestion (see Table 5.1) Surgery: indicated especially if emboli has occurred and left ventricular function is adequate (see Appendix A for cardiac surgery)

Right-sided heart failure secondary to chronic increased left atrial pressure and pulmonary hypertension; see heart failure section

Increased left atrial pressure and PAWP (see "Mitral Valve Regurgitation")

Atrial fibrillation (see "Mitral Valve Regurgitation")

Thromboemboli 80% of patients have atrial fib that promotes blood stasis and clot formation

Heart sounds: loud S_1 and normal S_2 and opening snap heard with diaphragm of the stethoscope due to blood flow impedance; diastolic murmur in mitral area: low pitched rumbling at apex with no radiation

ECG: widened, notched, or flat topped P wave (P mitrale) due to enlarged left atrium; right axis deviation secondary to right heart hypertrophy

Chest X-ray: enlarged pulmonary artery and right ventricle

Echocardiogram: degree of calcification

Cardiac catheterization: severity of obstruction and left ventricular function

Closed mitral commissurotomy: a transventricular dilator increases valve opening; used if no mitral valve regurgitation; no atrial thrombosis, or serious calcification

Open mitral commissurotomy requires cardiopulmonary bypass; splitting of the fused chordae or papillary muscles and removal of left atrial thrombi

Mitral valve replacement also uses bypass and is indicated for immobile and extremely calcified rheumatic valves

Valvuloplasty may be indicated for patients that are high risk for surgery, refuse surgery, or >80 years; dilates stenotic heart valves (see Appendix A)

Aortic regurgitation

Etiology: incomplete aortic valve closure allows the backflow of blood into the left ventricle caused by inflammation from rheumatic fever or syphilis; congenital malformation; acquired injury from trauma, endocarditis, or hypertension

PAP, PAWP, and CVP (preload) increases from volume overload in the left ventricle created by the backflow from the aorta

Chest pain secondary to increased myocardial oxygen demand to compensate for volume overload

Heart failure due to volume overload and left ventricular failure (see section on CHF)

Cardiac output is decreased due to left ventricular dysfunction

Diastolic blood pressure is very low and may even reach zero due to incomplete closure of the valve; this results in a widened pulse pressure in the chronic regurgitation patient; no dicrotic notch seen in A-line or pulmonary artery waveform

Heart sounds auscultation will demonstrate a decreased S_1 because of premature closure of the mitral valve due to increased left ventricular pressure; S_3 is common and represents left ventricular failure; diastolic murmur heard in aortic area: high pitched, blowing and radiates to left sternal border

IABP is contraindicated in aortic regurgitation because the increase in diastolic pressure created by the pump will directly increase the work of the left ventricle because the aortic valve has incomplete closure

Surgery: see Appendix A for the care of cardiac surgery patients

Aortic valve replacement is indicated for most patients with adequate left ventricular contractile function

Table 5.5 *Continued*

Valvular Disorder and Etiology	Assessment: Signs and Symptoms	Valve-Specific Treatment
Aortic regurgitation (cont.)	ECG: large-amplitude waveforms, especially in precordial leads (V_1–V_6) due to hypertrophy (large muscle mass to depolarize); may have sinus tachycardia to compensate for fall in CO Cardiac catheterization to determine severity of regurgitation and to estimate left ventricular function	Diuretics are used with caution to avoid hypovolemia that will drop left ventricular end-diastolic pressure, thus decreasing CO IABP may be indicated to enhance diastolic coronary filling pressure; see Appendix A Surgery valve replacement will improve left ventricular function (see Appendix A for care of the postoperative cardiac surgery patient) Valvuloplasty dilates the valve opening and is indicated for stenotic valves in patients that are poor surgical risks, refuse surgery, or are >80 years
Aortic stenosis Etiology: Stiff or incompetent aortic valve impedes the forward flow of blood caused by congenital malformations that include unicuspid, bicuspid, or unequal valve leaflets causing turbulent blood flow resulting in calcification fibrosis and stenosis.	Left ventricular hypertrophy Increased chamber pressure: obstruction of blood flow from left ventricle to aorta causes wall stretch and thickening PAP and PAWP elevated from impedance of left ventricular emptying; PAWP with prominent A wave Chest pain: tremendous increase in myocardial oxygen demand to overcome ejection resistance Syncope: abrupt decrease in CO without increase in SVR; decrease in SVR without increase in CO, dysrhythmias, or increase in left ventricular pressure stimulates baroreceptors that cause peripheral vasodilation, thereby decreasing BP Heart failure: decreased left ventricular contractile function Heart sounds: crescendo-decrescendo systolic ejection murmur after the S_1 is loudest at the second intercostal space, right sternal edge radiating toward the carotid artery due to impeded blood flow Widened pulse pressure: rise in systolic blood pressure with a constant diastolic pressure ECG: conduction abnormalities (ie, heart blocks, delays) common due to left ventricular hypertrophy influencing the AV node Chest radiography: dilated aorta, calcified valve, hypertrophic left ventricle, or cardiomegaly Echocardiogram: dilated aorta and left ventricular wall thickening Cardiac catheterization: can determine severe obstruction, left vent. contractile function, and coronary circulation	

Abbreviations as defined in text.
Adapted from Kinney, M. R., Packa, D. R., and Dunbar, S. B. (eds.). *AACN's Clinical Reference for Critical-Care Nursing* (3rd ed.). St. Louis: Mosby–Year Book, 1993, Pp. 598, 605.

iv. Continuously monitor for ECG changes and dysrhythmias that could interfere with CO such as conduction disorders and ectopic beats; collaborate with physicians to treat specific rhythms.

v. Continuously monitor HR, BP, mean arterial pressure (MAP), CVP, PAPs, and $S\bar{v}O_2$, if parameters are available; monitor CO, CI, SVR, and PAWP every 1–4 hours depending on drug titrations and other interventions.

vi. Administer positive inotropic agents to enhance left ventricular function, decrease left ventricular volume, and increase ejection fraction; choices should include digoxin, dopamine, dobutamine, and amrinone (see Table 5.1).

vii. Continuously monitor fluid status by assessing breath sounds, respiratory status, urine output, and PAPs; administer diuretics to maintain optimal fluid volume; collaborate with physician for drug choice (see Table 5.1).

viii. Administer vasodilators to decrease preload and afterload caused by decreased left ventricular function (nitroprusside and nitroglycerine) (see Table 5.1).

ix. Encourage and teach patient to maintain a low-sodium diet to prevent further overload.

x. Plan with patient and family to limit patient activity to avoid unnecessary myocardial workload.

xi. Administer oxygen as needed to enhance blood oxygenation.

xii. Prepare patient and family for possible valvular repair or replacement surgery (see Appendix A).

c. Desired outcome

i. Enhanced left ventricular function as evidenced by normal CO, PAWP, and left ventricular end-diastolic pressure

ii. Absence of pulmonary congestion as evidenced by normal breath sounds and absence of dyspnea

iii. Urine output greater than 30 mL/h

iv. Adequate pulses and warm skin

v. Normal mentation

2. Impaired gas exchange related to pulmonary congestion secondary to decreased left ventricular function

a. Problem: Impaired gas exchange decreases blood oxygenation and interferes with tissue perfusion possibly resulting in cellular injury.

b. Intervention

i. Administer oxygen 2–4 liters via nasal cannula to maintain PaO_2 greater than 80 mm Hg to support perfusion efforts; be prepared to provide mechanical ventilation if necessary.

ii. Monitor oxygen saturation by pulse oximetry and maintain greater than 94%.

iii. Continuously monitor $S\bar{v}O_2$ and attempt to maintain between 70% and 80%.

iv. Obtain arterial blood gases as needed to monitor adequate oxygenation; collaborate with physicians for changes needed in oxygen therapy.

        v. Assess breath sounds every 4 hours for crackles, rhonchi, or wheezing; collaborate with physician and respiratory therapy for needed treatments based on assessment findings.

       vi. Assist patient to a position that maximizes chest expansion.

      vii. Encourage patient to cough frequently to expel sputum.

     viii. Prevent pneumonia and atelectasis by encouraging patient to cough and deep breathe or use incentive spirometer every hour while awake.

       ix. If intubated, suction as needed to control secretions.

  c. Desired outcome: Arterial blood gas results within normal limits; RR 12–20 breaths/min; vesicular breath sounds; adequate tissue perfusion

C. Discharge planning

  1. Teach patient to share information about valve defect with all health care providers with whom they come in contact.

  2. Prophylactic penicillin or other antibiotic must be given before any dental or surgical procedure. The nonfunctioning valve provides an optimal environment for infection colonization.

  3. Educate patient and family on how to maintain a low-sodium diet.

  4. Teach patient importance of limiting activity and avoiding overexertion.

  5. Teach patient how to care for valve if patient has undergone surgical repair.

  6. Ensure that patient has adequate knowledge of medications and realizes the importance of medication regime.

Cardiomyopathy

I. Definition: Cardiomyopathy is a disease of the myocardium from an unknown cause that interferes with diastolic and/or systolic functioning. Cardiomyopathies are commonly categorized into three groups: dilated, hypertrophic, and restrictive. Table 5.6 [6] lists the characteristics of each category.

II. Etiology: The etiology of cardiomyopathy is unknown. Primary damage to the myocardium due to known pathologic conditions such as MI, CAD, or valvular dysfunction can be distinguished from cardiomyopathy.

III. Nursing process

A. Assessment

  1. Signs and symptoms

    a. *SV* and ejection fraction are reduced secondary to poor ventricular contractility.

    b. *Sinus tachycardia* greater than 100 beats per minute to compensate for decreased SV.

    c. *CO* is initially normal due to compensatory increase in HR, but it will fall with stress and/or exercise due to poor cardiac reserve.

    d. *Chest pain:* Myocardial oxygen consumption increases as the atria and ventricles dilate; dilation causes increased myocardial workload and increased wall tension.

Table 5.6 Characteristics of the three types of cardiomyopathy

Type of Cardiomyopathy	Function and Structural Characteristics
Dilated cardiomyopathy (associated with alcohol consumption, pregnancy, hypertension)	Most common type Dilation of both ventricular chambers Cardiomegaly Impaired systolic function Low ejection fraction due to poor contractile function High end-systolic ventricular volume
Hypertrophic cardiomyopathy, also known as idiopathic, hypertrophic, subaortic stenosis (associated with heredity, hypertension)	Disorganization of myocardial fibers, especially in the septum Massive ventricular hypertrophy with resulting reduced inner chamber size Decreased end-systolic ventricular volume Supernormal ejection fraction
Restrictive cardiomyopathy (associated with endomyocardial fibrosis, neoplastic tumor)	Endomyocardial fibrosis restricts the filling capabilities of the ventricles Similar to restrictive endocarditis

Adapted from Laurent-Bopp, D. Cardiomyopathies and Myocarditis. In Underhill, S. L., et al. (eds.). *Cardiac Nursing* (2nd ed.). Philadelphia: J. B. Lippincott, 1989. Pp. 924–933.

    e. *Dyspnea* initially on exertion, but worsens over time; caused by progressive heart failure and resultant pulmonary congestion

    f. *Fatigue/Weakness* related to poor ventricular function

    g. *Right-sided heart failure* signs appear as left ventricular function declines; signs include JVD, hepatomegaly, ascites, and edema. (See section "Congestive Heart Failure/Pulmonary Edema.")

    h. *Heart sounds* include auscultation of S_3 and S_4 as a result of left heart failure.

    i. *Hypotension:* SBP less than 90 mm Hg may occur if SV is significantly reduced.

  2. Diagnostic tests

    a. Serum

      i. No findings particular to pathology

    b. Urine

      i. No significant changes

    c. Other

      i. *ECG* almost always abnormal, but usually nonspecific; may display conduction disorders or various ectopy; atrial fibrillation is common secondary to atrial wall tension; PVCs also are common.

      ii. *Chest radiography* reveals ventricular enlargement and a possible pleural effusion caused by left-sided heart failure.

      iii. *Echocardiography* may reveal poor wall motion in the ventricles and thrombi in the chambers from blood stasis.

      iv. *Cardiac catheterization* demonstrates elevated pressures in both ventricular chambers; obtaining a biopsy sample during catheterization may support diagnosis of hypertrophic cardiomyopathy.

B. Patient management

    1. Alteration in cardiac output related to poor ventricular function and complex dysrhythmias

        a. Problem: Decreased tissue perfusion leads to cellular injury and alterations in heart, brain, and other organ functioning.

        b. Intervention

            i. See ACLS algorithms in Appendix C for the treatment of complex ventricular dysrhythmias.

            ii. Administer medications in collaboration with physicians to include the following (see Table 5.1):

- *Vasodilators:* Morphine decreases venous return and myocardial oxygen consumption; nitrates increase venous capacity, thus reducing venous blood return, which decreases CVP, RAP, PAS, PAD, PAWP (preload); nitroprusside dilates arterial vessels, thus reducing SVR and myocardial workload.
- *Inotropes* enhance myocardial contractility and ventricular ejection of blood volume (digitalis, dopamine, dobutamine, and amrinone).
- *Diurectics* reduce actual circulating blood volume (furosemide, bumetanide, and ethacrynic acid).
- *Beta-adrenergic blocking agents* block the effects of catecholamines and decrease contractility and rate, thus decreasing myocardial oxygen demand (labetalol and propranolol).
- *Calcium channel blockers* vasodilate coronary arteries to supply more blood and decrease contractility, thus reducing myocardial workload (diltiazem, nifedipine, and verapamil).
- *ACE inhibitors* decrease preload and afterload while increasing CO by preventing angiotensin I from converting to angiotensin II (captopril and enalapril).

            iii. Continuous heparin infusion may be required to prevent thromboemboli caused by frequent episodes of atrial fibrillation (see Table 5.1).

            iv. Monitor and report changes in CVP or PAP measurements every hours, as needed or with every drug titration.

            v. Monitor BP closely for hypotension; notify physician; and titrate drugs to keep SBP greater than 90 mm Hg.

            vi. Continuously monitor $S\bar{v}o_2$ and attempt to maintain between 70% and 80%.

            vii. Monitor I&O hourly; maintain urine output greater than 30 mL/h; limit fluid intake to support reducing circulating volume.

            viii. Weigh patient every day; 1 kg = 1 liter of fluid.

            ix. Limit patient activity to conserve myocardial oxygen utilization.

            x. Assess physical signs of fluid retention every 4 hours: pedal (pitting) edema, jugular vein distention, S_3 heart sound.

            xi. Continuously monitor for cardiac dysrhythmias, and treat according to ACLS guidelines (see Appendix C).

            xii. Maintain patent IV/central lines for medication administration.

            xiii. Monitor digitalis levels to maintain in therapeutic range; assess for digitalis toxicity even if level is within normal range especially in the presence of electrolyte imbalances and acidosis.

xiv. Maintain serum potassium greater than 4.5 mEq/L, especially if administering digitalis and diuretics.

xv. May administer heparin 5000 U SC twice daily if patient undergoing bed rest to prevent thrombus formation.

xvi. Monitor and control chest pain (ischemia secondary to inadequate myocardial perfusion).

xvii. Heart transplantation may be the only option available to improve quality of life; donor availability and careful crossmatching required (see Chap. 14).

c. Desired outcome

i. Patient will maintain adequate cardiac output and tissue perfusion as evidenced by HR, BP within normal limits; PA, SVR, CI, and $S\bar{v}O_2$ within normal range; JVD diminished; lung fields clear; appropriate mentation; normal organ functioning; urine output greater than 30 mL/h; palpable pulses; and warm/dry skin.

2. Alteration in gas exchange related to ventricular failure and resultant pulmonary congestion

a. Problem: Decreased oxygen delivery to the tissues causes cellular injury and possible cellular death.

b. Intervention

i. Administer oxygen 2–4 liters via nasal cannula to maintain PaO_2 greater than 80 mm Hg to support perfusion efforts; be prepared to provide mechanical ventilation if necessary.

ii. Monitor oxygen saturation by pulse oximetry and maintain greater than 94%.

iii. Continuously monitor $S\bar{v}O_2$ and attempt to maintain between 70% and 80%.

iv. Obtain arterial blood gases as needed to monitor adequate oxygenation; collaborate with physicians for changes needed in oxygen therapy.

v. Assess breath sounds every 4 hours for crackles, rhonchi, or wheezing; collaborate with physician and respiratory therapist for treatment needs based on assessment.

vi. Assist patient to a position that maximizes chest expansion.

vii. Encourage patient to cough frequently to expel sputum.

viii. If intubated, suction as needed to control secretions

ix. Prevent pneumonia and atelectasis through encouraging patient to cough and deep breathe or use incentive spirometer every hour while awake.

c. Desired outcome: Arterial blood gas results within normal limits; RR 12–20 breaths/minute; vesicular breath sounds; adequate tissue perfusion

C. Discharge planning

1. Ensure that patient understands actions and need for medication regimen.

2. Instruct patient and family to limit activities and to take frequent rest periods to preserve cardiac function.

3. Ensure patient and family understand the importance of follow-up care.

Aneurysm/Acute Aortic Dissection

I. Definition: Atherosclerosis, cystic medial necrosis, and hypertension lay the foundation for the development of an aortic aneurysm. A false aneurysm may develop whereby blood accumulates in the media; a disruption of the intima occurs, but the adventitia remains intact. True aneursyms are typically categorized as fusiform or saccular, and they involve the entire wall of the artery. A diffuse area of weakness in the wall of the aorta causing a spindlelike deformity is called a fusiform aneurysm. Saccular aneurysms are described as a ballooning out of the wall of the aorta. Aneurysms are commonly associated with individuals having Marfan's syndrome or those suffering from autoimmune disease or chest trauma. Acute aortic wall dissection or rupture of the aneurysm are real concerns, and they are most commonly seen in individuals with hypertension.

II. Etiology: Acute aortic dissection or rupture starts with a laceration or tear of the intimal (inner) layer under the high arterial pressure that is present in the aorta and causes blood to enter the media. This causes further damage to the layers of the aorta and increases the chance for complete rupture. Dissecting aneurysms are divided into three types based on the location of the disruption: DeBakey type I involves the ascending aorta and the aortic arch extending throughout the thoracic aorta, DeBakey type II involves the ascending portion of the aorta only, and DeBakey type III begins near the subclavian artery and extends distally.

III. Nursing process

A. Assessment

 1. Signs and symptoms (for acute aortic dissection)

 a. Note: True aortic aneurysms may be asymptomatic, or they may be present with chronic pain or thromboembolic complications to the extremities and/or cerebrovascular ischemia.

 b. Pain: the abrupt onset of excruciating pain, reaching a peak almost immediately, differentiating itself from that of a myocardial infarction, whereby pain develops over a few minutes; pain may occur in the chest or back or migrate into different areas as the dissection extends; pain is seldom completely absent

 c. Syncope: along with neurologic changes that may result from ischemia to the brain, spinal cord, or a peripheral nerve; stroke develops in 10% of these patients

 d. Hypertension: severe in most patients accompanied by pale and clammy skin from extreme vasoconstriction

 e. Hypotension: if aortic rupture has occurred (hypovolemia) or if cardiac tamponade has developed

 f. Aortic diastolic murmur: (medium-pitched and harsh sound heard between S_1 and S_2) occurs in some patients and is extremely significant, since it indicates aortic valve insufficiency secondary to the proximal extension of the aneurysm into the valve itself

    g. Unequal carotid or subclavian pulses: may occur from the asymmetric compression of these vessels and the narrowing aortic lumen size due to the dissection of the aortic wall

    h. Delayed capillary refill, cool skin, and other signs of decreased tissue perfusion: results from hypovolemia (rupture), cardiac tamponade, narrowing aortic lumen, and extreme peripheral vasoconstriction

2. Diagnostic tests

    a. Serum

        i. Elevated BUN and Cr if renal dysfunction is present from disruption in renal blood flow

        ii. Cardiac enzymes may be elevated if dissection involves the coronary arteries and results in an AMI.

    b. Urine

        i. No significant changes

    c. Other

        i. Chest x-ray: a widened mediastinum or a left pleural effusion from extravasation of blood; radiography may be normal in some patients

        ii. Electrocardiography: should be normal or show signs of left ventricular hypertrophy; useful in distinguishing from MI

        iii. Computerized axial tomographic (CAT) scan: noninvasive imaging technique that can clearly demonstrate the presence of a true and false lumen and its extension into the proximal and distal aorta

        iv. Ultrasound: easily performed noninvasive imaging technique that may distinguish the true and false aortic lumens as well as the presence of blood clots

        v. Aortography: may outline the double lumen; most definitive diagnostic procedure; crucial for diagnosis and can be used as a "road map" in planning surgical intervention

B. Patient management

1. Maintain adequate tissue perfusion by preventing further dissection or possible rupture of aneurysm

    a. Problem: further dissection, rupture, and possible exsanguination

    b. Intervention

        i. Control hypertension and decrease left ventricular contractility and blood ejection velocity

            ▪ Sublingual nifedipine may be used to decrease BP emergently (see Table 5.1).

            ▪ Administer sodium nitroprusside (see Table 5.1) to decrease BP.

            ▪ Administer beta-adrenergic blocking agents (see Table 5.1) to decrease left ventricular work and aortic wall stress.

            ▪ Administer agents to decrease anxiety such as diazepam.

---

diazepam
Action Anxiolytic.
Administration Guidelines 2–10 mg every 4–6 hours IV as needed.
Special considerations Monitor for respiratory depression.

- Titrate drugs by continuously monitoring BP, HR, and urine output (> 30 mL/h) to establish responsiveness to therapy and ensure continued adequate perfusion.
  - ii. Prepare patient and family for emergency surgery for aortic resection and grafting by providing information, education, and support.
  - iii. Obtain cardiac enzymes and continuously monitor the ECG to detect ST-segment changes; myocardial ischemia may result if aneurysm involves coronary arteries or from underlying CAD.
  - iv. Continuously monitor for symptoms of CHF (crackles, S_3 or S_4, tachycardia), since this is evidence that the aneurysm involves the aortic valve.
  - v. Assess extremities hourly for bilateral pulse equality, color, capillary refill, and temperature; notify physician of any significant finding immediately; this may be a sign of further dissection or thromboembolic complications.
  - vi. Monitor urine output hourly; sudden drop in output may signify renal artery dissection.
  - vii. Administer oxygen as needed to maintain adequate blood oxygenation.
  - viii. Limit patient activity (bed rest) to prevent further stress on the aneurysm and cardiovascular system.
  - c. Desired outcome
    - i. Aneurysm will not dissect further.
    - ii. Hypertension will be controlled while adequate perfusion is maintained as shown by BP within 20 mm Hg of baseline, HR within 20 beats of baseline, urine output greater than 30 mL/h, normal mentation, and adequate pulses.
    - iii. Patient and family able to cope with surgical intervention as shown by addressing appropriate concerns and participating in decisions.
- 2. Pain related to dissecting aneurysm
  - a. Problem: further dissection from increased BP, anxiety, stress, and activity; inability to cope with situation
  - b. Intervention
    - i. Explain the cause of pain to patient and that pain will probably not worsen.
    - ii. Assess pain using an objective pain scale and document.
    - iii. Instruct patient to notify nurse with any changes in pain intensity or location; notify physician with significant changes.
    - iv. Explain all procedures and therapies to patient and family to decrease anxiety.

      v. Provide as quiet an environment as possible; the emergent nature of the surgical intervention will create tremendous stress.

      vi. Allow family members maximum access to patient.

      vii. Administer analgesics with physician collaboration and with extreme caution; usually withheld so that further dissection can be monitored.

   c. Desired outcome

      i. Pain is decreased as evidenced by objective pain scale rating.

      ii. Patient will participate in decision making appropriately.

      iii. Patient will verbalize that pain is understood and bearable.

C. Discharge planning

   1. Discuss with patient the need to control BP and ensure that patient and family support and understand medication regimen.

   2. Explain the importance of returning for follow-up observation of the development of another aneurysm.

References

1. Malseed, R. T. *Pharmacology Drug Therapy and Nursing Considerations* (3rd ed.). Philadelphia: J. B. Lippincott, 1990.

2. Underhill, S. L., et al. (eds.). *Cardiovascular Medications for Cardiac Nursing*. Philadelphia: J. B. Lippincott, 1990.

3. Stillwell, S. *Quick Critical Care Reference*. St. Louis: C. V. Mosby, 1990.

4. Drew, B. Bedside electrocardiographic monitoring: State of the art for 1990s. *Heart Lung* 20: 610–623, 1991.

5. Drew, B., and Tisdale, L. ST segment monitoring for coronary artery reocclusion following thrombolytic therapy and coronary angioplasty: Identification of optimal bedside monitoring leads. *Am. J. Crit. Care* 2: 280–292, 1993.

6. Muirhead, J. Pericardial Disease. In Underhill, S. L., et al. (eds.). *Cardiac Nursing* (2nd ed.). Philadelphia: J. B. Lippincott, 1989. P. 915.

7. Kinney, M. R., Packa, D. R., and Dunbar, S. B. (eds.). *AACN's Clinical Reference for Critical-Care Nursing* (3rd ed.). St. Louis: Mosby–Year Book, 1993. Pp. 586–605.

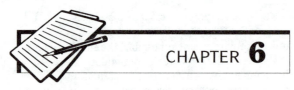

CHAPTER 6

Endocrine Disorders

Merrily A. Kuhn

Adrenal Crisis (Addisonian Crisis)

I. Definition: Adrenal crisis is an acute onset of a lack of adrenal hormones, usually occurring during stress (trauma, sepsis, surgery). There are two types, primary and secondary. Primary adrenal insufficiency occurs from destruction of at least 90% of adrenocortical tissue. As the gland is destroyed, there is a combined glucocorticoid and mineralocorticoid deficiency.

Secondary adrenal insufficiency is due to adrenocorticotropic hormone (ACTH) deficiency. Corticosteroids maintain the responsiveness of the vasculature to catecholamines, and cortisol deficiency results in hypotension. Long-term administration of corticosteroids suppresses the hypothalamic–pituitary–adrenal axis, which can result in ACTH deficiency.

II. Etiology: Primary adrenal insufficiency is associated with autoimmune adrenalitis (80% of cases), mycobacterium tuberculosis (> 20% of cases), and adrenal hemorrhage associated with sepsis (Waterhouse-Friderichsen syndrome). Patients with human immunodeficiency virus infection may also develop primary adrenal insufficiency due to destruction of the adrenal gland resulting from cytomegalovirus infection. Tumor metastasis to the adrenal gland may also occur from cancers of the lung, breast, melanoma, or lymphoma, but it is rare, since over 90% of the gland must be destroyed.

Secondary adrenal insufficiency is associated with cessation of steroid therapy, vascular lesions, pituitary surgery, head trauma, autoimmune conditions, and sarcoidosis. Careful assessments are required in patients who have received exogenous steroids in the previous 2–3 months. When the hypothalamic–pituitary axis is depressed from steroid replacement, it may take 12–18 months to recover.

III. Nursing process

  A. Assessment findings

  1. Signs and symptoms

  a. Unexplained hypotension: related to mineralocorticoid-aldosterone deficiency resulting in decreased Na^+ and decreased extracellular fluid balance; may be impaired cellular response to catecholamine due to decreased cortisol.

b. Fatigue, weakness: Lack of cortisol decreases gluconeogenesis, thus decreasing glucose metabolism and reducing liver glycogen stores.

c. Nausea, vomiting, diarrhea, abdominal pain: due to decreased secretion of digestive enzymes and dehydration.

d. Weight loss: Decreased mobilization of fat and proteins leads to sluggish energy generation.

e. High-grade 39°C (102°F) or low-grade fever: due to changes in temperature control center in hypothalamus and dehydration.

f. Confusion, coma: related to hypoglycemia and severe dehydration; decreased Na^+, increased K^+, and decreased extracellular fluid balance due to mineralocorticoid deficiency.

g. Costovertebral angle tenderness (in adrenal hemorrhage only): related to collection of blood and pressure on nerve endings.

h. Hypoglycemia: Lack of cortisol decreases gluconeogenesis.

i. Hyperpigmentation: Increased secretion of melanocyte-stimulating hormone plus the melanocyte stimulatory effects of ACTH (as seen in primary insufficiency) contribute to abnormal deposition of melanin in skin, leading to brown-copper coloring.

j. Hypovolemia: due to mineralocorticoid-aldosterone deficiency and decreased Na^+ and decreased extracellular fluid balance; poor skin turgor.

2. Diagnostic parameters

a. Serum test

  i. Hyperkalemia: greater than 5.0 mEq/L due to aldosterone deficiency; may predispose to dysrhythmias.

  ii. Hypoglycemia: less than 75 mg/dL due to cortisol deficiency; may predispose to mental confusion and fatigue.

  iii. Blood urea nitrogen (BUN): greater than 15 mg/dL due to hypovolemia and impaired free water clearance.

  iv. Hyponatremia: less than 135 mEq/L due to aldosterone deficiency.

  v. Hypercalcemia: greater than 10.5 mg/dL; due to lack of cortisol to counteract intestinal calcium absorption.

  vi. Acidemia: impaired secretion of K^+ and H^+.

  vii. Increased eosinophil count: due to autoimmune reaction.

  viii. Cortisol level: less than 20 μg/dL, due to decreased or no production; less than 10 μg/100 mL at 8:00 AM, less than 5 μg/100 mL at 4:00 PM.

b. Urine

  i. Decrease 17-ketosteroids and decrease urine cortisol: due to lack of cortisol secretion.

c. Other: Rapid ACTH stimulation test—draw basal levels of cortisol, aldosterone, and ACTH. Administer 250 μg of synthetic ACTH. Draw levels again after 30 and 60 minutes. Cortisol less than 20 μg/dL indicates insufficiency.

B. Patient management

1. Decreased cardiac output related to a reduced circulating blood volume and decreased venous return and dysrhythmias associated with hyperkalemia.

a. Problem: A decrease in cardiac output secondary to aldosterone deficiency results in volume depletion and affects total body supply of oxygen, nutritional products, and fluids and electrolytes. Tissue ische-mia, fatigue, cardiac dysrhythmias may cause a crisis for the patient.

b. Intervention

　　i. Correct and monitor fluid and electrolyte balance. IV therapy: 5% dextrose in normal saline (D5NS) or plasma expanders to restore volume and treat hypovolemia. Administer vasopressors like do-butamine to relieve hypotension and restore renal function. (Re-store fluid volume before administering any vasopressor.)

　　ii. Monitor input and output, renal function, gastrointestinal (GI) losses.

c. Desired outcome

　　i. Patient will maintain the following:

- Usual mental status
  - Alert, oriented to person, place, date
- Effective cardiovascular function
  - Heart rate 60–100 beats/minute.
  - Cardiac rhythm: regular sinus, no dysrhythmias.
- Hemodynamic parameters (central venous pressure [CVP], pulmonary artery occlusion pressure [PAOP], cardiac output, arterial blood pressure) return to normal.
- Renal status
  - Urine output greater than 30 mL/h.
- Respiratory status
  - Respiratory rate normal.

2. Fluid volume deficit related to hyponatremia associated with hyposecre-tion of aldosterone.

a. Problem: Fluid volume deficit could result in hypotension and hypo-perfusion of all organs.

b. Intervention

　　i. Intravenous (IV) therapy: D5NS solution or plasma expanders to restore volume.

　　ii. Monitor Na^+; restore Na^+ as needed.

　　iii. Monitor level of consciousness (LOC).

c. Desired outcome

　　i. Patient will maintain effective fluid and electrolyte balance.

- Neurologic status
  - Alert, oriented to person, place, date.
  - Behavior appropriate.
  - Usual personality (as per family).
  - Deep tendon reflexes brisk.
- Hemodynamic status
  - Near normal.

3. Electrolyte imbalance related to hyponatremia, and hyperkalemia associ-ated with hyposecretion of mineralocorticoids (eg, aldosterone) and glu-cocorticoids (eg, cortisol).

a. Problem: Electrolyte imbalance may lead to cardiac dysrhythmias and dehydration. Glucocorticosteroid deficit may also contribute to hypoglycemia.

b. Intervention

   i. Immediate therapy.

      • Replace corticol hormones (Table 6.1). Steroids are more than 90% protein bound; monitor serum proteins and replace as necessary.

---

steroids

Action Enhance reabsorption of Na^+ and Cl^-, and enhance excretion of K^+ and H^+ in distal tubule of kidney.

Administration Guidelines Never discontinue abruptly or without checking with physician. Obtain an order for parenteral form if unable to take orally. Massage topical drugs into area thoroughly and gently. Apply sparingly. Wear gloves when applying. Apply occlusive dressing only if ordered. Inject intramuscularly (IM) deeply into dorsal gluteal or ventrogluteal of buttock. Rotate injection sites and record. Dilute IV solutions according to package direction.

Special Considerations Encourage patient to carry identification card or wear a bracelet or necklace if on long-term therapy. Weigh patient regularly, and check urine for glucosuria. Patient should take antacids as prescribed; avoid aspirin; take oral drugs with food. Teach patient at what time of day drug is to be taken. Teach patient that dose will need to be increased with physiologic stress and that doctor should be consulted. Store in a dry, tightly closed container; protect from light.

Table 6.1 Glucocorticoid/Mineralocorticoid Replacement

Generic Name (Trade Name)	Gluco-corticoid Potency	Mineralo-corticoid Potency	Dose and Route	Administration Guidelines
Hydrocortisone (Solu Cortef)	1.0	1	100 mg IV, PO	Very slowly IV: 100 mg over 20–30 minutes
Methylprednisolone (Medrol)	5	0.5	20 mg IV, PO	Inject IM deeply into dorsal gluteal or ventrogluteal of buttock; rotate sites
Dexamethasone (Decadron)	25.0	2	4 mg IV, PO	With food to decrease GI upset; avoid aspirin
Prednisolone (Deltasone)	4.0	0.7	25 mg PO	With food to decrease GI upset; avoid aspirin

  ii. Correct hypoglycemia.
   ▪ Administer 5%–10% dextrose solution as ordered.
   ▪ Conserve energy, minimize stress, provide frequent rest.
 c. Desired outcome
  i. Renal status returns to normal. Urine output (hourly) greater than 30 mL/h.
  ii. Respiratory status
   ▪ Respiratory rate less than 25–30 breaths/minute.
   ▪ Breath sounds clear.
  iii. GI status
   ▪ Absence of anorexia, nausea, vomiting, diarrhea, bleeding.
  iv. Laboratory data: All values return to normal.
   ▪ Serum osmolality, Na^+, K^+, glucose.
   ▪ Hematology.
   ▪ Urine—specific gravity returns to normal.

4. Altered cerebral tissue perfusion related to fluid volume deficit, electrolyte disturbance, hyponatremia, hyperkalemia.
 a. Problem: Altered perfusion to the brain may lead to confusion and impaired neurologic function.
 b. Intervention
  i. Correct and monitor fluid and electrolyte balance. IV therapy: D5NS or plasma expanders to restore volume and treat hypovolemia. Administer vasopressors like dobutamine to relieve hypotension and restore renal function. (Always restore volume before administering a vasopressor.)
  ii. Monitor input and output, renal function, GI losses.
 c. Desired outcome
  i. Neurologic status returns to normal.
   ▪ Exhibits intact LOC and mentation.
   ▪ Demonstrates intact sensorimotor function.
   ▪ Deep tendon reflexes brisk.
  ii. Respiratory status returns to normal limits.

5. Alteration in nutrition less than body requirements, related to catabolic state.
 a. Problem: As LOC decreases, nutritional intake is reduced. Utilization of nutrients is also decreased due to deficit of glucocorticoids. Body proteins are catabolized for energy.
 b. Intervention
  i. Monitor level of nutrition; increase carbohydrate, protein, and Na^+.
  ii. Reduce risk of infection; steroids suppress immune response. Prevent complications of immobility. Encourage early ambulation, deep breathing and coughing, turn, reposition often.
 c. Desired outcome
  i. Patient's body weight will stabilize within 5% of baseline.
  ii. Serum proteins will be maintained within acceptable physiologic range including serum albumin, prealbumin, transferrin, total lymphocyte count. Serum glucose will return to normal.
  iii. Urine negative for glucose and acetone.

C. Discharge planning
  1. Review all treatments and activities to prevent complications.
  2. Discuss body image alterations: Hirsutism due to increased testosterone (particularly in women) should decrease with therapy. Changes in fat distribution (in face and back) may begin as glucocorticoids are administered.
  3. Continue to encourage and teach nutritional support. Severe hypoglycemia may result from fasting or delaying meals. Hypoglycemic reactions may occur from increased sensitivity to insulin and low serum glucose.
  4. Protect from crowds to decrease chance of infection. Steroids suppress the immune response.
  5. Discuss need for follow-up appointments to monitor progress.
  6. Review medications, their action, dosage, and side effects.

Diabetes Insipidus

  I. Definition: Diabetes insipidus (DI) is a disorder of impaired renal/water conservation due to inadequate and/or impaired antidiuretic hormone (ADH) synthesis, secretion, or activity. ADH secretion is decreased either from the hypothalamus nuclei or from the axonal ending in the posterior pituitary. ADH antibodies may be present in the body and accelerate ADH breakdown. Defective chemoreceptors may require higher serum osmolarity levels to elicit a response. Inability to concentrate urine results in chronic polyuria (4–12 L/d), increased plasma osmolarity, low urine osmolarity, and specific gravity.

  A. Types: complete, partial, or transient.
  B. Forms
  1. Neurogenic (central)—insufficient amounts of ADH being produced or released secondary to CNS depression/injury.
  2. Nephrogenic—inadequate response to ADH due to kidney disease (rarely seen and does not usually present with massive polyuria).
  3. Psychogenic—extremely large fluid intake resulting in decreased ADH levels.

  II. Etiology

  A. Hypothalamic or central DIs is associated with recent illness, head injury, head surgery (particularly transphenoidal hypophyseal surgery), any cerebral vascular insult such as a cerebrovascular accident (CVA) or bleeding, pituitary tumors, cerebral edema, and brain infections.
  B. Nephrogenic DI may result from any condition that impairs the responsiveness of the collecting ducts to ADH including drugs (alcohol, phenytoin, and others), obstruction in the urinary tract, hypercalcemia, or congenital defects. Intrinsic renal disease, protein malnutrition, or diuretic therapy may also limit renal concentrating ability. Forty-five percent to 50% of all cases are idiopathic.
  C. Psychogenic DI occurs with massive increases in water consumption.

III. Nursing process

A. Assessment findings
  1. Signs and symptoms
     a. Polyuria (4–12 L/d or more): due to lack of ADH and inability to concentrate urine.
     b. Polydipsia (extreme thirst): due to massive fluid loss; often craves cold drinks.
     c. Hydronephrosis (enlarged bladder capacity in long-term DI): related to increased urine production.
     d. Dehydration, sunken eyeballs, poor skin turgor, dry mucous membranes, hypotension, rapid pulse—all related to severe cellular dehydration.
     e. Decreased mentation, LOC, deep tendon reflexes, and possibly even seizure activity—related to cerebral intracellular dehydration and cell shrinkage.
  2. Diagnostic parameters
     a. Serum tests
        i. Plasma osmolarity elevated (greater than 300 mOsm/kg water): plasma constriction and concentration related to increased excretion of fluid volume.
        ii. Hypernatremia: related to excretion of water without concomitant excretion of Na^+.
     b. Urine tests
        i. Low osmolarity and low specific gravity: related to increased urine production and dilution.
B. Patient management
  1. Fluid volume deficit related to decreased ADH synthesis and or secretion, defective osmoreceptors, altered immunologic function (presence of ADH antibodies), and unresponsiveness of cells in the late distal tubules and collecting ducts to action of ADH (nephrogenic DI).
     a. Problem: Fluid volume deficit leads to dehydration and hypotension.
     b. Interventions
        i. Assess for signs and symptoms of DI (as earlier).
        ii. Monitor for neurologic dysfunction.

---

vasopressin (Pitressin)

Action Vasopressor activity by stimulating smooth-muscle contraction, particularly in the hepatic and splanchnic beds; acts in the kidney in the distal tubules and collecting ducts to increase the cellular permeability to water, thus decreasing urine output and increasing water absorption.

Administration Guidelines Warm ampule and shake vigorously to disperse tannate uniformly. Administer with one to two glasses of water to minimize side effects.

Special Considerations Be alert for signs of water toxicity, and withdraw drug and restrict fluid intake until urine specific gravity is at least 1.015.

lypressin (Diapid)

Action Mainly antidiuretic activity as above.

Administration Guidelines Drug should not be inhaled. Allergic rhinitis or upper respiratory infections may affect absorption. Hold bottle upright, and patient should be in a vertical position with head upright. Do not use more than three sprays.

desmopressin acetate (deamino-D-arginine vasopressin)

Action Antidiuretic effect, increase factor VIII levels.

Administration Guidelines Drug should not be inhaled. Allergic rhinitis or upper respiratory infections may affect absorption. Hold bottle upright, and patient should be in a vertical position with head upright. Do not use more than three sprays.

    iii. Administer ADH replacement therapy for central DI.
    iv. Monitor respiratory function for tachypnea, dyspnea, adventitious sounds, cough, which may indicate hypervolemia.
  c. Desired outcome
    i. Patient will maintain stable
      • Hydration status
      ○ Body weight within 5% of baseline.
      ○ Balanced intake and output.
      • Laboratory studies (serum osmolarity and urine specific gravity) will return to normal.
      • Neurologic status
      ○ Alert, oriented to person, place, and date.
      ○ Visual fields at baseline.
      ○ Motor function: muscle tone and strength intact; absence of twitching or seizure activity.
      ○ Deep tendon reflexes brisk.
2. Alteration in cardiac output related to severely contracted intravascular volume
  a. Problem: A reduction in cardiac output compromises total body function.
  b. Interventions
    i. Monitor cardiac status, hemodynamic pressures.
    ii. Monitor for and prevent complication venous stasis, pressure-sore formation.
  c. Desired outcome
    i. Hemodynamic status
      • Blood pressure within 10 mm Hg of baseline.
      • Pulse is strong: heart rate 60–100 beats/minute.
    ii. Hemodynamic parameters return to normal: CVP, PAOP, CO, pulmonary artery pressure (PAP).
3. Electrolyte imbalance related to excess water loss with hypernatremia
  a. Problem: Electrolyte imbalances can precipitate cardiac dysrhythmias, hematologic problems, and disturbances in neurologic function.

b. Interventions
  i. Replace fluids as ordered (hypotonic solutions).
  ii. IV fluids may be replaced hour by hour to match urine output.
  iii. Administer thiazide diuretics as ordered for nephrogenic DI.

---

chlorothiazide (Diuril, Diachlor)
hydrochlorothiazide (Esidrix, HydroDIURIL)
trichlormethiazide (Naqua)
polythiazide (Renese)
Action Inhibit tubular reabsorption of Na^+ and Cl^- by direct action on distal tube.
Administration Guidelines Take with food to avoid GI upset. Administer early in day to avoid sleep disruption. Best not to administer after 3:00 PM. Hyperglycemia may affect diabetes mellitus; insulin dose may need to be adjusted.

---

c. Desired outcome
  i. Renal status
    ▪ Hourly urine outputs: greater than 30, less than 200 mL/h.
  ii. Laboratory studies return to normal: BUN and creatinine, serum Na^+, and urinary Na^+.
    ▪ Hematology profile within acceptable range (hematocrit, hemoglobin).
  iii. Respiratory status
    ▪ Respiratory rate less than 25–30 breaths/minute.
    ▪ Respiratory rhythm: eupneic.
    ▪ Breath sounds: clear to auscultation.

IV. Discharge planning
A. Review all medications dosages, administration techniques, and side effects.
B. Review symptoms that indicate worsening of condition.
C. Implement nutritional regimen to restore nutritional balance.
  1. Provide sufficient calories to prevent protein catabolism.
  2. Provide sufficient protein to ensure tissue healing and to prevent breakdown.
  3. Limit Na^+ intake until fluid and Na^+ balance return to normal.
D. Assist with coping of patient and family to current needs.

Diabetic Ketoacidosis

I. **Definition:** Diabetic ketoacidosis (DKA) is an acute, complex, multisystem metabolic disorder due to an absolute or relative lack of insulin usually with a compromise of basal requirements and often with an excess of the counterregulatory hormone glucagon. DKA is a serious, life-threatening condition. Eighty percent to 90% of cases of DKA occur in someone with previously diagnosed diabetes. DKA is characterized by hyperglycemia; osmotic diuresis causing cellular dehydration, ketosis, fluid and electrolyte imbalance; and a negative nitrogen balance and is associated with severe, uncontrolled diabetes type 1 (insulin-dependent diabetes mellitus [IDDM]). The development of DKA always requires an explanation, such as interruption of insulin therapy, nonadherence to a diabetic meal plan, an inappropriate exercise routine, or a precipitating stress that increases basal insulin needs. Although the condition is typically considered a metabolic problem, pathologic involvement of all major body systems is evident. Mortality ranges between 5% and 10%. However, in young patients with IDDM, DKA and its complications result in 30%–50% mortality. Women outnumber men in incidence of DKA and death rate.

II. Etiology: Cells are unable to use glucose as a source of energy even though hyperglycemia is evident. Therefore, fatty cells and protein are used for energy and converted to ketones. DKA can be the first presentation of IDDN or occur when insulin is omitted (severe stress is experienced without appropriate insulin and diet management); when calories are increased; when medication (thiazides, furosemide, anti-inflammatory agents, psychotropic agents, glucagon, glucocorticoids, analgesics) that impair glucose metabolism are used; when beta-blockers are used that may mask symptoms; when another illness is present such as acute pancreatitis, thyroid crisis, or Addison's disease; when salicylate or alcohol intoxication is present; when total parenteral nutrition is being used; or when (in 25%–30% of cases) no precipitating factor may be found.

III. Nursing process

A. Assessment findings

1. Signs and symptoms

   a. Profound dehydration, poor skin turgor, tachycardia, flushed dry skin, orthostatic hypotension, dry mucous membranes, pleuritic chest pain, friction rub: related to osmotic diuresis.

   b. Fatigue, altered LOC, and visual disturbances: most consistently correlated with serum osmolarity changes rather than pH, which results in brain cell dehydration.

   c. Coma: results from brain cell dehydration and results in a mortality rate of 15%–20% [1].

   d. Weakness, anorexia, vomiting, altered mental status: related to volume depletion.

   e. Fruity odor of breath: because of increased acetones.

   f. Kussmaul breathing: results from respiratory compensation for metabolic acidosis.

   g. Nausea, vomiting, abdominal pain or cramps: may be related to ileus secondary to electrolyte abnormalities or hepatic congestion (more likely in those < 40 yr old).

   h. Weight loss: due to lack of glucose body begins to catabolize protein to remain stable. Body protein is lost for several days, and then fat is used for energy requirements.

   i. Polydipsia: Thirst mechanism is increased due to osmotic diuresis and fluid loss occurring in the kidney.

    2. Diagnostic tests

      a. Serum tests

        i. Hyperosmolarity: greater than 300 mOsm/L due to hyperglycemia and excessive water loss.

        ii. Metabolic acidosis: pH less than 7.35, HCO_3^- less than 15 mEq/L; related to conversion of fats to ketoacids and acetone and dissociation of H^+.

        iii. Arterial CO_2: low due to compensatory hyperventilation.

        iv. Hematocrit and total protein: elevated related to dehydration.

        v. Hypophosphatemia less than 1.0 mg/100 mg results from phosphate shifting from in the cell to outside the cell and then being lost by kidney due to the osmotic diuresis.

        vi. Leukocytosis: due to severe dehydration, may mask signs of underlying infection.

        vii. Liver function tests (elevated): actually may have no specific correlation to DKA but are often seen.

        viii. Hyperkalemia: greater than 5.0 mEq/L (early); K^+ moves out of cells in exchange for H^+ and is not yet excreted by kidney.

        ix. Hypokalemia: less than 3.5 mEq/L (late); total body deficit; K^+ is lost by kidney, since serum K^+ is above normal.

        x. Hyperglycemia: greater than 250 mg/dL (average 675 mg/dL but rarely reaches 1000 mg/dL); related to inability to utilize glucose due to lack of insulin. As excessive glucose is seen by the kidney, an osmotic diuresis results.

        xi. BUN: greater than 20 mg/dL; slowed perfusion in the kidney and volume depletion.

      b. Urine tests

        i. Ketonuria (moderate to large amount): due to excessive production and decreased metabolism of ketone bodies.

        ii. Polyuria: related to hyperglycemia, hyperosmolarity, and osmotic diuresis.

        iii. Glucosuria: due to excessive serum level of glucose that is above urine threshold for glucose and, thus, is excreted.

        iv. Urine Na^+ and Cl^-: both decreased due to excessive loss related to osmotic diuresis.

        v. Specific gravity: greater than 1.025 due to increased amount of solute being lost.

  B. Patient management

    1. Actual (total body dehydration) fluid volume deficit related to osmotic diuresis caused by extreme glycosuria associated with hyperglycemic state, and ketosis and ketonemia associated with enhanced lipolysis caused by insulin insufficiency.

      a. Problem: Hypovolemia leads to hypotension and decreased tissue perfusion to organs. As fluid level falls, cardiac output and all hemodynamic values become abnormal.

      b. Intervention

        i. Treat the underlying cause.

    ii. Monitor fluid status (skin turgor, urinary output, vital signs), neck veins.

    iii. Administer IV fluids as ordered. First to restore vascular volume-isotonic-solution 0.9% normal saline. Hypotonic solutions (0.45 normal saline) are then infused. One half of the calculated fluid deficit is restored in the first 12 hours with the remainder restored during the next 24 hours. Fluids may be ordered at 500 mL/h. When blood glucose reaches 250 mg/dL, IV infusion of 5% dextrose in water is usually begun to prevent hypoglycemia from occurring.

    iv. Monitor lungs for adventitious lung sounds, which may indicate developing congestive heart failure from too rapid fluid replacement.

    v. Record intake and output and weigh daily.

  c. Desired outcome

    i. Laboratory data indicating hemoconcentration returning to normal BUN, Na^+, and plasma osmolarity.

    ii. Increased hydration evidenced by the following:
- Moist oral mucous membranes.
- Improved skin turgor.

    iii. No cold perspiration usually associated with shock will be evident.

    iv. Skin integrity maintained.

    v. Neurologic status
- Alert, oriented to person, place, and date.
- Appropriate behavior.
- Usual personality (per family).
- Sensorimotor function intact.
- Deep tendon reflexes brisk.

2. Decreased cardiac output in severe volume depletion with reduced venous return.

  a. Problem: A decreased cardiac output results in decreased tissue perfusion to all organs. Cardiac output may be decreased secondary to dysrhythmias, dehydration, and electrolyte imbalances.

  b. Intervention

    i. Monitor cardiovascular status as fluid is administered, particularly CO, cardiac index, PAP, PAOP, CVP. If there is a rapid rise in any measure, reduce the IV rate.

  c. Desired outcome

    i. Hemodynamic status returns to normal including PAOP, cardiac output, PAPs, CVP; blood pressure within 10 mm Hg of patient's usual pressure; pulse rate within 15 beats of patient's usual pulse.

    ii. Cardiac rhythm—regular.

    iii. Urine output greater than 30 mL/h, and there is a normal urine specific gravity.

3. Electrolyte imbalance related to profound osmotic diuresis caused by extreme glycosuria, acidemia, and ketonemia associated with enhanced lipolysis; lactic acidosis associated with tissue hypoxia; and profound dehydration and hypovolemia.

a. **Problem:** Electrolyte imbalance may lead to renal, neurologic, and cardiac complications.
b. Intervention
   i. Return and maintain all electrolytes to normal.
   ii. Monitor body weight and vital signs.
   iii. Monitor input and output.
   iv. Monitor skin turgor and signs of dehydration.
   v. Monitor for GI losses and diarrhea.
   vi. Monitor electrolyte and urine often during therapy.
   vii. Restore fluid balance to normal.
   viii. Monitor for K^+ levels of hyperkalemia; ECG finding; prolonged QRS complex; tall, tented T waves; and depressed J-point. Cardiac dysrhythmias, including ventricular tachycardia. Hypokalemia usually occurs within 2–4 hours after insulin therapy is started. On ECG, monitor for low T waves, developing U waves, and lengthening of QT interval.
   ix. Monitor for hypophosphatemia; phosphorus is a major constituent of adenosine triphosphate (ATP), so as phosphorus goes down, muscle weakness becomes profound and may also depress contractility. In addition, phosphorus is a part of 2,3-diphosphoglycerate so there is a shift in the oxyhemoglobin dissociation curve to the left, thus reducing the amount of oxygen delivered to cells.
   x. Administer insulin as ordered. Usually 6–10 units IV stat and then 6–10 units/h. Decrease insulin dosage as blood glucose is lowered.

---

insulin

Action Replaces endogenous insulin deficiency: increases glucose transport across muscle and fat cell membranes; promotes conversion of glucose to glycogen; triggers amino acid uptake and conversion to protein in muscle cells; inhibits protein breakdown; stimulates triglyceride formation and inhibits release of free fatty acids from adipose tissue; and stimulates lipoprotein lipase activity, thereby converting lipoproteins to fatty acids.

Administration Guidelines Bolus dose 0.1–0.2 units/kg, followed by 0.1–0.2 units/kg per hour. Blood glucose is lowered to about 250–300 mg/dL.

Special Considerations As insulin is administered, it moves K^+ into the cell. Therefore, it is important to monitor for early signs and symptoms of hypokalemia.

---

   c. Desired outcome
      i. Laboratory status
         ▪ Serum levels return to normal including osmolality, Na^+, K^+, Cl^-, Ca^{2+}, and phosphorus.

- Glucose returns to normal.
- Hematology profile, total protein returns to normal.
- Urine, sodium, and specific gravity return to normal.
- Urine is negative for glucose and acetone.

4. Alteration in acid–base balance related to ketoacidosis associated with insulin insufficiency, enhanced lipolysis, and lactic acidemia associated with reduced tissue perfusion and tissue hypoxia.

  a. Problem: Acid–base imbalance may lead to changes in LOC and cardiac dysrhythmias.
  b. Intervention
      i. Restore and maintain normal pH.
      ii. Calculate anion gap: The major two anions are Cl^- and HCO_3^-. They account for all but 10–15 mmol/L of the total anion charge in the body. To calculate: Anion gap $= Na^+ - (Cl^- + HCO_3^-)$.
      iii. Normal anion gap: less than 15 mmol/L. If anion gap is above 15 mmol/L, another anion is present such as ketones, acetoacetic acid, beta-hydroxybutyric acid, and acetone.
      iv. Monitor ketonuria.
  c. Desired outcome
      i. Patient's arterial blood gases will normalize.
      ii. Anions will stabilize: HCO_3^-, Cl^-, and anion gap.

5. Alteration in cerebral, peripheral tissue perfusion related to hypovolemic state, severe dehydration, and extreme hyperosmolarity with hemoconcentration.

  a. Problem: Decreases in tissue perfusion may lead to neurologic, renal, and cardiac dysfunction. A decreased LOC may occur. Urinary output may be reduced, and cardiac ischemia, dysrhythmias, and even myocardial infarction may occur.
  b. Intervention
      i. Establish baseline neurologic function.
      ii. Maintain proper hydration level.
      iii. Monitor cardiac and renal function to assess hydration and tissue perfusion.
  c. Desired outcome
      i. Patient will maintain stable
          - Neurologic status.
          ○ LOC consistent with precrisis state.
          ○ Pupils equal in size and react briskly to light.
          ○ Moves all extremities consistent with precrisis mobility.
          ○ No seizure activity.
          - Hemodynamic status, as PAOP and CVP return to normal.
          - Renal status.
          - Laboratory parameters.
          - Respiratory rate and pattern, returning to normal for patient.
      ii. Patient safety maintained.

IV. Discharge planning

A. Teach patient the reasons for DKA and how to prevent in the future.

B. Review dietary and insulin therapy, and provide teaching materials for patient to take home.
C. Teach patient the importance of stress reduction, routine meals, and exercise.
D. Teach the concepts of diabetes.
E. Teach the need for routine medical follow-up, hygiene, and foot care.

Hyperglycemic Hyperosmolar Nonketotic Coma

I. Definition: Hyperglycemic hyperosmolar nonketotic coma (HHNK) is a syndrome associated with a relative insulin deficit, occurring most often in older adults over 50 years of age with non–insulin-dependent diabetes mellitus (type II) who have been exposed to severe stress. Often this is the first presentation of diabetes. Patients with HHNK have sufficient insulin levels to prevent excessive lipolysis but not to use glucose properly. Glucose levels are considerably higher in HHNK than in DKA and may rise above 1000 mg/dL. High serum osmolarity may prevent the liver from producing free fatty acids; therefore, the patient is nonketotic or has a very small amount of ketones and minimal acidosis. Levels of free fatty acids are consistently lower than those found in DKA. Symptoms often develop over days to weeks. Mortality rate varies from 40% to 70%.

II. Etiology: Gradual onset with sufficient insulin to prevent lipolysis (fatty acid breakdown) but insufficient amounts for carbohydrate metabolism. May be associated with:

A. Acute illness: conditions such as infections, trauma, thyrotoxicosis, myocardial infarction, cerebrovascular accident, hypothermia, anesthesia, stress. Most often the precipitating factor is a stressful environment.
B. Chronic illness: renal disease, cardiovascular dysfunction.
C. Drugs: propranolol, steroids, thiazides, furosemide, phenytoin, diazoxide.
D. Procedures: dialysis, total parenteral nutrition.

III. Nursing process

A. Assessment findings
  1. Signs and symptoms
    a. Hypovolemia/Dehydration: due to profound osmotic diuresis resulting in contraction of intra- and extracellular fluid compartments. Water losses may reach 8–12 liters.
    b. Alteration in LOC, possibly seizures, aphasia, confusion, extensor plantar reflex, visual hallucinations, stupor and coma: related to high serum osmolarity and intercellular dehydration of the brain. These neurologic symptoms generally clear as serum osmolarity is reduced.
    c. Hypotension, tachycardia, decreased PAOP, and decreased CVP and PAP: all related to extreme reduction in circulating volume.
    d. Tissue dehydration, dry mucous membranes, poor skin turgor, and dry axillae: all related to severe dehydration. (The extent of dehydration often is 20–25% of total body water.)

e. Possibly polydipsia: The thirst mechanism may be lost due to the high serum osmolarity, which impairs the thirst center in the hypothalamus.

2. Lab data

a. Serum tests

i. Hyperglycemia: due to relative insulin deficiency. Blood glucose is above 650 mg/dL and has been reported up to 4800 mg/dL. Reduced volume also decreases kidneys' ability to excrete glucose.

ii. Hyperosmolarity: greater than 295 mOsm/kg due to high level of glucose.

iii. BUN: greater than 10 mg/dL as circulating blood volume is reduced due to hyperglycemia and polyuria; glomerular filtration rate (GFR) may decrease by 50%. Thus, blood stays in the kidney for longer periods of time and reabsorbs more urea.

iv. Creatinine: greater than 1.5 mg/dL as GFR decreases; creatinine, which is produced in the body each time muscles move, begins to increase in the serum, since it is no longer being filtered.

v. Hyperkalemia (early): greater than 5.0 mEq/L K^+ shifts from the cells into the serum during early acidosis (in exchange for H^+) and dehydration.

vi. Hypokalemia (late): less than 3.5 mEq/L increased aldosterone stimulates the distal tube to reabsorbed Na^+; therefore, K^+ is lost in increasingly large quantities. In addition, as treatment is begun, insulin is administered, which forces K^+ back into the cell.

vii. Hypernatremia: greater than 145 mEq/L, related to severe dehydration. Because of severe hyperglycemia, Na^+ levels may seem deceptively low. To correct Na^+ levels, add 2.8 mmol to patient's reported Na^+ level for every 100-mg/dL increase in blood glucose [1].

viii. Hemoconcentration and hypercoagulopathy: due to severe osmotic diuresis. These symptoms may lead to embolic complications.

ix. pH normal to mildly acidotic: pH is often not altered because ketones are not produced.

b. Urine tests

i. Glycosuria: results when glucose in proximal renal tubule is greater than 225 mg/minute.

ii. Polyuria: results from the high serum osmolality and glucose causing more fluid to be lost.

iii. Ca^{2+} greater than 8.5 mg/dL; phosphate greater than 4 mg/dL; all related to osmotic diuresis and loss through the urine.

iv. Normal to low ketones: mechanism is not fully understood; however, possibly the hyperglycemia and hyperosmolarity decrease lipolysis in liver.

B. Patient management

1. Actual fluid volume deficit related to osmotic diuresis induced by hyperglycemia; inadequate oral intake

a. Problem: Water losses are generally between 4.8 and 12.6 liters, which are associated with the extreme loss of glucose, as much as 19 g/h. The glucose loss leads to an osmotic diuresis. As volume is lost, this may contribute to renal, neurologic, and cardiac dysfunction.

b. Intervention

    i. Treat the underlying cause.

    ii. Monitor fluid status (skin turgor, urinary output, vital signs), neck veins.

    iii. Administer IV fluids as ordered. First, to restore vascular volume, administer isotonic solution: 0.9% normal saline. Hypotonic solutions (45% normal saline) are then infused. One half of the calculated fluid deficit is restored in the first 12 hours with the remainder restored during the next 24 hours. Fluids may be ordered at 500 mL/h. As blood glucose approaches 250 mg/dL, 5% dextrose 45% saline may be started to prevent a rebound hypoglycemia.

    iv. Monitor cardiovascular status as fluid is administered, particularly cardiac output, cardiac index, PAP, PAOP, and CVP. If there is a rapid rise in any measure, reduce the IV rate.

    v. Monitor lungs for adventitious lung sounds which may indicate developing congestive heart failure from too rapid fluid replacement.

    vi. Record intake and output and weigh daily.

c. Desired outcome

    i. CVP and PAOP return to normal.

    ii. Urine output greater than 30 mL/h.

    iii. Blood pressure within 10 mm Hg of patient's usual pressure.

    iv. Heart rate within 15 beats of patient's usual rate.

    v. Normal urine specific gravity.

    vi. Laboratory data indicating hemoconcentration (BUN, hematocrit, plasma osmolarity) returning to normal.

    vii. Increased hydration evidenced by the following:

       ▪ Moist oral mucous membranes.

       ▪ Improved skin turgor.

    viii. No cold perspiration usually associated with shock will be evident.

    ix. Skin integrity maintained.

2. Hyperglycemia related to insufficient secretion of insulin, effects of insulin-antagonistic hormones, medications that aggravate diabetic control, preexisting renal or cardiovascular problems, and impaired secretion of renal glucose.

a. Problem: Hyperglycemia leads to hyperosmolality and a resultant decreasing LOC. Seizures and a positive Babinski's sign may result. The neurologic signs and symptoms disappear as the serum osmolality is reduced.

b. Intervention

    i. Administer regular insulin. See p. 136 for administration guidelines.

    ii. As serum glucose approaches 250–300 mg/dL, the insulin should be stopped and an infusion of 5% dextrose in 45% saline started to prevent hypoglycemia.

  c. Desired outcome
    i. Blood glucose less than 300 mg/dL
    ii. Intake exceeds output.
3. Electrolyte imbalances related to osmotic diuresis, preexisting cardiac or renal problems, and previous medications.
  a. Problem: Electrolyte imbalances, particularly K^+, may lead to cardiac dysrhythmias.
  b. Intervention
    i. Replace K^+ as soon as normal renal function is restored. Often 20–40 mEq/KCl is added to each IV bottle. Monitor ECG for hypokalemia (flat T waves, U waves, prolonged QT interval) and for hyperkalemia (peaked T waves and ST-segment changes). When insulin is administered, K^+ is returned to the cell, so hypokalemia may be seen 2–4 hours after starting insulin.
  c. Desired outcome
    i. Electrolyte laboratory data are returning to normal.
4. Altered levels of consciousness related to cellular dehydration in central nervous system from increased plasma osmolarity, impaired oxygen dissociation in the central nervous system (hypophosphatemia), cerebral edema induced by rapid fluid shifts, and electrolyte imbalance (Na^+).
  a. Problem: A depressed level of consciousness related to hyperosmolarity may result in seizures and neurologic dysfunction.
  b. Intervention
    i. Assess and monitor neurologic symptoms. Protect from injury if seizures occur.
    ii. Monitor fluid status (skin turgor, urinary output, vital signs), neck veins.
    iii. As serum glucose approaches 250–300 mg/dL, the insulin should be stopped and an infusion of 5% dextrose in 45% saline started to prevent hypoglycemia.
    iv. Monitor lungs for adventitious lung sounds, which may indicate developing congestive heart failure from too rapid fluid replacement.
    v. Record intake and output and weigh daily.
  c. Desired outcome
    i. LOC consistent with precrisis state.
    ii. Pupils equal in size and react briskly to light.
    iii. Moves all extremities consistent with precrisis mobility.
    iv. No seizure activity.
    v. Patient safety maintained.
    vi. Respiratory rate and pattern returning to normal for patient.

IV. Discharge planning

A. Teach about disease, etiology, prevention, and management. Teach about diet and drug therapy.
B. Encourage activity (walking and exercise) but provide for frequent rest periods.
C. Teach skin care: cleaning, drying, lubrication, avoidance of very hot water when bathing.
D. Stress importance of regular rest, sleep, exercise, and control of stress.

Hypoglycemia (Insulin Shock, Insulin Reaction, Insulin Coma)

I. Definition: Hypoglycemia is a symptom complex associated with a lowered blood glucose. Hypoglycemia is not a disease but a symptom of disturbance in glucose homeostasis. Serum glucose levels are insufficient to meet the metabolic demands of the body, particularly the nervous system. Hypoglycemia is most often a complication of diabetes mellitus and needs to be investigated as to its cause.

The diagnosis of hypoglycemia requires a blood glucose of less than 55 mg/100 mL (normal 80–110 mg/100 mL). Three criteria are required for the diagnosis of hypoglycemia (Whipple's triad): signs and symptoms compatible with hypoglycemia, low blood glucose level, and relief of symptoms as blood glucose returns to normal.

II. Etiology: Hypoglycemia may be associated with underproduction of glucose by the liver during a fasting state, excess of insulin, excessive antidiabetic medications, or too rapid glucose uptake and utilization.

The most common cause associated with underproduction of glucose by the liver is heavy alcohol ingestion. Alcohol (ethanol) directly blocks several pathways in hepatic gluconeogenesis and thus reduces available glucose to the body. Drugs, such as aspirin, disopyramide (Norpace), haloperidol (Haldol), propoxyphene (Darvon), and others reduce glucose production. The patient may also have an insufficient dietary intake that will decrease availability of necessary substrates for glucose synthesis in the liver.

The patient may also be taking too much antidiabetic medication or may have insufficient dietary intake of nutrients. Concurrent drugs such as beta-blockers and oxytetracycline may prolong or potentiate antidiabetic medications or inhibit glycogenolysis. Beta-blockers also mask the signs of hypoglycemia by blocking the normal adrenergic response. Patients with kidney disease and diabetes have impaired inactivation of insulin in the kidney, thus leading to the increased likelihood of hypoglycemia. Some patients may have insulin-binding autoimmune antibodies present that may result in the liberation of excessive amounts of insulin.

Patients with pancreatic tumors or GI disease or requiring surgical intervention such as gastroenterostomy may increase their glucose uptake and utilization, which can lead to hypoglycemia.

III. Nursing process

A. Assessment
  1. Signs and symptoms
    a. Increasing nervousness, "fight or flight" symptoms, dilated pupils, profuse diaphoresis, apprehension, general weakness, palpitations, circumoral numbness: occur secondary to activation of the sympathetic nervous system, which releases epinephrine in an attempt to raise blood glucose level. These symptoms begin to occur when blood sugar is less than 70 mg/dL.

b. Headache, restlessness, difficulty in thinking and speaking, emotional instability, aggression, maniacal behavior, catatonia, visual disturbances: occur due to a reduction in blood glucose and, thus, a reduction in brain glucose. Glucose level is approaching 60 mg/dL.

c. Hemiplegia, paraplegia, seizures and LOC: occur as blood glucose level approaches approximately 55 mg/dL.

d. Hypothermia, coma: Blood glucose is reduced to such a critical level that the brain loses its ability to function. Heat conservation begins as the hypothalamus control center reduces its function.

2. Diagnostic parameters

   a. Serum tests

      i. Hypoglycemia (less than 55 mg/dL): related to a decreased serum glucose level.

   b. Urine tests

      i. None significant.

B. Patient management

1. Alteration in cerebral function related to hypoglycemia

   a. Problem: As serum glucose level is reduced, the level of this primary energy substrate of the brain is reduced, and brain function deteriorates from confusion and lethargy to seizures and coma.

   b. Intervention

      i. Draw blood to measure baseline glucose level.

      ii. Stabilize serum glucose level.

      iii. If patient is conscious, he or she should eat fast-acting carbohydrates, such as bread with cheese, crackers, milk. Establish that protective reflexes (gag, swallowing, cough) are intact before administering oral intake.

      iv. If patient is unconscious, administer glucagon.

---

glucagon

Action Stimulates the release of glucogen by the liver, which in turn increases blood glucose. If there has been no response to glucogen, administer 10%–15% *dextrose IV.*

Administration Guidelines Administer 0.5 mg by any route; 0.5–1 mg IV, subcutaneously (SC), or IM if no response; administer again in 15 minutes. If no response occurs, it is likely that glucogen in the liver has been utilized. Alcohol-induced hypoglycemia is often unresponsive to glucogen therapy.

dextrose IV

Action Dextrose rapidly restores the blood glucose level.

Administration Guidelines Administer over 5 minutes, undiluted into a large vein. Elevate and maintain blood glucose level between 100 and 200 mg/dL.

---

      v. Establish baseline neurologic function.

      vi. Monitor changes in neurologic function from baseline such as

mental status, cranial nerve function, sensory/motor function, deep tendon reflexes, cerebellar function.
  vii. Monitor all vital signs.
  c. Desired outcome
    i. Neurologic status
      ▪ Mental status: oriented to person, place, date.
      ▪ Level of consciousness: arousal and awareness intact.
      ▪ Cranial nerve function intact.
      ▪ Sensorimotor function intact.
      ▪ Deep tendon reflexes brisk.
    ii. Vital signs
      ▪ Arterial blood pressure within 10 mm Hg of patient's baseline.
      ▪ Heart rate: greater than 60, less than 100 beats/minute.
      ▪ Cardiac rhythm: regular sinus.
      ▪ Respirations: less than 25–30 breaths/minute.
    iii. Serum glucose: stable at 70–110 mg/100 mL.
2. Potential injury from seizures related to altered neuronal cellular metabolism associated with hypoglycemia.
  a. Problem: As blood glucose falls to a critical level, neurologic function deteriorates, and seizures occur, since there is an absence of glucose to maintain cerebral function. Seizure activity may lead to permanent neurologic dysfunction or even death.
  b. Intervention
    i. Implement seizure precautions.
    ii. Monitor seizure activity.
      ▪ Record time, precipitating event, description of seizure.
      ▪ Note any changes in pupil size and reactivity; urinary or bowel incontinence.
      ○ Duration of apneic periods if generalized seizure.
      ○ Duration of seizure activity.
      ○ Patient's postseizure behavior.
      ▪ Equip room with oxygen and suction equipment.
  c. Desired outcome
    i. Patient will remain without seizures or injury.
3. Alteration in nutrition less than body requirements related to altered glucose metabolism.
  a. Problem: The hypoglycemic episode may be associated with a lack of nutritional intake or may actually precipitate a nutritional deficit. It is important for the diabetic to maintain a near-normal weight and a near-normal blood glucose level.
  b. Intervention
    i. Assess nutritional intake.
    ii. Teach patient about proper nutrition.
  c. Desired outcome
    i. Patient's condition will stabilize
      ▪ Serum glucose levels maintained within normal physiologic range.

- Body weight will stabilize within appropriate range; positive nitrogen balance will be maintained.
- Patient will have an increase in strength and improved appetite.
- Patient will verbalize the effects of alcohol on glucose metabolism.

IV. Discharge planning

A. Assess patient and family knowledge of diabetes.
B. Teach patient and family about diabetes and its complications.
C. Assess patient and family attitude regarding chronic diabetes.
D. Teach patient and family the importance of continued follow-up care.
E. Identify risk factors for hypoglycemia and teach patient and family how to avoid them.
F. Stabilize serum glucose.

Syndrome of Inappropriate Antidiuretic Hormone Secretion

I. Definition: The syndrome of inappropriate antidiuretic hormone secretion (SIADH) is the most common cause of hyponatremia in hospitalized patients. The syndrome is characterized by the continued secretion of ADH in the absence of a physiologic stimulation for its release such as hypovolemia, hypotension, or dehydration. As a result of the increased ADH release, electrolyte-free water excretion is limited, allowing even a moderate water intake to lead to progressive hypotonicity (water intoxication). Serum osmolarity is below 280 mOsm/L, and serum sodium is reduced.

II. Etiology: SIADH is commonly associated with many conditions seen in critically ill patients. It is often a secondary occurrence in some forms of cancer (oat cell adenocarcinoma of the lung, cancer of the duodenum/pancreas, leukemia, lymphoma, Hodgkin's disease, sarcoma, and squamous cell carcinoma of the tongue). It may follow pituitary surgery, may be associated with psychiatric disorders, or may follow drug therapy (anesthesia, barbiturates, diuretics, morphine, nicotine, synthetic hormones, thioridazine, vincristine). SIADH may also be associated with Gullian-Barré syndrome and positive pressure ventilation. To be diagnosed as SIADH, both adrenal and thyroid function must be normal.

III. Nursing process

A. Assessment
   1. Signs and symptoms
      a. Severe GI symptoms (vomiting, abdominal cramps): due to serum Na^+ less than 130 mEq/L. Na^+ is needed for normal function of the GI cell.
      b. Confusion, lethargy, muscle twitching, seizures: due to serum Na^+ less than 115 mEq/L. Na^+ is necessary for neuromuscular function.
      c. Water retention and an increase in total body water: related to increased release of ADH.
      d. Hypertension, tachycardia: due to increased burden of extra water on the cardiovascular system

2. Diagnostic parameters
  a. Serum tests
   i. Hypo-osmolality: less than 280 mEq/L due to an increase in total body water.
   ii. Hyponatremia: below 115–125 mEq/L due to increased renin and aldosterone secretion and thus increased Na^+ loss.
  b. Urine tests
   i. Hyperosmolarity greater than 50–150 mOsm/L is greater than expected for concomitant serum osmolarity.
   ii. Urine sodium excretion elevated greater than 200 mEq/24 h or 20 mEq/L: Since there is depressed renin and aldosterone secretion, thus there is a decreased proximal tubular reabsorption of Na^+.

B. Patient management
 1. Excess fluid volume related to increased secretion of ADH in presence of low serum osmolality
  a. Problem: Excessive fluid volume leads to water intoxication of all cells, particularly brain cells. The acute hypotonicity results in an osmotic shift of water into the brain and cerebral edema. The degree of edema depends on the rate of development and the magnitude of hypotonicity. Cerebral edema can be so severe that brain stem herniation can result.
  b. Intervention
   i. Treat the underlying cause.
   ii. Administer diuretic therapy to assist with removal of free water.
   iii. Fluid restriction to 600–800 mL/d.
   iv. Monitor for confusion, disorientation, irritability, restlessness, lethargy, hyperreflexia.
   v. Monitor hemodynamic status.
   vi. Monitor for fluid overload in the lung (pulmonary congestion).
  c. Desired outcome
   i. Neurologic status
    ▪ Mental status: alert, oriented to person, place, and date.
    ▪ Appropriate behavior.
    ▪ Without seizure activity, tremors, weakness.
    ▪ Deep tendon reflexes brisk.
 2. Electrolyte imbalance related to hyponatremia (dilutional), water intoxication
  a. Problem: The primary electrolyte imbalance that occurs is hyponatremia. The severity and abruptness of the onset of hyponatremia will determine the extent of symptoms. Symptoms may range from (Na^+ 130–140 mEq/L) thirst, impaired taste, dyspnea, fatigue, dulled sensorium, seizures to irreversible neurologic damage when serum Na^+ is less than 115 mEq/L.
  b. Intervention
   i. Administer hypertonic saline (3% NaCl) solutions to restore serum Na^+ levels.
   ii. Monitor renal function, intake and output, body weight.
   iii. Assess pulmonary status, particularly for presence of adventitious lung sounds.

      iv. Monitor cardiovascular function, vital signs, and hemodynamics: PAOP, PAP, CVP.

  c. Desired outcome

      i. Hemodynamic status returns to normal (CVP, PAOP, cardiac output).

        ▪ Blood pressure within 10 mm Hg of baseline.

        ▪ Pulse strong: heart rate greater than 60 to less than 100 beats/minute.

      ii. Respiratory function returns to normal.

      iii. Renal status: hourly urine output greater than 30 mL/h.

      iv. Laboratory and urine studies return to normal: BUN, creatinine, serum osmolality, serum Na^+.

      v. Weight within 2%–5% of baseline.

3. Alteration in thought process related to hyponatremia (dilutional) and water intoxication

  a. Problem: Impaired thought processes are related to the osmotic shift of fluid into the brain and the dilutional hyponatremia. The patient may be mentally slow or actually develop seizure.

  b. Intervention

      i. Provide explanations that are short, clear, and concise.

      ii. Provide quiet environment.

  c. Desired outcome

      i. Demonstrate improved neurologic status:

        ▪ Alert and oriented to person, place, date.

        ▪ Longer attention span.

        ▪ Improved memory; speech intact.

IV. Discharge planning

A. Involve patient and family in decision making whenever possible.

B. Teach how to measure and record intake and output.

C. Teach how to administer medications in the proper dosage, and their side effects.

D. Teach patient why there is a need to restrict fluids until symptoms are brought under control.

E. Encourage foods with high sodium content.

F. Assist with coping of patient and family.

Thyrotoxicosis (Thyroid Storm)

  I. Definition: Thyrotoxicosis is a rare but acute medical emergency in which thyroid hormones are produced in excessive amounts, resulting in multisystem dysfunction and pyrexia. Severe hyperthyroidism results in excessive beta-adrenergic stimulation, which can result in dysrhythmias, high-output congestive heart failure, increased cardiac output, and increased oxygen consumption. The positive inotropic and chronotropic vascular effects of catecholamines are potentiated. The severe hypermetabolic state puts a burden on all organ systems. Beta-adrenergic antagonists are the first-line treatment, since they block the catecholamine effects by reducing cardiac rate and output and pulse pressure. Body temperature may rise to 41°C (106°F). The body literally "burns up." Death may ensue within 48 hours without treatment.

II. Etiology: May be spontaneous but usually occurs in patients who have diagnosed or undiagnosed hyperthyroidism and who are subjected to excessive stress (infection, surgery, dialysis, emotional stress, or inadequate preparation for thyroid surgery). It is important to determine the underlying cause and to begin treating the disease as well as current symptoms. Thyrotoxicosis is often precipitated by hyperthyroidism including Graves' disease, toxic multimodular goiter, thyroid cancer, and increased thyroid-stimulating hormone (TSH). Nonhyperthyroid causes include subacute thyroidism, ectopic thyroid tissue, and ingestion of excessive thyroid hormone.

III. Nursing process

  A. Assessment findings

    1. Signs and symptoms

      a. Hyperthermia, sweating, warm skin: related to hyperdynamic circulatory state

      b. Goiter, systolic or continuous bruit over thyroid (97%–99%): related to hyperactivity of thyroid gland metabolism.

      c. Diminished sensitivity to insulin: related to increased insulin degradation.

      d. Oligomenorrhea/amenorrhea in women; increased serum estrone radial and estrone but lower levels of freed products: due to the increase in sex hormone–binding globulin.

      e. Impotence/increased libido, gynecomastia: in men related to hypothalamic or pituitary disturbances.

      f. Weight loss, increased appetite: due to increased catabolism in an attempt to meet body demands.

      g. Increased peristalsis (may be diarrhea): related to increased GI activity and malabsorption of fats and other nutrients.

      h. Ocular changes (bulging eyes, elevated upper eyelid, decreased blinking, staring, tremor of lid, possible infiltrative ocular changes, edema of ocular muscles, damage to retina and optic nerves, exophthalmos, periorbital edema, extraocular muscle weakness leading to diplopia): related over activity of Müller's muscle in the eye.

      i. Increased cardiac output, tachycardia, decreased peripheral vascular resistance, loud heart sounds and third heart sound, superventricular dysrhythmias: related to hypermetabolic rate, the effects of beta-adrenergic stimulation of the thyroid hormones, and the need to dissipate heat.

      j. Congestive heart failure, crackles: relative to activation of $beta_1$ receptors in the heart by thyroid hormones.

      k. Dyspnea, reduced vital capacity: due to weakness of respiratory muscles.

      l. Restlessness, short attention span, fatigue, tremor, insomnia: possibly due to alterations of cerebral metabolism.

    2. Diagnostic parameters

      a. Serum tests

        i. Hypercalcemia: excessive bone resorption due to hyperactivity of the thyroid gland and disruption of parathyroid hormone–regulating mechanism.

ii. Decreased lipid levels: related to increased cholesterol excretion in feces and cholesterol conversion to bile salts.

iii. Decreased B vitamins: related to impaired conversion of B vitamins to their coenzymes.

iv. Decreased TSH and thyroid-releasing hormone: Due to overfunction of thyroid gland, there is a reduction in thyroid-stimulating hormones.

v. Increased iodine uptake: due to gland hyperactivity.

vi. Increased triiodothyronine (T_3), increased thyroxine (T_4): related to chronic hyperstimulation of thyroid gland. (T_3 and T_4 are largely affected by thyroid hormone transport proteins. Serum levels of thyroid hormones T_3 and T_4 more appropriately reflect thyroid hormones, since they are independent of transport proteins.)

vii. Increased alkaline phosphatase: due to increased metabolic activity.

viii. Hypokalemia: (below 3.5 mEq/L) due to increased cellular damage from hypermetabolism and heat production and increased urinary loss of K^+.

B. Patient management

1. Decreased cardiac output related to high-output cardiac failure associated with increased metabolic demand; and exaggerated adrenergic effect, cardiac dysrhythmias, and reduced circulating blood volume associated with excessive diaphoresis, vomiting, and diarrhea.

a. Problem: Excessive, prolonged increases in cardiac output ultimately precipitate high-output congestive heart failure. As the heart fails, there is a decreased perfusion of blood to the entire body, which can lead to shock and organ failure. Ineffective breathing patterns can lead to intercostal muscle weakness and a fall in oxygen delivery.

b. Intervention

i. Treat underlying cause.

ii. Maintain cardiovascular function: Assess rate, rhythm, occurrence of chest pain. Arterial oxygen-saturation within normal limits.

iii. Administer beta-blockers such as propranolol. See Table 5.1.

iv. Administer digitalis as ordered.

---

digitalis

Action Increases force of contraction and controls symptoms of high-output failure (positive inotrope, negative chronotrope).

Administration Guidelines IV: 0.25–0.50 mg q4–6h to total 1.0 mg, then 0.125–0.500 mg daily. PO: 0.50–0.75 mg followed by 0.5 mg q6–8h to total 1.0 mg, then 0.125–0.500 mg daily. Administer bolus dose diluted or not, but over at least 10 minutes. Too rapid administration may precipitate a hypertensive episode.

Special Considerations Monitor for digitalis toxicity (nausea, vomiting, visual disturbances, dysrhythmias), especially if acidotic or electrolytes imbalanced.

      v. Monitor for cardiac dysrhythmias. Supraventricular tachycardias and premature ventricular contraction often occur. Treat with appropriate antiarrhythmic agents—calcium channel blockers (verapamil) or procainamide (Pronestyl). Patients may have a sudden episode of possible lethal dysrhythmias.

      vi. Administer antithyroid drug. (These drugs take days to weeks to be effective.)

---

propylthiouracil

Action Blocks synthesis of thyroid hormones and inhibits conversion of T_4 to T_3. Only available in oral form.

Administration Guidelines Take at regular intervals, usually every 8 hours.

sodium iodide

Action Blocks thyroid secretion. Full therapeutic effects take 10–14 days.

Administration Guidelines Dilute dose with water or juice to improve bitter taste.

---

      vii. Monitor thyroid laboratory studies. Serum levels do not change for several days. Initial response is probably due to diminished adrenergic response. Cardiac symptoms should subside. Mental status should clear, and temperature should be reduced.

      viii. Administer oxygen as needed during hypermetabolic state.

      ix. Maintain respiratory function.

   c. Desired outcome

      i. Patient will maintain the following:

- Usual mental status: alert, oriented, deep tendon reflexes brisk
- Adequate cardiovascular function
- Cardiac rate and rhythm: heart rate greater than 60 to less than 100 beats/minute; rhythm: regular sinus without dysrhythmias.

      ii. Hemodynamic status returns to normal: CVP, PAOP, cardiac output.

      iii. Arterial blood pressure within 10 mm Hg of baseline supine and upright.

      iv. Renal status: urine output greater than 30 mL/h.

      v. Respiratory status: respiratory rate and breathing pattern—less than 25–30 breaths/minute; eupnea.

2. Fluid volume deficit related to hypermetabolic state with hyperpyrexia associated with profuse diaphoresis.

   a. Problem: Fluid volume deficit may lower cardiac output and further compromise organ perfusion.

   b. Intervention

      i. Monitor for and prevent fluid imbalance by assessing and evaluating changes in the following:

- Lung sounds.

- Cough.
- Neck veins (flat: hypovolemia; distended: hypervolemia).
- Urinary output.
- Intake and output.

   ii. Administer volume: crystalloids or colloids depending on need, to prevent dehydration from sweating. Keep mucous membranes moist. Monitor skin turgor.
   iii. Administer nutrition: Increase calories, increase carbohydrates, increase protein, increase fats. Enteral nutrition is best.
   iv. Administer glucocorticoids to assist with stressed state.

  c. Desired outcome
   i. Patient will maintain effective fluid and electrolyte balance.
   - Neurologic status: alert, oriented.
   - Hemodynamics return to normal: cardiac output, arterial blood pressure with 10 mm Hg of baseline supine and upright, CVP, PAOP.
   - Renal status: urine output greater than 30 mL/h.
   - Body weight will stabilize within 5% of patient's baseline.

3. Electrolyte imbalance, related to severe dehydration, hemoconcentration with hypernatremia.
  a. Problem: Electrolyte imbalance may precipitate ECG changes, cardiac dysrhythmias, and neurologic signs and symptoms.
  b. Intervention
   i. Monitor for hyperglycemia. Increased thyroid hormones enhance glycogenolysis and reduce insulin levels. In addition, increased adrenergic activity may impair insulin secretion and decrease tissue response to insulin.
   ii. Administer K^+ (20–40 mEq/L IV), Na^+, and Ca^{2+} as needed.
   - Hypokalemia
   ○ Monitor the ECG for signs of hypokalemia: U wave.
   ○ Additional signs of hypokalemia: fatigue, anorexia, nausea, vomiting, diarrhea, abdominal cramps, hyporeflexia
   - Hyponatremia: Assess for headache, mental confusion, seizures, or coma.
   - Hyperkalemia: Drowsiness, fatigue, nausea, vomiting, thirst, hypotonic muscle response, central nervous system depression, lethargy, coma. Monitor ECG for short QT interval (<0.34 seconds). Bone reabsorption may occur due to increased activity of osteoclasts, so monitor for pathologic fractures.
  c. Desired outcome
   i. Respiratory status
   - Respiratory rate and breathing pattern: less than 25–30 breaths/minute; eupnea
   ii. GI status
   - Absence of anorexia, nausea, vomiting, and diarrhea.
   iii. Laboratory data returns to normal: serum osmolality, sodium, potassium, glucose, BUN, creatinine, and hematology profile at optimal levels for patient.

4. Hyperthermia related to hypermatabolic rate and enhanced adrenergic activity.
- **a.** Problem: Hyperthermia increases the metabolic rate increasing requirements for oxygen and nutrients. Extreme hyperthermia may cause an increase in intracranial pressure.
- **b.** Intervention
  - **i.** Assist with body cooling to decrease metabolic needs. Cool environment, cooling blankets. Do not allow patient to shiver from over cooling. (Wrap both arms and legs in four layers of bath blankets when patient is placed on cooling blanket. This technique usually prevents shivering.) May administer acetaminophen to reduce temperature. (Do not administer aspirin products because aspirin pushes thyroid hormone off protein binding site, which increases thyroid hormone level in serum.)
  - **ii.** Protect skin from injury. Do not rip tape off. (Skin is often thin and friable.) Scrupulous skin care: frequent tepid baths and careful skin drying. Egg-crate mattress; turn frequently.
- **c.** Desired outcome
  - **i.** Patient's body temperature will stabilize at 37°C (98.6°F).

IV. Discharge planning

- **A.** Discuss etiology and treatment plan with client.
- **B.** Stress importance of taking medications as ordered. Teach about side effects of medications.
- **C.** Monitor weight weekly.
- **D.** Continue with increased caloric requirements until symptoms are brought under control.
- **E.** Encourage frequent rest and stress reduction.
- **F.** Encourage good skin care.
- **G.** Teach the importance of following care that may include iodine 131 or surgery.
- **H.** Encourage patient and family to discuss symptoms and treatment. (Condition may be chronic and need continued care and monitoring.)

Reference

1. Saurie, D., and Kessler, C. Hyperglycemia emergencies. *AACN Clinical Issues* 3:350–360, 1992.

CHAPTER 7

Gastrointestinal Disorders

Nancy Dodd

Abdominal Injuries

I. Definition: Any injury that involves the abdominal cavity and compromises the integrity of the abdominal viscera and surrounding organ systems. Abdominal injury is rarely one organ or just the gastrointestinal system. Most injuries to the abdomen also involve related injuries to the chest, pelvis, ribs, and spinal cord. For this reason, injuries to the abdomen may be more difficult to diagnose and treat.

II. Etiology

A. Blunt trauma

    1. Acceleration: force against an immovable object, ie, punch to abdomen.

    2. Deceleration: movement within the abdominal cavity, ie, movement of liver against fractured ribs.

    3. Compression: crush injury, ie, abdominal contents crushed between the anterior chest and spinal cord while wedged against a steering wheel.

B. Penetrating trauma

    1. Gunshot wounds: dependent on caliber of weapon, length from body, structures hit, energy released, and entrance and exit sites.

    2. Stab wounds: dependent on size of knife or weapon, strength of assailant, angle of injury, number of stab wounds and structures involved.

    3. Impalement injuries: usually a result of high velocity onto or into a foreign object, ie, motorcycle or skiing accidents.

III. Nursing process

A. Assessment

    1. Signs and symptoms

        a. Pulmonary

            i. Airway obstruction secondary to pulmonary injuries such as rib fractures, pulmonary contusions, pneumothorax, hemothorax, or facial fractures. Suspect hypoxia in any patient with abdominal injuries, since the abdomen and chest are both in the torso. Observe for flail chest, asymmetric breathing, absence of breath sounds, or laryngospasm.

        b. Cardiovascular

        i. Shock and hypovolemia caused by massive blood losses may become irreversible if not treated immediately and aggressively. Observe for hypotension, tachycardia, impaired perfusion, and cold, clammy skin.

    c. Neuro: Glasgow coma score less than 8; confusion to unresponsiveness; spinal cord injury should be suspected in any patient with abdominal injuries; note motor or sensory deficits if patient is alert.

    d. GI

2. Primary inspection

    a. General appearance.

    b. Location of wounds.

    c. Entrance or exit sites.

    d. Symmetry.

    e. Distention.

3. Other inspection parameters

    a. Auscultation: presence or absence of bowel sounds.

    b. Palpation to identify tenderness, rigidity, or guarding.

    c. Genitourinary: Renal injury should be suspected; insertion of Foley catheter to determine amount, color, and protein in urine.

    d. Skin: Note any lacerations, contusions, abrasions that would help identify underlying organ injury.

4. Diagnostic parameters

    a. Serum

        i. CBC with differential.

           • Red blood cell (RBC) count less than $4.7/mm^3$ in men, less than $4.2/mm^3$ in women; may be low from blood loss.

           • Hemoglobin less than 14 g/dl in men, less than 12 g/dl in women from blood loss.

           • Hemotocrit less than 42% in men, less than 37% in women; hemotocrit should be three times hemoglobin.

           • WBC count, normal $5000–10,000/mm^3$; a rise will be seen with injury; infection indicated by a sharp rise from baseline.

       ii. Thrombocytopenia secondary to severe hemorrhage.

      iii. Potassium: Crush injuries will elevate K^+ greater than 5.5 as myoglobin is released from muscle damage, which can lead to renal failure.

      iv. Calcium will be depleted when more than 5–10 U of banked blood are used, because citrate in banked blood binds with calcium.

       v. Sodium: elevated level greater than 145 mEq/L seen with excessive blood loss due to hemoconcentration.

      vi. Prothrombin time (PT) and partial thromboplastin time (PTT) should be drawn initially for a baseline; will be elevated in hepatic injury or with massive transfusions as clotting factors are depleted.

    b. Urine test

        i. Urinalysis to rule out protein in urine.

       ii. Drug screen to test for any alcohol, medications, or recreational drugs that would impair patient's level of consciousness, vital signs, or other assessment parameters.

c. Other tests

    i. Abdominal flat plate to rule out free air, which would indicate a perforated viscous or bowel associated with abdominal distention or pain.

    ii. Peritoneal lavage may be done in patient after inserting Foley catheter to prevent bladder rupture and nasogastric tube to empty stomach.

- Trocar inserted into peritoneal cavity if frank blood is returned—immediate laparotomy.
- Infusion of 1 liter of warmed normal saline solution (NSS).
- Drainage of fluid, examine for the following:
  ◦ Contaminants of feces or bile.
  ◦ Blood cell count: RBCs greater than 100,000/mL.

    iii. CT scan

- Solid organ injury: liver, spleen, kidneys, pancreas.
- Free air perforation of viscous or bowel.

    iv. Angiography to rule out aortic injury, usually with associated chest injuries and widening mediastinum.

B. Patient management

1. Potential for hemorrhage and/or rupture secondary to splenic injury.

    a. Problem

        i. Hypovolemic shock requiring early, aggressive intervention.

        ii. Hypotension.

        iii. Spleen enlargement on CT scan.

        iv. Kehr's sign: left shoulder pain due to diaphragmatic irritation.

        v. Left upper quadrant fullness and tenderness, which would indicate hemorrhage or rupture of spleen.

    b. Intervention

        i. Aggressive treatment in the patient with hypovolemic shock: establish two large-bore intravenous (IV) lines with rapid-flow tubing, rapid replacement of volume losses with warm lactated Ringer's (LR) solution or NSS; transfuse to replace blood losses, serial hemoglobin and hematocrit (H & H).

        ii. Conservative treatment: Observe, transfuse to replace blood losses, assist with serial CT scans to observe hematoma size; splenic capsule can become up to four times normal; bed rest, monitor hemodynamic values, monitor NG tube output.

        iii. Support patient and family

- Surgical removal will impair immune response, since antibodies and lymphocytes are manufactured in the spleen.
- Splenorrhaphy vs splenectomy: Every effort to save all or part of spleen is made before removal, dependent on extent of injury, blood supply, and patient's condition; arteriogram may be done to help determine extent of injury.
- Splenectomy requires observation for overwhelming postsplenectomy infection (OPSI); pneumococcal vaccine (Pneumovax) should be administered within 72 hours.

---

pneumococcal vaccine (Pneumovax)
Action Promotes immunity to infections caused by *Streptococcus pneumoniae.*
Administration Guidelines 0.5 ml IM or SC.
Special Concerns Contraindicated in patients who have previously received any polyvalent pneumococcal vaccine; local area soreness.

- Autotransplantation may be attempted if organ can be safely moved, repaired, and transplanted into pelvic cavity.
  c. Desired outcome
    i. Restore normal hemodynamics and fluid volume.
    ii. Systolic BP greater than 90 mm Hg.
    iii. Heart rate less than 100 beats/minute.
    iv. H & H within normal range.
    v. Adequate end organ perfusion as noted by normal mentation, skin turgor, and urine output.
    vi. Prevention of secondary infections.
2. Potential for hemorrhage, pancreatitis, or rupture secondary to pancreatic injuries.
  a. Problem
    i. Hypovolemic shock: Since the pancreas lies directly in front of the aorta, assessment of possible aortic injury should be done.
    ii. Hypotension.
    iii. Septic shock related to release of pancreatic enzymes especially trypsin, which can cause a chemical peritonitis.
    iv. Examination for diffuse abdominal tenderness, guarding, low-grade fever, Grey-Turner's sign (ecchymosis of flank) or Cullen's sign (ecchymosis of umbilicus), which indicate hemorrhage from the pancreas.
  b. Intervention
    i. Assist with peritoneal lavage or CT scan to determine extent of injury.
    ii. Support measures to control bleeding, monitor hemodynamic values including BP, heart rate, and central venous pressure (CVP); if patient does not respond to volume replacement, hypovolemic shock is persistent, and/or septic shock is suspected, a pulmonary artery (PA) catheter should be inserted, and further support with volume and vasopressors should be considered.
    iii. Support measures to control pancreatic secretions: keep patient NPO, insert and monitor nasogastric drainage, administer morphine for pain control and promethazine hydrochloride (Phenergan) for vomiting, document response to pain intervention using a standardized pain scale.
    iv. Support patient and family through possible surgical resection: distal pancreatectomy, pancreatoduodenectomy, Roux-en-Y; surgical resection can remove up to 80% with no loss of function.

    v. Observe for the following complications:
- Pancreatitis.
- Glucose imbalance.
- Hypokalemia.
- Acid–base imbalances: Large loss of bicarbonate is associated with pancreatic drainage.
- Delayed hemorrhage.
- Abscesses.
- Fistulas.
- Pseudocysts.

  c. Desired outcome
    i. Restore normal hemodynamics and fluid volume; systolic BP greater than 90 mm Hg; heart rate less than 100 beats/minute; H & H within normal range; adequate end organ perfusion as noted by normal mentation, skin turgor, and urine output.
    ii. Prevention of secondary infections.
    iii. Control of glucose, calcium, magnesium.
    iv. Control of pain.
    v. Nutritional needs met.

3. Potential for life-threatening hemorrhage related to hepatic injury.
  a. Problems
    i. Massive hemorrhagic losses leading to profound hypovolemic shock.
    ii. Injury to chest, ribs, and spinal cord; liver capsular injury with leakage of bile and blood leading to peritonitis.
    iii. Subcapsular hematoma causing delayed hemorrhage.
    iv. Injury to hepatic vessels leading to necrosis; associated injury to the vena cava.
    v. Associated hemopneumothorax could be associated with liver laceration.

  b. Intervention
    i. Insert two large-bore IV lines.
    ii. Use rapid infusion IV tubing to administer warmed NSS or lactated Ringer's solution wide open until systolic BP is 90 mm Hg; administer blood products per physician order.
    iii. Assist with peritoneal lavage or CT scan.
    iv. Prepare patient and family for probable laparotomy that may include surgical repair of lacerations, removal of damaged tissue, lobectomy, or packing abdomen for tamponade, depending on the extent of injury.
    v. Monitor serial lab studies including H & H every 4 hours, electrolytes.
    vi. Prepare for endotracheal intubation and mechanical ventilation.
    vii. Support measures to control bleeding; monitor hemodynamic values including BP, heart rate, and CVP; if patient does not respond to volume replacement, hypovolemic shock is persistent, and/or septic shock is suspected, a PA catheter should be inserted, and further support with volume and vasopressors should be considered.

       viii. Observe for the following complications:
- Peritonitis.
- Jaundice.
- Coagulopathies.
- Nutritional deficits.
- Abscess formation.

    c. Desired outcome

       i. Restore normal hemodynamics and fluid volume; systolic BP greater than 90 mm Hg; heart rate less than 100 beats/minute; H & H within normal range; adequate end organ perfusion as noted by normal mentation, skin turgor, and urine output.

       ii. Prevention of secondary infections.

       iii. Prevention of pulmonary complications associated with intubation.

       iv. Pain control.

       v. Prevention of complications.

C. Discharge planning

  1. Patient and family understand the need for gradual return to activities.

  2. Patient and family understand the need for follow-up visits.

  3. Patient and family know what signs and symptoms point toward complications: fever, abdominal tenderness, loss of appetite.

  4. Patient and family understand medication and dosage schedules.

  5. Patient and family understand any drainage systems that may be with patient upon discharge.

Acute Gastrointestinal Hemorrhage

I. Definition: Any acute bleeding in the GI tract presenting a potential life-threatening situation. Up to 90% of GI bleeding can be controlled with medical management and fluid resuscitation. Stress ulceration may occur in up to 100% of critically ill patients; therefore, the emphasis should be on prevention.

II. Etiology

A. Peptic ulcers: an excavation found in the mucosal lining of the esophagus, stomach, pylorus, or duodenum caused by hypersecretion of hydrochloric acid.

B. Mallory-Weiss tear: a linear, nonperforating tear of the gastric mucosa near the juncture between the stomach and esophagus; it may be the result of violent vomiting.

C. Gastritis: inflammation of the stomach lining; it may be from irritation of a nasogastric tube or secondary to medications.

D. Esophagitis: inflammation of the esophagus from a nasogastric tube or reflux of stomach acid.

E. Esophageal varices: dilated, tortuous veins found in the submucosa of the lower esophagus, secondary to portal hypertension, which causes increased collateral circulation and elevated venous pressures in the esophageal veins.

F. Stress ulcers: more commonly not ulceration but gastritis and inflammation in the stomach, which, left untreated, could result in ulceration.
  1. Curling's ulcers: found in burn patients secondary to hypermetabolic needs combined with acute stress.
  2. Cushing's ulcers: found in brain-injured patients; associated with high levels of serum gastrin and hypersecretion of gastric acid and pepsin.
  3. Drug-induced: related to a therapeutic regimen such as corticosteroids, salicylates, or nonsteroidal anti-inflammatory drugs (NSAIDs).
  4. Other risk factors include sepsis, multiple trauma, hepatic failure, adult respiratory distress syndrome (ARDS), renal failure, and major surgery.
G. Aortic fistula: a leak found between the aorta and peritoneum secondary to erosion of the vessel.
H. Neoplasms
  1. Carcinoma: usually an adenocarcinoma of the stomach that causes erosion of the blood vessels from invasion by the tumor.
  2. Lymphoma can be found in the stomach or the colon; caused by hyperplasia of lymph tissues.
  3. Polyps are tissue masses that can be attached to the bowel wall itself or attached with a stem; most do not cause bleeding; they are usually removed to prevent them from developing into cancer.
I. Lower GI bleeding
  1. Diverticulitis: an inflammation of the wall of a diverticulum (a herniation of intestinal tissue that causes a sac to form) causing fever and left lower quadrant pain, which can lead to abscess formation.
  2. Carcinoma: 95% of colon cancers are adenocarcinomas and occur in the cecum, ascending colon, and sigmoid colon; most involve intestinal obstruction and/or bleeding from tumor invasion.
J. Inflammatory bowel disease
  1. Ulcerative colitis: a chronic inflammatory disorder of the mucosal lining of the colon causing ulceration, hemorrhage, and congestion of the lower colon.
  2. Crohn's disease: Recurrent inflammatory disease of the entire intestine causing mucosal disruption, fistulas, strictures, and severe pain.
  3. Meckel's diverticulum: a congenital anomaly; blind tube opens into the distal ileum causing painless rectal bleeding or intestinal obstruction.
  4. Hemorrhoids: vascular masses that may be internal or external leading to rectal pain and bright red bleeding; caused by straining, hardened stools, and pregnancy.
  5. Aortointestinal fistula: rare complication of abdominal aortic aneurysm.

III. Nursing process

A. Assessment
  1. Signs and symptoms
    a. Pulmonary: hypoventilation secondary to guarding of abdominal muscles, hypoxia secondary to loss of large volumes of blood and hemoglobin, which affects oxygen-carrying capacity.
    b. Cardiovascular (CV): tachycardia secondary to hypovolemia, hypotension, and dizziness secondary to hypovolemia, or may present in shock (may remain asymptomatic until 1000 mL or more is lost).

    c. Neuro: may be confusion, agitation, anxiety, or depression secondary to low cerebral perfusion.

    d. GI

        i. Nausea and vomiting from irritation of the stomach lining.

        ii. Hematemesis: bright red from a recent bleeding or a ruptured varice; note color, clots, and amount; coffee ground emesis from bleeding that is several hours old.

        iii. Melena: dark, tarry stools from upper GI bleeding; the color and consistency of stools will be altered by the speed of motility.

        iv. Pain caused by a breakdown in the mucosal barrier from hypersecretion of acid that leads to edema and release of more acid over inflamed area.

    e. Genitourinary: decreased urine output consistent with hypovolemia.

    f. Skin

        i. Jaundice: secondary to hepatic impairment or biliary tract obstruction.

        ii. Pallor: secondary to decreased hemoglobin.

        iii. Edema: secondary to fluid shifts that cause third spacing.

        iv. Petechiae and ecchymosis: secondary to coagulopathies from hemorrhage or hepatic dysfunction.

2. Diagnostic parameters

    a. Serum

        i. Hemoglobin and hematocrit decrease secondary to bleeding.

        ii. Electrolytes: may be altered by vomiting or profuse nasogastric drainage; hypokalemia (K^+) from vomiting, nasogastric suction, or diarrhea; hyponatremia (Na^+) from vomiting, nasogastric suction, or diarrhea.

        iii. Coagulation profile: to determine if blood and clotting factors are needed for transfusion; especially important in anyone with hepatic impairment.

        iv. BUN and creatinine may be elevated from dehydration, shock, and/or renal impairment secondary to hepatic impairment.

    b. Urine: Urine urea nitrogen (UUN) may be elevated.

    c. Other studies

        i. Endoscopy: A scope is passed via the mouth into the esophagus, stomach, and duodenum, visualizing the site of bleeding and degree of ulceration or tissue injury. *Caution:* Rupture of vessels can occur requiring massive blood replacement; blood products should be made available prior to beginning endoscopy; due to the high possibility of aspiration of gastric contents, elective intubation is recommended.

            ▪ Sclerotherapy: injection of a sclerosing solution into a bleeding varice.

            ▪ Ligation: placement of a rubber band or ring on target vessels.

            ▪ Biopsy: Any suspicious areas can be biopsied to rule out carcinoma.

ii. Radiologic studies: Critically ill patients may be too hemodynamically unstable for these studies.
- Upper GI series: may show any ulceration, reflux, or inflammation.
- Small bowel swallow through: may show duodenal or jejunal ulceration, strictures, or motility problems.
- Barium enema: may show ulcers, tumors, diverticuli, and inflammation.

iii. CT scan: diagnosis and extent of malignancies

iv. Nuclear medicine: Radioactive nucleotide is used to determine site of bleeding.

B. Patient management

1. Fluid volume deficit related to GI bleeding and fluid loss.

  a. Problem: hypovolemic shock and decreased tissue perfusion, may lead to cellular death.

  b. Intervention

   i. Emergent period
   - Fluid resuscitation: replacement of blood loss with blood products; large-bore IV lines to provide quick volume replacement.
   - Decrease bleeding.
   - Administer vasopressin to constrict bleeding vessels.

---

vasopressin
Action Enhances contraction of the vascular and nonvascular smooth muscle resulting in decreased peripheral blood flow and mesenteric blood flow.
Administration Guidelines IV or intra-arterially 50 U/250 mL physiologic saline solution (PSS) at 0.2–0.4 U/mL per minute.
Special Concerns May cause cardiac ischemia secondary to coronary artery disease; may decrease cardiac output; may increase systemic vascular resistance; nitroglycerine or nitroprusside infusions may be used to counteract this effect.

   - Administer histamine blockers to decrease hydrochloric acid secretion.

Histamine blockers

Action Decrease the hydrochloric acid in the stomach by blocking the release of histamine.

Administration Guidelines May be given PO or IV by continuous or intermittent dosing; continuous infusion is usually given to stop acute bleeding while the patient is being hemodynamically stabilized. *Cimetadine:* PO 300 mg three to four times daily, IV 300 mg every 6–8 hours, or 900–1200 mg in 250 mL over 24 hours. *Ranitidine:* PO 150 mg twice daily, IV 150 mg every 12 hours, or 300 mg in 250 mL over 24 hours.

Special Concerns May interfere with the absorption of other drugs; may cause headache, dizziness, diarrhea, and constipation. May cause hepatotoxicity, hallucinations, and agitation.

- Gastric lavage to wash blood and secretions from the stomach, prepare the stomach for endoscopy, evaluate the amount and characteristics of bleeding. Saline or sterile water may be used; iced solution may be used, but room temperature is as effective. *Caution:* Vigorous lavage may dislodge clots causing further bleeding.
- Administer antacids to neutralize hydrochloric acid in stomach.

Antacids

Actions Neutralize hydrochloric acid and relieve ulcer pain; keep pH greater than 4.5.

Administration Guidelines See Table 7.1.

Special Concerns May cause diarrhea or constipation; may cause metabolic alkalosis. Interfere with the absorption of many drugs.

- Angiography: may be used to locate feeding vessel and embolize; usually used in patients who are high surgical risks.
- Surgery: oversew or resection of bleeding area; tumor resection; partial or total gastric resection.

  c. Desired outcomes

    i. Restore normal hemodynamics and fluid volume; systolic BP greater than 90 mm Hg; heart rate less than 100; H & H of 10/30% or within patient's normal range; adequate end organ perfusion as noted by normal mentation, skin turgor, and urine output.

    ii. Prevent further bleeding and pain; gastric pH greater than 4.5; cardiac ischemia is avoided.

2. Potential for airway obstruction, aspiration, or impaired gas exchange related to decreased level of consciousness, nasogastric tubes, and vomiting.

  a. Problem: hypoxia secondary to pneumonia, ARDS, or respiratory arrest.

  b. Intervention

Table 7.1 Antacid Guidelines

Antacid	Special Concerns	Administration Guidelines
Aluminum hydroxide (Gaviscon)	Contraindicated with tetracycline Contraindicated on a sodium-restricted diet May cause constipation May cause hypophosphatemia	2 to 4 tablets PO 4 × /d
Aluminum OH$^+$; magnesium OH$^+$ simethicone (Mylanta, Maalox)	Contraindicated in renal insufficiency May cause hypermagnesemia, constipation, or diarrhea	30 mL every 2–4 h, PO or NG
Calcium carbonate (Tums)	May cause constipation May cause hypercalcemia May cause hyperphosphatemia	Chewable tablets as needed
Magnesium hydroxide (Milk of Magnesia)	Contraindicated in renal insufficiency	30 mL daily PO
Malgaldrate (Riopan)	Contraindicated in renal insufficiency Contraindicated with tetracycline	30 mL every 2–4 h, PO or NG

   i. Emergent period
      - Maintain adequate airway: auscultate lungs for rales, rhonchi, decreased breath sounds; note respiratory pattern trends along with level of consciousness.
      - Support patient's breathing with oxygen or mechanical ventilation as needed.
      - Monitor arterial blood gases and oxygen saturation.
      - Aspiration precautions: Have suction readily available at all times; observe for coughing, vomiting, or gagging; keep gastric tube patent. *Caution:* This is very important during endoscopy when IV sedation may impair patient's gag and cough reflexes.
   c. Desired outcome
      i. Patient will have support of respiration as needed for maintaining adequate airway protection.
      ii. Aspiration will be prevented.
      iii. Serial arterial blood gases within normal limits.
C. Discharge planning
   1. Prepare for discharge
      a. Patient and family learn to recognize signs of GI irritation and bleeding.
      b. Patient and family understand the role and dosage of histamine blockers.
      c. Patient and family understand the role and dosage of antacids.
      d. Patient and family understand dietary restrictions: avoid spicy foods, caffeine, chocolate.
      e. Patient understands the need to abstain from or limit alcohol intake.
      f. Stress management techniques are discussed with the patient and family.
      g. Patient and family understand the need for follow-up visits.

Pancreatitis

I. Definition

A. Pancreatitis is a sterile inflammation of the pancreas that can lead a mild or fulminant course. The pancreatic enzymes overcome their normal inhibitory and control mechanisms resulting in activation of pancreatic enzymes within the pancreas that leads to autodigestion.

B. Acute edematous pancreatitis occurs when interstitial edema within the pancreas causes an escape of pancreatic enzymes into the surrounding tissue and peritoneal cavity, resulting in peritoneal fluid accumulation causing abdominal pain, back pain, nausea, and vomiting. Recovery may occur; however, progression to acute hemorrhagic pancreatitis often results.

C. Acute hemorrhagic pancreatitis (also called necrotic pancreatitis) causes enzymatic destruction of the pancreas, causing blood to escape into the pancreatic tissue and retroperitoneum. This leads to severe abdominal pain and peritonitis. The patient may lose 5–6 liters of fluid into the peritoneum. There can be up to a 50% mortality with necrotic pancreatitis.

II. Etiology

A. Biliary tract disease that causes a physical obstruction of bile or pancreatic fluids.

B. Alcohol use or abuse theories of causes include hypersecretion of gastric acid, leading to bicarbonate fluid release from the pancreas; partial obstruction of the ampulla of Vater and sphincter of Oddi, leading to a backflow of pancreatic enzymes; protein deposits occurring in the pancreatic ducts, causing extravasation of pancreatic enzymes; and hypertriglyceridemia, leading to toxic levels of free fatty acids that damage the acinar cells.

C. Peptic ulcer disease from increased gastric acid.

D. Trauma, surgery, pregnancy that make the patient hypermetabolic.

E. Medications: The exact mechanism of medications causing pancreatitis is unknown, although toxic levels will cause damage to the acinar cells, and normal level may impair secretory functions.
   1. Azathioprine.
   2. Estrogens.
   3. Corticosteroids.
   4. Thiazides.

F. Metabolic disorders.
   1. Hyperlipoproteinemias.
   2. Hypercalcemia.

G. Infectious agents: viral or bacterial.

H. Carcinoma.

I. Shock, sepsis.

III. Nursing process

A. Assessment
   1. Signs and symptoms
      a. Pain: persistent and unrelenting in the epigastric area and radiating to the back.

b. Pulmonary: hyperventilation; patient may have to sit up and lean forward in order to get comfortable; secondary to diaphragmatic irritation from pancreatic enzyme leakage, crackles may be heard at the lung bases, and a left pleural effusion secondary to lymphatic leakage into the pleural space.

c. CV: hypovolemia secondary to large fluid losses; tachycardia; hypotension secondary to septic shock; or hypertension related to pain; slight fever.

d. Neuro: may be confused or disoriented secondary to hypovolemia or sepsis.

e. GI: nausea, vomiting, abdominal distention, left upper quadrant rebound tenderness with guarding, hemorrhagic or interstitial ascites, and a paralytic ileus with decreased bowel sounds.

f. GU: glycosuria secondary to injury to the alpha and beta cells of the islets of Langerhans, which produce insulin and glucagon; decreased urinary output from hypovolemia or shock.

g. Skin is slightly jaundiced from biliary tree inflammation or blockage.

h. Gray-Turner's sign: ecchymosis of the groin and flank region caused by retroperitoneal hemorrhage secondary to tissue damage from activated pancreatic enzymes (proteases).

i. Cullen's sign: ecchymosis of the periumbilical region also related to retroperitoneal hemorrhage.

2. Diagnostic parameters

  a. Serum

    i. Glucose level may be elevated, may become very unstable secondary to injury to the alpha cells, which make glucagon, or the beta cells, which make insulin. The patient may require an insulin drip and glucose monitoring every hour in the acute phase.

    ii. Potassium (K^+) less than 3.5 mEq/L secondary to vomiting, NG drainage, and loss into the peritoneum.

    iii. Amylase increased to more than twice normal for 2–3 days, then tapers off; normal 60–180 U/mL; it is released by damaged pancreatic cells.

    iv. Lipase elevates after 3–7 days, then tapers off; normal 1.5 U/mL; released by damaged pancreatic cells.

    v. Calcium (Ca^{2+}) less than 8 mg/dL is a result of several factors. Calcium binds to the areas of fat necrosis within the pancreas; colloid (albumin) leakage from the intravascular compartment; hyperglucagonemia; thyrocalcitonin levels due to lack of feedback mechanism to release calcium from bone.

    vi. Magnesium (Mg^{2+}) less than 1.2 mEq/L is a result of several factors: will be lowered by malnutrition; loss in the GI tract; pancreatic insufficiency with steatorrhea (fatty stools); sequestration of magnesium in the inflamed pancreas; chronic alcoholism, which leads to a poor diet, GI losses related to diarrhea; and renal loss from alcohol's effect on renal tubular absorption.

    vii. Phosphate less than 3.0 mEq/L associated with decreased intake and metabolism; greater than 4.5 mEq/L in connection with low potassium and magnesium levels.

   viii. Acid–base balance may be altered in many ways: Most commonly a metabolic acidosis is seen and may be in conjunction with a respiratory alkalosis.

   ix. Alkaline phosphatase is elevated if there is obstruction of the biliary tree.

b. Other studies

   i. Ultrasound will be able to detect stones in the gallbladder or common bile duct.

   ii. CT scan will allow for visualization of any tumor, abscesses, or pseudocysts.

   iii. Endoscopic retrograde cholangiopancreatography (ERCP) uses endoscopy to cannulate either the common bile duct or the duct of Wirsung (main pancreatic duct); this can then be used for removing stones or a dye study of the pancreatic ducts to diagnose blockage or inflammation. A sphincterotomy may also be done at this time to decrease congestion of the bile duct. *Caution:* Mechanical manipulation during this study can cause pancreatitis.

   iv. Chest x-ray will show any left pleural effusions and atelectasis.

B. Patient management

1. Fluid volume deficit related to hemorrhage, pancreatitis, peritonitis, and third spacing (NG tube may drain 1–2 liters per shift initially).

a. Problem: hypovolemic shock, decreased tissue perfusion, and cellular injury.

b. Intervention

   i. Fluid resuscitation; replacement of blood loss with blood products; replace fluid losses with crystalloid solutions; large-bore IV lines to provide rapid volume replacement; monitor fluid volume status by trends in vital signs and end organ perfusion; patient may need a pulmonary artery catheter for fluid management assessment of impending septic shock.

   ii. Serial H & H studies to ensure there is no drop in blood counts secondary to massive retroperitoneal hemorrhage; the abdomen can hold several liters of fluid, and retroperitoneal hemorrhage can be insidious.

   iii. Surgery may be needed if fevers continue and necrosis and abscesses are present; this may involve a partial or total pancreatectomy.

c. Desired outcome

   i. Restore normal hemodynamics and fluid volume; systolic BP greater than 90 mm Hg; heart rate less than 100 beats/minute; H & H of 10/30% or within patient's normal range; adequate end organ perfusion as noted by normal mentation, skin turgor, and urine output.

   ii. Prevention of secondary infections.

2. Impaired gas exchange related to elevated diaphragm from ascites and pain, related to infiltrates and atelectasis, related to decreased level of consciousness, risk of aspiration from NG tube or vomiting, sedation.

a. Problem: decreased tissue, cerebral and myocardial oxygenation.
b. Intervention: emergent period
   i. Maintain adequate airway: Auscultate lungs for rales, rhonchi, and decreased breath sounds; note respiratory pattern along with level of consciousness.
   ii. Support patient's breathing with oxygen or mechanical ventilation as needed.
   iii. Monitor arterial blood gases and oxygen saturation.
   iv. Monitor pulmonary artery pressures: Hypoxia can increase sympathetic tone and increase pulmonary vasoconstriction.
   v. Use sedation carefully: Amount of sedation needed to control pain may impair respirations; this may be especially true in the alcoholic or drug abuser; patient-controlled analgesia works well in this patient population. Demerol may be used in place of morphine, since morphine may induce spasms at the sphincter of Oddi, although this remains controversial.
   vi. Positioning: The patient may need to have the bed elevated 45–90 degrees to improve chest expansion and provide comfort.
c. Desired outcome
   i. Patient will have support of respiration as needed for maintaining adequate airway protection.
   ii. Aspiration will be prevented.
   iii. Serial arterial blood gases within normal limits.
3. Potential for further injury related to glucose and electrolyte imbalances.
a. Problems
   i. Alteration in glucose metabolism.
   ii. Alteration in calcium metabolism.
   iii. Alteration in magnesium.
   iv. Alteration in potassium.
b. Intervention
   i. Monitor glucose every hour or as needed; patient may require D50W.

---

dextrose 50% in water
Action Restores serum glucose to normal levels when glucose less than 40 mg/dL or patient is symptomatic.
Administration Guidelines 1 amp IV push bolus.
Special Concerns Patient's glucose may rise suddenly and fall again suddenly from an overcompensation of insulin; this is called the Symogi effect.

---

   ii. Patient may require an insulin drip.

Insulin drip
Action Keeps serum glucose less than 250. Enhances glucose
transport across cell membranes to reduce blood glucose level.
Administration Guidelines Usually mixed 1:2; 125 U/250 mL NS
(0.5 U/mL) and titrated to glucose level.
Special Concerns Glucose should be monitored every hour while
patient is receiving an insulin drip.

---

    iii. Monitor ionized calcium, since this is the more metabolically
active form; note serum albumin, since most calcium is bound to
albumin; replace calcium.

---

calcium
Action Replaces calcium.
Administration Guidelines Calcium chloride 1–2 g IV push
in critical situations such as dysrhythmias or shock. Calcium
gluconate, 1–2 g IV piggyback (PB) over 0.5 hour.
Special Concerns Use caution in patients with renal failure.

---

    iv. Monitor magnesium; administer magnesium sulfate replacement.

---

magnesium sulfate
Action Decreases acetylcholine release.
Administration Guidelines 1–2 g of magnesium sulfate over 1–2
hours IV.
Special Concerns Patient with a low serum magnesium may have
ventricular irritability; monitor cardiac rhythm.

---

    v. Monitor potassium frequently (every 2–4 hours); administer po-
tassium replacement.

---

potassium
Action Enhances conduction of excitable cells; replaces serum
potassium.
Administration Guidelines Potassium should be repleted via IV
replacement not to exceed 10 mEq/h in as large a volume as
possible; ie: 10 mEq in 100 mL NS infused over 1 hour.
Special Concerns Monitor for cardiac dysrhythmias associated
with hypokalemia. *Never* administer IV push.

---

  c. Desired outcome
    i. Repletion of electrolytes without complications.
    ii. Control of glucose within normal therapeutic range.

C. Discharge planning
   1. Patient and family understand the need for total abstinence from alcohol.
   2. Patient and family understand the need for follow-up lab studies and visits to doctors.
   3. Patient and family understand the role of glucose and insulin, monitoring of glucose, and prevention of hypoglycemia or insulin shock vs hyperglycemia; if patient is receiving insulin, full instruction will be given before discharge.
   4. Patient may require oral ingestion of pancreatic enzymes to allow for metabolism of food; education related to this medication should be discussed with the patient and family.
   5. Patient and family know the possible complications and will observe patient for fever, abdominal pain, ascites, abdominal distention, and signs and symptoms of shock.

Hepatic Failure

I. Definition

A. Hepatic failure: injury or dysfunction of units of the liver; failure may be acute or chronic; extent of failure can vary widely from slightly elevated enzymes to hepatic coma. Cases of alcoholism and hepatitis represent the largest number of patients seen in the critical care unit.

II. Etiology

A. Hepatitis (Table 7.2) [1]
   1. Hepatitis A is a viral, inflammatory disease that has a 4-week incubation period; noninfectious when jaundice appears; symptoms include loss of appetite, weakness, fatigue; often patients think they have a flu-type illness; route of transmission is oral-fecal; sources are water and shellfish; prevention gamma globulin shot prior to travel to endemic areas.
   2. Hepatitis B has a more prolonged clinical course. Appearance of the surface antigen occurs several weeks after exposure with clinical hepatitis, ie, 4 weeks later (incubation 12–14 weeks). Patient is considered infectious while hepatitis B surface antigen (HBsAg) is in blood, usually 1–3 months. Outcome can vary greatly; 90% recover fully; less than 10% have a chronic infection that can lead to cirrhosis; less than 1% develop fulminant hepatitis. Route of transmission is blood and body fluids; sources are needles, blood products, and IV drug abuse. Prevention is three injections over 6 months of hepatitis B immunoglobulin (Heptovax, Recombivax). Prophylaxis is recommended for patient's family, health care workers, and immunosuppressed patients.
   3. Hepatitis C occurs worldwide and has a more insidious path. The incubation period can vary greatly from weeks to months. In 60% of patients, no exposure history is found. Transmission is thought to be primarily parenteral. The hepatitis C antibody (HCVAb) is usually detected late in the course of the illness, if it is detected at all. Acute (at time of onset of symptoms) and convalescent (every 2–3 weeks) specimens should be

Table 7.2 Clinical and Epidemiologic Features of Hepatotrophic Viruses

Organism	Hepatitis A	Hepatitis B	Hepatitis C	Hepatitis D	Hepatitis E	NANB
Incubation	2–6 wk	1–6 mo	2 wk–6 mo	3 wk—3 mo	3–6 wk	2 wk–6 mo
Transmission	Fecal/oral Blood Sexual	Blood Sexual Perinatal	Sporadic Blood Sexual Perinatal	Blood Sexual Perinatal	Fecal/oral	Sporadic Blood ?Sexual ?Perinatal
Risk groups	Military personnel Children in day care and their care providers	IVDA Homosexuals Native Asians Health care workers Transfusion recipients	IVDA Health care workers Transfusion recipients	IVDA Anyone with hepatitis B	Travelers to endemic areas	IVDA Health care workers Transfusion recipients
Fever	Common	Uncommon	Uncommon	Uncommon	Common	Uncommon
Nausea/vomiting	Common	Common	Common	Common	Common	Common
Immune complex disease	Uncommon	Common	Common	Common	Common	Unknown
Severity	Mild	Mild to moderate	Mild to moderate	Moderate to severe	Mild to moderate	Mild to moderate
Diagnosis Acute	Anti-HAV IgM	Anti-HBc IgM HBsAg	Clinical	Anti-HDV IgM HDAg	Clinical[a]	Diagnosis of exclusion in appropriate clinical setting
Chronic	NA	Anti-HBc Total HBsAg	HCVAg RIBA II PCR for HCV RNA	HDAg	NA	Diagnosis of exclusion in appropriate clinical setting

Sequelae						
Fulminant	0.1–0.2%	<5%	<5%	5–20%	1–2%; 10–30% in pregnant women	<5%
Carrier	No	Yes	Yes	Yes	No	Unknown but likely
Chronic hepatitis	No	Yes	Yes	Yes	No	Yes
Prophylaxis						
Adults	ISG[b]	HBIG[c] + vaccine[d]	?ISG	None available[e]	None available	?ISG[b]
Perinatal	ISG[b]	HBIG[f] + vaccine[g]	?ISG[b]	None available[e]	None available	?ISG[b]

NANB = non-A, non-B hepatitis; IVDA = intravenous drug abusers; NA = not applicable; RIBA II = recombinant immunoblot assay II; PCR = polymerase chain reaction; ISG = immune serum globulin.

[a]Testing available from the hepatitis branch of the Centers for Disease Control.

[b]Immune serum globulin, 0.02 mL/kg IM. Use in NANB and HCV unsubstantiated.

[c]Hepatitis B immunoglobulin, 5 mL IM.

[d]Vaccine is either Engerix B, 20 µg IM, or Recombivax, 10 µg IM at 0, 1, and 6 months.

[e]Vaccination against hepatitis B will protect individuals from hepatitis D. No specific vaccine for hepatitis D is available.

[f]Hepatitis B immunoglobulin, 0.5 mL IM within 12 hours of birth.

[g]Vaccine is either Engerix B, 10 µg IM, or Recombivax, 5 µg IM at 0, 1, and 6 months.

From Ewald, G. A., and McKenzie, C. R., *Manual of Medical Therapeutics* (28th ed.). Boston: Little, Brown and Company. 1995. Pp. 366–367.

drawn. Fulminant hepatitis results in fewer than 5% of cases. There is no vaccine at this time. Blood and body fluid precautions are recommended.

4. Hepatitis D or delta agent is found only in patients with hepatitis B. It is difficult to know if patients are infected with hepatitis B and hepatitis D at the same time or if hepatitis D follows as a superinfection. Hepatitis D increases the virulence and severity of hepatitis B. Acute and convalescent specimens are recommended. Source is parenteral, in the United States most patients are IV drug abusers or patients with multiple transfusion histories. Fulminant hepatitis secondary to hepatitis D occurs in 30% of acute hepatitis B patients and in 70% of chronic hepatitis B patients.

5. Hepatitis E is the epidemic type of non-A, non-B hepatitis. Hepatitis E is especially virulent and frequently progresses to fulminant hepatitis. It is associated with a high number of fatalities in pregnant women. Hepatitis E is prevalent in underdeveloped countries. The route of transmission is oral-fecal and is diagnosed by exclusion of other types of hepatitis.

6. Other causes of hepatitis
   a. Herpes simplex virus.
   b. Epstein-Barr virus.
   c. Cytomegalovirus.
   d. Adenovirus.
   e. Amoebic infection.
   f. Malaria.

B. Toxic hepatic failure is a poisoning that causes injury to the hepatic cells. The two most common are acetaminophen (Tylenol) overuse or overdose and poisonous mushrooms. These can be fatal unless hepatic transplantation takes place as soon as possible.

C. Cirrhosis causes the replacement of the architecture of the liver with fibrous tissue.
   1. Laennec's cirrhosis is a result of alcohol's direct toxic effect on the liver.
   2. Primary biliary cirrhosis is found in young women and is usually idiopathic; damage causes an inability to drain bile into the ducts; most patients are chronically ill; some are eventually transplanted.
   3. Postnecrosis cirrhosis is usually secondary to hepatitis.
   4. Cardiac cirrhosis is a result of right-side heart failure that causes retrograde pressure gradient (a backflow that engorges the liver) and damages the liver.

D. Obstructive processes and subsequent damage can cause a mechanical hepatic blockage (such as cholelithiasis or tumor).

E. Hepatic failure can result from hemodynamic causes, ie, shock, sepsis, and hypoxia.

F. Metabolic disease
   1. Wilson's disease is associated with a high serum copper level and may present in a fulminant or progressive pattern resulting in hepatic transplantation.
   2. Alpha$_1$ antitrypsin deficiency is confirmed by liver biopsy, and transplantation is usually indicated.
   3. Fatty liver can be caused by alcoholic liver disease in a chronic form and pregnancy or Reye's syndrome in an acute form.

G. Vascular disorders

    1. Budd-Chiari syndrome, hepatic vein thrombosis, accompanied by hypercoagulation or malignancy.

    2. Portal vein thrombosis can occur secondary to other phenomena such as vena caval syndrome, trauma, or intra-abdominal sepsis.

III. Nursing process

A. Assessment

    1. Signs and symptoms

        a. Early changes include fatigue, anorexia, weight loss, abdominal discomfort, weakness, constructional apraxia (inability to draw figures clearly because of loss of fine motor coordination), and asterixis (a decrease in fine motor control seen in the hand when the arm is extended; also called liver flap, since the hand flaps uncontrollably).

        b. Late changes

            i. Neurologic: minor personality changes to coma, toxic effects of ammonia and other metabolic waste products on the CNS.

            ii. CV: development of collateral circulation causes a hyperdynamic, hypertensive system with bounding pulses; this is seen mostly in the patient with chronic hepatic disease.

            iii. Pulmonary: hypoventilation related to ascites; pleural effusions from ascites traveling through the lymphatic system; and hypoxemia related to coma, sepsis, or shock.

            iv. GI: extensive collateral circulation related to the hepatic changes both mechanical and pressure related; the blood will flow to the areas of least resistance, ie, spleen, kidneys, esophagus, intestine, resulting in esophageal varices, ascites, and splenomegaly. This causes malnutrition, since the liver can no longer metabolize fats, proteins, and starches. Ascites is formed by the leakage of fluid into the abdominal cavity from impaired colloid osmotic pressure and decreased manufacturing of albumin. As much as 5 liters of ascites can easily occupy the abdominal cavity. Stools may become gray or white as a result of impaired bilirubin metabolism.

            v. GU: renal impairment related to decreased perfusion; urine will become rust-colored to brown as a result of impaired bilirubin metabolism.

            vi. Skin: jaundice ranging from slight yellow discoloration to gray-green appearance; ecchymosis, bruising, petechiae related to hypercoagulability and thrombocytopenia.

        c. Specific changes

            i. Portal hypertension is a result of elevated portal pressures by obstruction of blood flow through the liver.

            ii. Esophageal varices usually occur *secondary* to portal hypertension, which causes gastroesophageal engorgement; this results in venous masses forming around the gastroesophageal junction.

            iii. Hepatic encephalopathy is a neurologic disorder of altered sensorium including abnormal behavior, impaired intellect, and disturbed neuromuscular function caused by ammonia and other metabolic waste products; may be acute or gradual.

    iv. Hepatic coma is any condition where there is sufficient damage to permit blood to enter the circulation without detoxification resulting in mental, biochemical, and neurologic disturbances; progresses from stupor to coma.

    v. Hepatorenal failure is associated with 100% mortality. Transplantation of both organs simultaneously has been attempted with limited success.

B. Diagnostic parameters

  1. Serum

    a. Glucose: affected by the ability to perform gluconeogenesis and glucogenolysis; glucose less than 50 mg/dL is a poor prognostic indicator (usually seen when death is imminent).

    b. Sodium: Although there is a total body retention of Na^+ and water, a dilutional hyponatremia is common.

    c. Potassium: commonly, serum K^+ is low (< 3.5 mEq/L) in association with acid-base disorders, affected by metabolic acidosis, losses from vomiting or nasogastric drainage, renal losses, and affected by *ammonia metabolism*; may, however, be elevated in renal failure or hepatorenal failure.

    d. Calcium is usually measured as ionized Ca^{2+}; this is the more metabolically active and is usually *bound to albumin;* therefore, if the patient has a low calcium, look also at the albumin level. *Caution:* Calcium can drop secondary to binding with citrate in stored blood products; if your patient is receiving multiple transfusion, monitor Ca^{2+}.

    e. Magnesium is usually low in conjunction with hypokalemia, hypocalcemia, and malabsorption.

    f. Phosphate may be low: associated with decreased intake and metabolism in acute hepatic failure or high in connection with low potassium and low magnesium levels of chronic hepatic failure.

    g. Albumin is affected by the inability of the liver to metabolize proteins and make albumin; albumin is vital in maintaining colloid osmotic pressure and in the clotting cascade. A serum albumin of less than 2 is a poor prognostic indicator.

    h. Acid–base balance may be altered in many ways; massive hepatic necrosis will cause a metabolic acidosis; elevation of bicarb levels will cause a metabolic alkalosis; hyperventilation will cause a respiratory alkalosis; hypoventilation will cause a respiratory acidosis.

    i. Serum glutamic-oxaloacetic transaminase (SGOT) and serum glutamic-pyruvic transaminase (SGPT): Aminotransferases are monitored to detect elevation trends that indicate hepatocellular injury.

    j. Alkaline phosphatase (AP) elevation usually indicates cholelithiasis or obstruction of the biliary tree.

    k. Gamma-glutamyl transpeptidase (GGT) is an enzyme that elevates with certain ingested agents (barbiturates, alcohol).

    l. Bilirubin measures the degradation of hemoglobin; direct (conjugated) bilirubin and indirect (unconjugated or free) bilirubin represent parts of the bilirubin pathway. Elevated direct bilirubin is found in hepatocellular dysfunction or biliary tract obstruction. Elevated indirect bilirubin is found in hemolysis.

m. PT, PTT, and platelet count are altered by the inability to make albumin, vitamin K, fibrinogen, and globulin and other vital proteins.

n. Ammonia is a metabolic waste product resulting from the deamination of proteins and excretion via the urea cycle. Elevated serum ammonia levels may indicate hepatic failure. *Caution:* Ammonia is not the only metabolic waste product; therefore, a patient may clinically be in coma with a normal or only slightly elevated ammonia.

o. Presence of hepatitis antibodies.

2. Other studies
   a. Imaging studies
      i. Ultrasound is used to diagnose cholelithiasis; may also be used to determine vessel flow, amount of ascitic fluid, and solid versus cystic tumors.
      ii. CT scan indicates tumor growth or abscesses.
      iii. Magnetic resonance imaging (MRI) visualization of tumor or abscesses.
   b. Endoscopy is usually used in the critical care setting to determine the exact site of bleeding; also for biopsy, curtory (ablation of the site of bleeding), and polypectomy.
      i. Sclerotherapy is used when bleeding esophageal varices are present; a sclerosing agent is injected directly into the varix; this may stop the acute bleeding and allow hemodynamic stabilization of the patient.
      ii. ERCP is a direct dye study of either the biliary tree or pancreatic duct; can also be used pre- and postultrasonic lithotripsy.
   c. Angiography
      i. Transjugular intrahepatic portosystemic shunts (TIPS) may be diagnostic or therapeutic; used to determine intrahepatic pressures with stent placement to decrease portal pressure; and, therefore, to relieve esophageal and collateral pressures.

C. Patient management
   1. Fluid volume deficit related to gastrointestinal bleeding.
      a. Problem: alteration in hemodynamic status secondary to bleeding esophageal varices and blood loss. Although bleeding esophageal varices do not always occur secondary to hepatic failure, their development alters the course of treatment. An esophageal varice that ruptures can cause exsanguination due to the higher pressures from portal hypertension (see Acute Gastrointestinal Hemorrhage).
      b. Intervention
         i. Fluid resuscitation; replacement of blood loss with blood products; large-bore IV lines to provide rapid volume replacement.
         ii. Decrease bleeding with vasopressin infusion.

vasopressin

Action Enhances contraction of the vascular and nonvascular smooth muscle resulting in decreased peripheral blood flow and mesenteric blood flow.

Administration Guidelines IV or intra-arterially 50 U/250 mL PSS at 0.2–0.4 U/mL per minute.

Special Concerns May cause cardiac ischemia, may decrease cardiac output, may increase systemic vascular resistance; nitroglycerine or nitroprusside infusions may be used to counteract this effect.

iii. Administer histamine blockers.

Histamine blockers

Action Decrease the hydrochloric acid in the stomach by blocking the release of histamine.

Administration Guidelines May be given PO or IV by continuous or intermittent dosing; continuous infusion is usually given to stop acute bleeding while the patient is being hemodynamically stabilized. *Cimetadine*: PO 300 mg three to four times daily, IV 300 mg every 6–8 hours, or 900–1200 mg in 250 mL over 24 hours. *Ranitidine*: PO 150 mg bid, IV 150 mg every 12 hours, or 300 mg in 250 mL over 24 hours.

Special Concerns May interfere with the absorption of other drugs; may cause headaches, dizziness, diarrhea, and constipation; may cause hepatotoxicity, hallucinations, and agitation.

iv. Gastric lavage to maintain patency of nasogastric tube, to clear stomach of clots so endoscopy can be performed.

v. Administer antacids.

Antacids

Actions Neutralize hydrochloric acid and relieve pain; keep pH greater than 4.5.

Administration Guidelines See Table 7.1.

Special Concerns May cause diarrhea or constipation; interfere with the absorption of many drugs; may cause metabolic alkalosis.

vi. Angiography may be used to locate feeding vessel and embolize, usually used in patients who are high surgical risk; TIPS procedure to place stent between the portal vein and hepatic vein, to decrease portal pressures.

vii. Endoscopy to sclerose the bleeding varices. *Caution:* To protect patient's airway and prevent aspiration, endotracheal intubation and mechanical ventilation should be considered.

viii. Balloon tamponade to control bleeding mechanically; usually used when other methods of stopping bleeding are not successful. *Caution:* The nurse should be familiar with individual hospital policy regarding procedure in the placement and care of the patient with a balloon tamponade device, ie, pressure limits for the balloon, how often balloons are to be deflated to prevent ischemia, and the method for safely doing this; how traction is applied to the device (football helmet or overhead traction), emergency precautions to be taken, ie, having scissors available to deflate all balloons if airway obstruction occurs, having suction available, having blood available in case of hemorrhage.

ix. Surgery: It is important to determine if the patient is a candidate for liver transplantation before abdominal surgery is done. If a liver transplant is not an option for this patient, then a palliative shunt may be considered. If, however, a liver transplant is a viable option, shunting will only complicate the surgery. (This does not include TIPS, since it is within the liver itself.) Vascular shunts include portacaval shunt, splenorenal shunt, and mesocaval shunt. *Caution:* Shunting may cause encephalopathy to worsen; the decrease in pressure may impair circulation within the liver.

c. Desired outcome
  i. Control of bleeding.
  ii. Hemodynamic stability.
  iii. Improved hepatic and neurologic status.

2. Malnutrition related to the inability to metabolize proteins, fats, and starches
  a. Problem: increased risk for infection, skin breakdown, and decreased healing.
  b. Interventions
    i. Limit ingestion of proteins, ie, meat, cheese; substitute simple carbohydrates, ie, hard candy, ie, 40-gm protein diet.
    ii. Calorie counts to determine if metabolic needs are being met.
    iii. Intake and output; daily weights.
    iv. If patient is on hyperalimentation, decrease amount of amino acids.
    v. Administer lactulose to promote osmotic diarrhea in order to decrease metabolic waste products in the colon.
    vi. Neomycin enemas may be used to decrease bacteria and metabolic waste products in the colon.
    vii. Monitor serum glucose frequently and support as needed; D10W infusion may be needed in the terminal phase.
  c. Desired outcome
    i. Patient will maintain nutritional balance and receive at least the minimum caloric requirements per day.
    ii. Patient will maintain or improve neurologic status.
    iii. Patient will maintain serum glucose above 50 mg/dL.

3. Ascites related to impaired hepatic functioning, decreased albumin production, and impaired colloid osmotic pressure, which causes capillary leakage.

   a. Problem: Intravascular hypovolemia with increased tissue pressure from ascitic fluid causes decreased tissue perfusion and cellular injury.

   b. Intervention

   i. Paracentesis to drain excess fluid from the abdominal cavity. *Caution:* Do not drain more than 2 liters per day; may cause hypovolemic shock.

   ii. Sodium and water restriction to decrease free water and capillary leak.

   iii. Administer diuretics.

---

aldactone

Action Potassium sparing diuretic.

Administration Guidelines Dosage starts at 25–50 mg PO and can increase to 250 mg/d.

Special Concerns Do not give if potassium level above 5.5 mEq/L; may cause severe hyperkalemia.

---

   iv. Administer albumin as ordered to replace losses and improve colloid osmotic pressure; failure to maintain normal albumin will lead to third-space losses and peripheral edema, normal 3.5–5.5 g/dL.

   v. Peritoneal-venous shunt (LeVeen shunt) may be placed as a palliative method of controlling ascites. *Caution:* Peritoneal-venous shunting may cause fluid shifts and hypovolemic shock in the immediate postoperative phase.

   c. Desired outcome

   i. Control of ascites will be assessed by decreased need for paracentesis.

   ii. Patient will maintain hemodynamic status; systolic BP greater than 90 mm Hg; HR less than 100 beats/minute.

   iii. Serum albumin will remain within normal limits.

   iv. Decrease in peripheral edema and third-space losses.

4. Impaired metabolic and neurologic functioning related to hepatic failure.

   a. Problem: Risk for death if hepatic failure not reversed secondary to fluid shifts, sepsis, and metabolic waste product poisoning.

   b. Intervention

   i. Administer lactulose.

Table 7.3 Grading of Hepatic Coma

Stage	
I	Mental slowness, mild impairment of coordination
II	Disorientation, mental confusion, asterixis, constructional apraxia
III	Progressive, markedly confused, periods of agitation mixed with periods of somnolence; patient may become violent when aroused; patient may bite, remove tubes, and lose inhibitions
IV	Patient cannot be aroused; associated with a 90% mortality

---

lactulose

Action Produces osmotic changes in the colon causing an influx of water, which results in diarrhea so that the colon can be emptied of metabolic waste products.

Administration Guidelines 20–30 g PO (NG) tid or qid, until two or three soft stools daily. May also be given as retention enema of 300 mL lactulose in 700 mL water.

Special Concerns Do not stop administration because of diarrhea; dosage adjustment is needed; may reduce serum ammonia levels by 25%–50%.

---

    ii. Airway protection (since patient will lose protective reflexes from neurologic impairment): Endotracheal intubation and mechanical ventilation may be needed; monitor respiratory patterns; monitor arterial blood gases; monitor oxygen saturation.

    iii. Blood product replacement as needed to maintain hematocrit of 30%, PT, PTT, and platelet count within normal limits; continuous infusion of fresh frozen plasma may be needed.

    iv. Serial lab tests including ammonia, electrolyte, enzyme, and coagulation studies.

    v. Neurologic assessment to assess and determine level of coma every 4 hours (Table 7.3).

    vi. Correction of alkalosis; serial arterial blood gases and electrolytes.

    vii. Control of intracranial pressure.

    viii. Use caution when administering medications; many are metabolized by the liver, ie, narcotics.

    ix. Prevent sepsis; dysfunction of Kupffer's cells prevents bacterial lysis.

    x. Hepatic transplantation may be done, but length of coma correlates with a poorer prognosis.

5. Knowledge deficit of family and significant others is related to preparation for possible surgery, transplantation, or terminal care.

    a. Problem: decreased decision-making and coping abilities.

    b. Preparation of family for future

        i. Patient/family assessment of support systems to provide long-term care and antirejection medications.

      ii. Discuss prognosis and possible outcomes, taking into account patient's specific issues: age, other diseases, infections.

     iii. Allow patient/family to decide on the level of care: Will care be aggressive, or will patient not be resuscitated?

     iv. Explain that shunts are palliative, not curative, and hepatic failure may reoccur.

     v. Provide emotional support as needed.

  6. Desired outcome

    a. Family members feel that all their questions were answered to their satisfaction.

    b. Family members feel comfortable with decisions made about patient's care.

D. Discharge planning

  1. For patients with hepatitis, family members will be given information about the disease to prevent further transmission of the disease and educate the community.

  2. Patient and family will understand that recovery will be slow and gradual. The patient will fatigue easily and will need time to rest.

  3. Patient and family will understand the need for follow-up care including medications, lab tests, and doctor visits.

  4. Patient and family must understand that hepatic disease may become chronic with a predisposition to bleeding, infection, and impaired metabolism.

  5. Support and education will be provided for withdrawal from alcohol consumption or other drug use.

Reference

1. Ewald, G. A., and McKenzie, C. R. *Manual of Medical Therapeutics* (28th ed.). Boston: Little, Brown and Company, 1995. Pp. 366–367.

CHAPTER 8

Hematologic Disorders

Brenda Shelton

Overview of Hematologic Disorders

Hematologic disorders are a group of disease processes involving red blood cells, immune function, and coagulation processes. Although labeled part of a single system, these are discrete processes that utilize components from the bone marrow, liver, spleen, and other lymphatic organs. Within this classification system, hematologic problems usually involve the red blood cells or coagulation system, and immunologic disorders affect the body's nonspecific and specific immune systems. This chapter discusses the most common primary hematologic problems in the critically ill patient. Primary disorders are those originating in the organ system, and therefore do not include secondary hematologic deficiencies such as GI bleeding. The most significant erythrocyte crises in the critical care setting are hemolytic anemia and sickle cell crisis. Life-threatening coagulopathies encompass platelet problems, hepatic coagulation protein deficiencies, and defibrination syndromes such as disseminated intravascular coagulation (DIC). An overview of these problems follows.

Hemolytic Anemia

I. Definition: Hemolytic anemia is a syndrome in which the red blood cells (RBCs) are abnormally hemolyzed and removed from the circulating blood. It is commonly a secondary disorder, arising as a complication of liver and spleen disease, autoimmune disorders, malignancy, bone marrow transplantation, and drug toxicity. Transfusion reactions may also cause hemolysis, although a persistent hemolytic anemia is unusual in these situations. Some patients present with only red cell lysis, while others have a combined syndrome that includes hemolysis and renal failure (hemolytic uremic syndrome [HUS]).

II. Etiology: The RBCs of the body are normally sensitized and removed by the spleen when they are senescent, deformed, or dysfunctional. The spleen can become oversensitized by the development of red cell autoantibodies. These autoantibodies interpret normal RBCs as foreign tissue and signal the splenic macrophages to remove the RBC and destroy it. In addition, the RBC autoantibodies may be circulating in the serum and initiate extrasplenic hemolysis. The physiologic consequence of hemolysis is the splitting of hemoglobin into the pigment heme and protein globin. Iron contained in the molecule is bound with circulating transferrin to be returned to the bone marrow for RBC production, and heme is bound to haptoglobin to be degraded into bilirubin for excretion. Both transferrin and haptoglobin are made by the liver and are dependent upon liver function for clearance. If the hemoglobin molecule is not properly degraded, free hemoglobin can cause renal damage, and unconjugated bilirubin accumulates in the systemic circulation.

III. Nursing process

A. Assessment
  1. Signs and symptoms
     a. Jaundice as evidenced as a yellowish skin tint or dark, tea-colored urine occurs as a result of the accumulation of unconjugated bilirubin when red cells are hemolyzed extrasplenically and are removed less efficiently.
     b. Enlarged and tender spleen and/or liver is the consequence of abnormal sequestration of senescent or damaged RBCs that are removed by the spleen or liver. Circulatory screening may occur due to truly abnormal cell structure or be the result of autoantibodies against the RBC.
     c. Respiratory distress, angina, or other symptom of reduced oxygen carrying capacity reflects the severity of oxygen deficit that occurs. It is usually demonstrated in patients with significant red cell loss without replacement.
     d. Oliguria is the result of renal insult from hemolyzed cells.
  2. Diagnostic parameters
     a. Serum tests
        i. Decreased haptoglobin, decreased transferrin: Since haptoglobin normally binds with heme, and transferrin binds with iron to facilitate removal from the circulation, free levels of these serum values decrease when extrasplenic hemolysis is occurring, since more heme and iron need transport back to the liver prior to removal or recirculation.
        ii. Increased total and direct bilirubin: When the demands for conjugation of RBC breakdown products exceed the body's ability to maintain a constant removal, hyperbilirubinemia is the result. More rapid onset of hemolysis is likely to produce higher levels of bilirubin. The bilirubin level correlates to the degree of jaundice; higher levels produce more jaundice.
        iii. Decreased hematocrit and hemoglobin are the result of RBC lysis and removal from the circulating RBC mass. Severity of deficit will depend on the rate of hemolysis.
        iv. Increased reticulocyte (immature RBCs) count occurs in response to blood loss. As the RBC mass decreases, the body's compensatory response is to release immature RBCs (called reticulocytes) to replace RBCs until stabilization occurs. Small amounts of reticulocytes are normal, but levels exceeding 4% of the total RBC mass indicate hemolysis.

       v. Evidence of schistocytes (fragmented RBCs) on RBC smear are evidence of sheared and damaged RBCs that occur during the hemolysis process.

      vi. Decreased platelets occur as platelets are trapped in small clots of hemolyzed RBCs and are due to excessive sensitivity of the spleen to remove cells.

      vii. Increased lactate dehydrogenase (LDH) is indicative of RBC breakdown. It is an enzyme released in RBC destruction.

      viii. Increased creatinine and BUN occur when the level of hemolysis is so significant that intravascular heme, globin, iron, and waste products cause toxic damage to the kidneys and induce renal dysfunction.

  b. Urine tests

    i. Increased urobilinogen occurs as the body attempts to excrete the excess circulating bilirubin.

  c. Other tests

    i. None

B. Patient management

  1. Impaired tissue perfusion related to decreased oxygen-carrying capacity from low hemoglobin, increased propensity for thromboses from hemolyzed cells.

    a. Problem: Lysis of RBCs produces circulating cell fragments that obstruct vascular flow, increase the tendency for thrombosis, and lead to decreased organ perfusion. In addition, lysis of RBCs decreases circulating RBC mass, which decreases oxygen-carrying capacity and decreases organ oxygenation.

    b. Interventions

      i. Periodically assess and maintain adequate vascular volume.

      ii. Assess specific tissue oxygenation such as evaluation of ECG for ischemic changes, notation of liver transaminase levels for evidence of hepatic ischemia, level of consciousness for neurologic perfusion.

      iii. Avoid excess vasoconstriction of the periphery.

      iv. Administer red blood cell replacement as ordered and monitor response to intervention.

      v. Administer oxygen therapy as ordered if the oxygen level is less than 60 mm Hg or oxygen saturation is less than 90%.

      vi. Perform active and passive range of motion or encourage movement of extremities to reduce stagnation of blood flow and a risk for thromboses.

      vii. Avoid hypothermia, which can worsen vasoconstriction and peripheral tissue perfusion.

      viii. Administer antiplatelet medications (eg, salicylic acid or indomethacin) as ordered to reduce ischemic damage.

      ix. If autoantibodies or abnormal splenic sequestration are implicated, immunosuppressive agents such as steroids, azathioprine, or cyclophosphamide are given as ordered.

    x. Provide supportive care while avoiding transfusion of RBCs, which trigger additional hemolysis, hypertension, hyperviscosity, and congestive heart failure.

    xi. Assess and monitor the patient during plasma exchange with staphylococcal protein A as needed throughout the course of 5–10 days of daily plasmapheresis treatments.

---

staphylococcal protein A

Action Staphylococcal protein A is a component of the cell wall of staphylococci and is capable of trapping IgG complexes which are thought to cause RBC autoantibodies.

Administration Guidelines Begin plasma reinfusion at a rate of 25 mL/h for 15 minutes, then increase to 100 mL/h.

Special Considerations Assess for hypersensitivity reactions. Assess for fluid shifts into the interstitial spaces during infusion or within 6–12 hours after infusion (eg, crackles in lungs, edema). Monitor for other adverse effects: vomiting, pain at infusion site, diarrhea.

---

  c. Desired outcome

    i. Have PaO_2 greater than 60 mm Hg and oxygen saturation greater than 90%.

    ii. Urine output exceeds intake on an hourly basis.

    iii. Absence of central cyanosis of acrocyanosis

    iv. Peripheral pulses are equal and normal strength.

    v. RBC levels are stable and without evidence of extrasplenic hemolysis (eg, LDH, reticulocytes, schistocytes).

2. Alteration in comfort related to splenic or hepatic enlargement or dry itching skin from jaundice

  a. Problem: Hemolysis of RBCs causes fragmented circulating cells, which are noted and removed by normal mechanisms in the liver and spleen. Engorgement of the liver and spleen with these damaged cells leads to enlargement of the organ and somatic pain.

  b. Interventions

    i. Assess patient's perception of comfort at least every shift using a quantitative scale that can reflect when the discomfort is worse or relieved by interventions (eg, visual analog scale).

    ii. Palpate the abdomen every shift to determine the degree to which abdominal organs are contributing to discomfort.

    iii. Assess the abdomen for splenic or hepatic enlargement.

    iv. If abdominal distention is present, obtain abdominal girths at least daily.

    v. Examine the sclera and skin for evidence of jaundice.

    vi. Apply lotion or mentholated creams to relieve itching as needed.

    vii. Administer antipruritus medications as ordered.

  c. Desired outcome

    i. Deny the presence of abdominal discomfort.

    ii. Have a nonpalpable spleen and liver.

    iii. Skin color is normal, without yellowish tint.

    iv. Denies itching skin.

3. Alteration in elimination: urinary; related to renal dysfunction from heme destruction of nephrons

  a. Problem: RBC hemolysis and immune complexes cause obstruction in the microvasculature of the kidneys. Ischemic damage leads to slowed glomerular filtration and acute renal failure.

  b. Interventions

    i. Insert Foley catheter as ordered.

    ii. Monitor urine output hourly, and report intake greater than output in 2 consecutive hours or according to other parameters as ordered.

    iii. Monitor free hemoglobin levels of the urine, urobilinogen, and urine specific gravity.

    iv. Monitor renal function through BUN and creatinine levels.

    v. Monitor electrolytes (especially K^+, Ca^+, phosphorus) and fluid balance as renal dysfunction progresses.

    vi. Intake and output totals every shift to evaluate fluid balance. Limit fluid intake by concentrating medications and blood products.

    vii. Daily weights to assess fluid balance.

    viii. Administer renal dose dopamine as ordered to improve renal perfusion.

    ix. Monitor peak and trough drug levels that may reflect effective renal clearance of medications.

    x. Administer antihypertensive medications as ordered.

    xi. Facilitate dialysis treatments and perform monitoring of fluids, electrolytes, and hemodynamic status with the treatments.

  c. Desired outcome

    i. Have normal BUN, creatinine, and electrolyte levels.

    ii. Have a urine output that exceeds intake.

    iii. Have a stable weight.

    iv. Blood pressure is within normal limits for the patient's preillness blood pressure.

Sickle Cell Crisis

  I. Definition: Sickle cell disease is a genetic malformation of the hemoglobin B strand (called hemoglobin S) that results in red blood cell sickling in the presence of hypoxia. The disease is most common in those of African or southern European descent, and since it is a protectant against malaria, it is most common in these tropical regions. It is estimated that 1 in 400–600 African-American children are afflicted with this disease. Sickle cell crisis is a condition in which large numbers of RBCs are sickled, producing decreased oxygen-carrying capacity, vascular obstruction, and depletion of hematologic cells.

  II. Etiology: In sickle cell disease, there is a genetic predisposition for amino acid substitution in the hemoglobin B chain. When the abnormal gene is inherited from both parents, sickle cell disease is the consequence. The disease can present with a wide variation of clinical syndromes. The triggers for sickle cell crisis are situations in which hypoxemia occurs. Common precipitating factors include decrease oxygen tension of the blood, acidosis, and hyperosmolarity. Clinical disorders that can cause these physiologic problems and precipitate crisis may include hemorrhage, hyperglycemia, hypernatremia, respiratory failure, pneumonia, excessive cold exposure, excessive exercise, dehydration (eg, due to diarrhea), and septicemia. Every individual has a threshold hypoxemia that precipitates sickling of circulating RBCs, which will predict the severity of symptoms.

III. Nursing process

A. Assessment

1. Signs and symptoms: Sickle cell anemia with crisis may present with a variety of common symptoms regardless of the type of crisis. These general clinical findings are outlined below. Additionally, sickle cell crisis has five major subtypes: (1) vaso-occlusive crisis, (2) anemic crisis, (3) aplastic crisis, (4) acute sequestration crisis, and (5) hemolytic crisis. These syndromes display unique clinical features which are described in Table 8.1.

Table 8.1 Types of Sickle Cell Crisis

Type of Crisis	Clinical Features	Management
Vaso-occlusive crisis	This is the most common form of crisis This crisis causes severe pain for the patient Microvasculature is obstructed by large amounts of sickle cells	Fluid resuscitation Aggressive pain management Oxygen therapy and correction of hypoxemia
Anemic crisis	Red cells are depleted due to hemolysis and splenic sequestration Folate deficiency due to hemolysis exacerbates problem	Oxygen therapy to maximize oxygenation RBC transfusions to replace oxygen-carrying capacity Folate supplements
Aplastic crisis	Bone marrow production of RBCs is suppressed Usually due to infection (especially viral) Rapid RBC turnover exacerbates problem	Transfusions Antimicrobials Oxygen therapy
Acute sequestration crisis	Occurs in age 8 mo–2 y Sudden enlargement of spleen or liver occurs Splenic and hepatic discomfort is severe Acute abdominal symptoms are present May lead to intra-abdominal sepsis and death	Fluid resuscitation Aggressive pain management Antimicrobials Possible surgery
Hemolytic crisis	Rare type of crisis May be due to precipitating factor such as infection rather than sickle cell disease Hemolysis continues even after hypoxia is corrected	Aggressive reduction of oxygen demands—mechanical ventilation, heavy sedation, or paralysis Transfusions Other symptomatic support

a. Swollen and painful joints occur when occlusion of the microvasculature in the joints produce an inflammatory reaction. The most common joints affected are the hands and feet, but others may occur. Due to prolonged ischemia, a long-term complication of aseptic necrosis of the joints may occur requiring surgical intervention.

b. Splenic enlargement with left-sided abdominal pain is a common complaint that represents the normal splenic response to the challenge of removing abnormal RBCs from circulation. The larger the number of sickle cells, the more severe this symptom may be initially; however, with repeated sickling episodes, the spleen will become so sequestered with RBCs that vascular obstruction and splenic infarction occurs. With repeated splenic infarctions, pain and swelling are reduced, but spleen function may be minimal.

c. Confusion and altered mental status occur due to reduced RBC-carrying capacity or ischemic damage from sickling of RBCs in the neurovasculature. Severe thrombosis with vessel rupture and intracranial hemorrhage may cause death, particularly in the young patient with frequent or severe crises.

d. Dyspnea, tachypnea, and respiratory distress reflect decreased oxygen-carrying capacity or sickle cell obstruction of the pulmonary circulation, leading to altered gas exchange. Over long periods of time, damage to the lung parenchyma leads to chronic pneumonias or chronic obstructive lung disease.

e. Chest discomfort occurs when sickle cells obstruct the coronary artery blood flow. Long-term or severe cardiovascular insufficiency can lead to ischemic heart disease, myocardial infarctions, and chronic congestive heart failure.

f. Hypertension is a common finding in patients who are experiencing acute vaso-occlusive crisis and hyperviscosity. Chronic hypertension and hyperviscosity leads to dilated cardiomyopathy and the risk of death from sudden dysrhythmias or congestive heart failure.

g. Jaundice is a symptom that reflects the tendency for intravascular hemolysis and subsequent difficulty in conjugation of bilirubin.

h. Heart murmurs, gallops, and shifted point of maximal impulse are symptoms of congestive heart failure that occurs due to chronic hyperviscosity, hypertension, and ischemic heart disease.

2. Diagnostic parameters
   a. Serum tests
      i. Abnormal serum protein electrophoresis is the definitive diagnostic test. It permits the clinician to detect hemoglobin S, which is present instead of hemoglobin B.
      ii. Decreased hematocrit, hemoglobin occur as the sickle cells are detected and removed from circulation from the spleen and liver.
      iii. Sickle cells on RBC smear demonstrate the severity of sickling that has occurred at any given time. Presence of sickle-shaped RBCs may trigger protein electrophoresis for definitive diagnosis.
      iv. Elevated bilirubin levels are the result of excess red cell lysis and decompensation in the conjugation of bilirubin.

    b. Urine tests

        i. Positive urine test for blood and urobilinogen are present because red blood cell lysis results in excretion of extra bilirubin via the renal system. Blood is in the urine when there is vascular occlusion with thromboses and rupture in the microcirculation of the kidney.

    c. Other tests

        i. None

B. Patient management

  1. Altered tissue oxygenation due to sickle RBCs and vascular occlusion

    a. Problem: Red blood cells become sickle shaped when exposed to a hypoxic environment. The sickle cells obstruct blood flow and increase blood viscosity, particularly in the microvasculature such as that of the lungs, joints, kidneys, and brain. Decreased vascular flow causes stagnation of blood and tissue ischemia.

    b. Intervention

        i. Treat all potential cries with oxygen supplementation as ordered to maintain a PaO_2 greater than 60 mm Hg and an oxygen saturation of greater than 90%.

        ii. Administer vigorous IV fluids (approximately 200–500 mL/h) to decrease blood viscosity and enhance tissue perfusion.

        iii. Avoid other potential stimulants of cellular hypoxia such as exposure to cold, excessive physical activity, acidosis, dehydration, infection.

        iv. Perform frequent or continuous assessments of oxygen saturation.

        v. Consider warming intravenous fluids or blood products to avoid additional sickling of cells.

    c. Desired outcome

        i. Patient is pain free and comfortable

        ii. Denies dyspnea, orthopnea

        iii. PaO_2 greater than 60 mm Hg, and oxygen saturation is greater than 90%

  2. Potential impaired gas exchange due to reduced oxygen-carrying capacity with sickle cells

    a. Problem: Sickling of red blood cells decreases the blood's oxygen-carrying capacity and can lead to symptomatic anemia or altered tissue perfusion.

    b. Intervention

        i. Administer oxygen therapy or assisted ventilation as ordered, for respiratory distress symptoms and when the oxygen saturation is below the ordered threshold (at least 90% unless ordered otherwise by physician).

        ii. Limit physical activity to conserve oxygen.

        iii. Position patient to optimize ventilation (high Fowler's or reverse Trendelenburg).

        iv. Provide sedation or pain medication if anxiety and pain are contributing to oxygen demands.

        v. Monitor oxygenation and ventilation status through arterial blood gases.

      vi. Administer blood products cautiously and monitor for increased symptoms of sickling or hemolysis.

  c. Desired outcome

      i. Absence of dyspnea, orthopnea.

      ii. PaO_2 greater than 60 mm Hg and oxygen saturation is greater than 90%.

3. Altered thought processes due to sickling, thromboses, and vascular rupture in neurologic vessels

  a. Problem: Vaso-occlusion of the microvasculature is particularly problematic in the neurologic vessels. Ischemic stroke, thrombotic stroke, and intracranial hemorrhage may occur.

  b. Interventions

      i. Perform neurologic assessments at least every shift.

      ii. Keep head of bed elevated 15–45 degrees.

      iii. Monitor blood pressure and report hypertension.

      iv. Administer sedating medications cautiously.

  c. Desired outcome

      i. Patient is alert, oriented, and appropriate and display no focal deficits.

4. Alteration in comfort, pain

  a. Problem: Vascular occlusion leads to tissue ischemia and necrosis. Ischemic tissue causes pain. The discomfort associated with sickle cell crisis may be peripheral or somatic. The most common sites are the joints, spleen (early in the disease before autosplenectomy occurs from infarction), liver, chest, and abdomen.

  b. Intervention

      i. Assess patient's perception of comfort at least every shift using a quantitative scale that can reflect when the discomfort is worse or relieved by interventions (eg, visual analog scale).

      ii. Administer pain and sedating medications to relax the patient and decrease oxygen consumption that may be contributing to the cellular hypoxia.

      iii. Palpate the abdomen every shift to determine the degree to which abdominal organs are contributing to discomfort.

      iv. Assess the abdomen for splenic or hepatic enlargement.

      v. If abdominal distention is present, obtain abdominal girths at least daily.

      vi. Apply warm compresses to painful joints.

  c. Desired outcome

      i. Patient is free of discomfort.

      ii. Has no splenic or hepatic enlargement.

5. Altered cardiac output, decreased due to hyperviscosity and increased workload on the heart

  a. Problem: Multiple cardiovascular problems occur when red blood cells sickle in the circulation: (1) Blood becomes more viscous and slows blood flow, increasing the propensity for thrombosis; (2) increased viscosity causes an increase in blood pressure; and (3) increased viscosity and blood pressure increase workload on the heart and cause heart failure.

b. Interventions
  i. Monitor blood pressure, cardiac rhythm, heart sounds, jugular venous pulsations (JVP), and pulse strength and equality frequently.
  ii. Administer antihypertensives as ordered.
  iii. Administer fluids and anticoagulants as ordered to establish normal viscosity, but not heart failure.
  iv. Monitor fluid status with intake and output measurements, and weights.
  v. Gradually increase physical activity while monitoring cardiac tolerance of increased workload.
c. Desired outcome
  i. Normal BP, heart sounds, and jugular venous pulsations.
  ii. Normal volume and bilaterally equal peripheral pulses.

6. Potential for infection due to decreased circulation related to sickle cells in vasculature
  a. Problem: Vascular occlusion by sickle cells leads to stagnant blood flow and a tendency for microorganisms to cause infection.
  b. Intervention
    i. Guard against infections by limiting invasive technologies, turning frequently and encouraging coughing, screening visitors, maintaining personal hygiene, and performing frequent oral care.
    ii. When the patient is febrile, perform a total body assessment and perform urine, sputum, blood, and cultures of the mouth, anus, nose as ordered to identify potential sources of infection.
  c. Desired outcome
    i. Patient afebrile and has negative cultures.

7. Potential for bleeding due to microvascular thromboses that deplete coagulation factors and cause vessel rupture
  a. Problem: Vascular occlusion and increased pressure will cause ruptured microvessels initially, but as more clotting factors are required to repair ruptured vessels, there is a risk of coagulopathy and a bleeding tendency.
  b. Intervention
    i. Monitor coagulation tests (prothrombin time [PT], partial thromboplastin time [PTT], fibrinogen, platelet count).
    ii. Administer coagulation products as ordered (see blood product transfusions in "Life-threatening Coagulopathies," p. 191).
    iii. Avoid invasive procedures when possible.
    iv. Administer anticoagulants cautiously.
    v. Hold pressure on a venipuncture site for at least 5 minutes.
    vi. Examine body for demarcated areas of cyanosis or frank necrosis.
    vii. Use topical remedies for bleeding as needed (eg, absorbable gelatin sponge [Gelfoam], topical thrombin).
    viii. Maintain good oral hygiene to prevent gum bleeding.
  c. Desired outcome
    i. Patient has no bleeding.

Life-threatening Coagulopathies

I. Definition: Disorders of coagulation in the critically ill may encompass a large number of potential etiologies and pathophysiologic effects. Disorders of quantity or quality of coagulation components will affect the body's ability to appropriately achieve hemostasis. With inadequate hemostasis, bleeding or life-threatening hemorrhage can occur.

II. Etiology: Using the pattern of coagulation, one can predict that disorders of hemostasis can occur at any one of the four coagulation processes of (1) vasoconstriction of local vessels to prevent blood loss, (2) platelet plug formation, (3) formation of a fibrin clot, or (4) lysis of an existing clot. An overview of the disorders which cause inadequate clotting included in Tables 8.2 and 8.3.

III. Nursing process

A. Assessment
   1. Signs and symptoms
      a. Petechiae, ecchymoses are tiny purple-red dots (petechiae) or bruises (ecchymoses) indicating capillary bleeding. They signify microvascular

Table 8.2 Platelet Disorder Etiologies

Bone marrow suppression
  Aplastic anemia
  Burns
  Cancer chemotherapy
  Exposure to ionizing radiation
  Nutritional deficiency (vitamin B12, folate)

Platelet destruction outside bone marrow
  Heat stroke
  Heart valves
  Heparin
  Infections: severe or sepsis
  Large-bore IV lines—eg, intra-aortic balloon pump
  Splenic sequestration of platelets
  Sulfonamides
  Transfusions
  Trimethoprim sulfamethoxazole

Immune response against platelets
  Idiopathic thrombocytopenia purpura
  Mononucleosis
  Thrombotic thrombocytopenia purpura
  Vaccinations
  Viral illness

Interference with platelet production (other than nonspecific marrow suppression)
  Alcohol
  Histamine 2 blocking agents
  Histoplasmosis
  Hormones
  Thiazide diuretics

Interference with platelet function
  Aminoglycosides
  Catecholamines—eg, epinephrine, dopamine
  Cirrhosis of the liver
  Dextran
  Diabetes mellitus
  Hypothermia
  Loop diuretics—eg, furosemide
  Malignant lymphomas
  Nonsteroidal anti-inflammatory agents
  Phenothiazines
  Salicylate derivatives
  Sarcoidosis
  Scleroderma
  Systemic lupus erythematosus
  Thyrotoxicosis
  Tricyclic antidepressants
  Uremia
  Vitamin E

Table 8.3 Coagulopathies

	Platelet Disorder	Hepatic Coagulation Protein Disorder	Disseminated Intravascular Coagulation
Definition	Thrombocytopenia—a reduced number of circulating and functional platelets for use in the body's clotting mechanism Immune thrombocytopenia—immunologic destruction of platelets after leaving the bone marrow. May be due to autoantibodies (immune thrombocytopenia purpura [ITP]), medication interference, or abnormal splenic sequestration	The liver is the production site of all coagulation proteins except factor VIII. When significant liver disease or malabsorption of vitamin K necessary for some protein production occurs, there is a failure to produce an adequate supply of functional coagulation proteins. Without coagulation proteins, a fibrin clot is not formed, and bleeding will go unchecked. Patients with hepatic-induced coagulopathies may have an intact platelet plug, but after the platelet plug dissolves, bleeding from the injured site will occur.	In normal circumstances, the clotting system is triggered by tissue injury, vessel injury, or a foreign body in the bloodstream. Hemostasis and fibrinolysis balance each other to produce a state of equilibrium between clot formation and dissolution. In severe disease, the stimulus to clot is overwhelming and does not remit, which leads to excess stimulation of clotting. This massive microvasculature clotting is the predominant feature; however, the clotting depletes coagulation factors, shears RBCs, and leads to fibrin clot breakdown products (fibrin degradation products [FDPs]) that all serve to increase the bleeding tendency. Thrombosed vessels also have a tendency to rupture, and depleted coagulation factors are unable to stave the flow of blood from the site (see Figure 8.1)
Etiology	See Table 8.2	Most common—liver disease. Central lobar damage such as seen with hepatitis, late cirrhosis, and end-stage hepatic disease must occur before coagulopathies are evident. Anticoagulant medications (eg, heparin, warfarin) achieve their therapeutic action through interference with these coagulation proteins; therefore, overtreatment with these medications may induce bleeding symptoms. Gastrointestinal malabsorption syndromes or limited oral intake diminish the amount of vitamin K absorbed from the GI tract and results in insufficient production of the vitamin K-dependent coagulation factors with a bleeding tendency.	Sepsis Trauma Burns Surgery, especially abdominal or prostate surgery Cancer Obstetric emergencies—amniotic fluid embolism, postpartum hemorrhage, eclampsia, HELLP syndrome Foreign bodies in the bloodstream—eg, fat embolism, sickle cell crisis

Etiology (cont.)	Certain broad-spectrum antibiotics destroy the normal GI flora that aid in vitamin K absorption, leading to coagulopathies (eg, beta-lactam antibiotics)		
Patho-physiol-ogy	Platelets may not be made adequately or normally signaling a bone marrow disease such as aplastic anemia, leukemia, or radiation injury to the marrow. Platelets may also be abnormally destroyed or rendered dysfunctional after leaving the marrow. Platelet problems are evident in capillary injury and early after injury, since the first line of coagulation after injury to the vessel has occurred	Lack of production of coagulation proteins results in the body's inability to form a stable fibrin clot after the platelet plug has dissolved. Initial platelet response may be adequate, but rebleeding will occur after the platelet plug dissolves in 20 min–2 h	
Signs/ Symp-toms	Petechiae Ecchymoses Occult blood in excrement Micro-organ hemorrhages—eg, kidneys—renal failure, brain—intracranial bleeds Mucous membrane bleeding—eg, oral cavity, urine Spontaneous infiltrative hemorrhage (especially dependent areas)—retroperitoneal, alveolar, intracerebral	Initial hemostasis with rebleeding from site of injury Occult blood in excrement Discrete bleeding from sites of injury (eg, a vessel punctured in earlier attempt to draw blood, small ulcerations in GI tract) May be asymptomatic in rare cases where no potential bleeding sites exist	Thrombotic presentation is usually earliest symptomatology—eg, oliguria, cyanosis, hypoxia, cardiac ischemia, deep vein thrombosis (DVT), altered level of consciousness Bleeding symptoms occur later in the process once clots have been made and are dissolving—eg, hematuria, GI bleeding, alveolar hemorrhage, intracranial bleeding, bleeding from every orifice and injured skin surface Symptoms of cell turnover such as jaundice or increased BUN vary among patients

Table 8.3 *Continued*

	Platelet Disorder	Hepatic Coagulation Protein Disorder	Disseminated Intravascular Coagulation
Diagnostic tests	Decreased platelet count Decreased platelet survival Prolonged bleeding time Positive platelet autoantibody	Prolonged prothrombin time (PT) Prolonged partial thromboplastin time (PTT) Prolonged thrombin time (TT) Decreased fibrinogen level	Decreased platelet count Prolonged PT Prolonged PTT Prolonged TT Decreased fibrinogen level Elevated fibrin degradation products Elevated D-dimer fibrin degradation product Decreased antithrombin III levels
Comments	Thrombocytopenia is the most common coagulation defect in the ICU Platelet are fragile cells easily damaged by a variety of problems experienced by ICU patients (eg, fever, dialysis filters, large-bore catheters, prosthetic heart valves)	Coagulation protein deficiencies are a late manifestation of most hepatic diseases Some anticoagulant medications that cause abnormalities in the coagulation cascade may be reversed by specific reversal agents, vitamin K, or administration of fresh frozen plasma Bleeding that persists despite replenishment of platelets and normalization of PT may require factor VIII replacement (cryoprecipitate), since this factor is not made by the liver	The most common causes of this syndrome are (1) sepsis, (2) trauma, (3) burns Mortality rate exceeds 50% Frequently occurs concomitantly with adult respiratory distress syndrome (ARDS) (it is uncertain which syndrome triggers which) May be acute or chronic symptomatology—slow tissue injury such as with malignancy more frequently presents with chronic symptoms Treatment of underlying etiology is essential for recovery Replacement of lost blood components essential while awaiting the patient's improvement

bleeding in the soft tissue. They may occur with minor injury, dependent pressure (eg, lying on area), or gravitational pressure (eg, limb hanging below body) in fragile vessels with inadequate coagulation factors.

b. Overt bleeding from wounds, body orifices, and around existing tubes occurs immediately if platelets are inadequate, since the platelet plug is the first step of the clotting cascade. Bleeding that is delayed 20 minutes to 2 hours indicates coagulation protein deficit. In many severe disorders, spontaneous and continuous bleeding occurs from open vessels.

c. Enlarged and tender liver or spleen is an indication that abnormal or fragmented cells are being captured by these organs. Excess removal can be a normal compensatory mechanism when there are cell fragments such as with massive thromboses.

d. Oliguria occurs when the microvasculature of the kidneys are thrombosed or ruptured, and the compromised blood flow to the kidneys causes slowed glomerular filtration.

e. Occult or overt bleeding in excrement (urine, feces, emesis): The mucous membranes of the body have capillaries close to the surface and, hence, are the earliest to bleed when coagulation mechanisms are inadequate. Bleeding may be occult and only detected by laboratory exam, or obvious. The mucous membranes of the body which tend to bleed include: nasopharynx, oral mucosa, GI tract, urinary tract, and the upper airways.

2. Diagnostic parameters are dependent upon the specific disorder of coagulation. Table 8.3 outlines distinctive diagnostic tests that are unique to each disorder.

    a. Serum tests

        i. Decreased hematocrit (HCT) and hemoglobin will occur with all coagulation disorders when a sufficient amount of blood is lost to demonstrate a functional anemia.

    b. Urine tests

        i. Guaiac positive test of urine: There is blood in the urine in most coagulation disorders, since the mucous membranes are the most sensitive to bleeding when there is coagulation deficit.

    c. Other tests

        i. None

B. Patient management

    1. Potential for bleeding related to low platelet count, decreased platelet quality, hepatic coagulation defects, or DIC

    a. Problem: Coagulopathies increase the risk of spontaneous bleeding as well as bleeding related to injury. The nature of the bleeding may be predicted based on the etiology, but severity is more dependent upon extent of the coagulation deficit and type of injury.

    b. Interventions

        i. Implement bleeding prevention strategies such as keep the head of bed elevated, avoid medications that induce coagulopathies (eg, aspirin), limit invasive procedures, pad bedrails and allow patient out of bed only with assistance and padding, avoid rectal procedures, maintain oral hygiene, or keep nares and lips softened.

   ii. Ensure that there is a stable blood-drawing access to avoid unnecessary venipunctures.

  iii. Use automatic BP cuff and clip on oxumeter probes cautiously to prevent injury.

  iv. Monitor all excrement for occult blood.

   v. Examine body (including cavities) every shift for bleeding, bruising, or petechiae.

  vi. Administer topical hemostatic agents when procedures must be performed.

 vii. Use paper tape and skin barrier on skin to prevent skin tears and bleeding.

viii. Administer blood components as ordered and monitor for transfusion reactions (Table 8.4) [1].

  ix. Monitor HCT, hemoglobin, RBC, platelets, PT, PTT, fibrinogen, fibrin degradation products, D-dimer, thrombin time as ordered.

   x. Estimate blood losses through excrement or exsanguination. If blood loss looks significant, run an HCT on drainage.

  xi. Monitor volume status (intake and output, central venous pressure) and blood pressure when actively bleeding to detect symptoms of hypovolemic shock.

  c. Desired outcome

    i. Have absence of bleeding.

   ii. Stable HCT and hemoglobin.

  iii. Normal coagulation studies.

2. Altered tissue perfusion due to intravascular clotting with ischemia, or rupture of vessels with hemorrhage

  a. Problem: In DIC, the etiology of bleeding is actually an excessive clotting stimulus that causes extensive microvascular clotting that depletes clotting factors to lead to bleeding (Fig. 8.1) [2]. Ischemic tissue injury is a common problem in this disorder. Other bleeding disorders will cause ischemic tissue damage when a large pocket of blood collects in a confined space and applies pressure to the normal tissue in the area.

  b. Interventions

    i. Maintain vascular volume with IV fluids and blood products.

   ii. Avoid vasoconstricting situations as much as possible (eg, excessive cold, overdiuresis, vasopressor agents).

  iii. Administer vasodilating agents if ordered (eg, nitroglycerin).

  iv. Administer renal dose dopamine (2–4 μg/kg per minute) through central venous access if ordered to improve renal perfusion.

   v. Monitor urine output and report output less than intake.

  vi. Administer heparin 100–800 U/h if ordered to stop the thrombotic stage of DIC. This therapy is rarely used if the patient has begun to display symptoms of bleeding.

Table 8.4 Blood Products

Blood Product	Description	Indications	Administration	Special Considerations
Whole blood	One 500-mL unit contains approximately 200 mL RBCs and 300 mL plasma	Massive blood loss Exchange transfusions	Large-gauge needle for administration Use 0.9% normal saline for starter fluid and flush Use blood administration set with filter pore size of 170 μm	Be certain blood is ABO and Rh compatible Monitor patient for fluid volume overload
Packed red blood cells	One 250-mL unit contains 200 mL RBCs and 50 mL plasma	Low hematocrit Inadequate oxygen-carrying capacity	Same as with whole blood, but surface area of filter may be larger to increase infusion rate	Be certain blood is ABO and Rh compatible Administer within 30 minutes of receipt
Washed red blood cells, buffy cells, leukocyte-poor cells	One 200-mL unit contains 50 mL normal saline solution and has few platelets or leukocytes	History of febrile or allergic blood reactions	Same as with whole blood but micro-aggregate filter is not necessary	Blood comes in special bag and connections are not as tight Premedication with Tylenol or Benadryl may be recommended
Frozen diglycerized RBCs	One 200-mL unit contains 50 mL normal saline; washed free of most WBCs and platelets	Rare blood types Special needs for oxygen-rich blood, as noncitrate preservative conserves 2,3-DPG better	Same as with red blood cells	Thawing process takes approximately 1 h Blood reactions should be decreased, but consult physician about premedication
Plasma (fresh, fresh-frozen, single-donor)	One 200- to 300-mL unit of fresh-frozen plasma contains all coagulation factors plus 400 mg fibrinogen; single-donor plasma contains less of factors V and VII	Coagulation deficiencies Dysfibrino-genemia Liver disease	Allow 45 minutes for plasma to thaw May infuse rapidly Smaller needle size may be used Microaggregate filter is not used	ABO compatibility is necessary, but Rh compatibility is not Administer within 6 h of thawing Febrile, allergic reactions are possible

Table 8.4 *Continued*

Blood Product	Description	Indications	Administration	Special Considerations
Platelets	35–50-mL unit contains 7 × 10^7 platelets	Thrombocyto-penia and thrombo-cytopathies Bone marrow aplasia	Use special platelet filter (not micro-aggregate) Administer 100 mL over approximately 15 minutes	ABO and Rh compatibility not necessary Febrile and aller-gic reactions are common Obtain post-platelet count to monitor effectiveness

From Shelton, B. K. Life-threatening coagulopathies and thrombotic disease. In J. E. Wright and B. K. Shelton (eds.), *Desk Reference for Critical Care Nursing*. Boston: Jones & Bartlett, 1993. P. 1181.

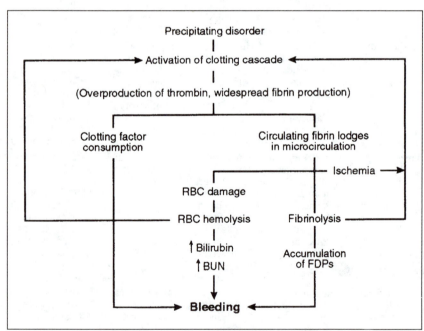

Figure 8.1 Pathophysiology of DIC. (From Shelton, B. K. Disorders of hemostasis in sepsis. *Crit Care Nurs Clin of North Am* 6:378, 1994.)

    vii. Assess patient every shift for symptoms of focal circulatory deficits. These are noted by demarcation cyanosis or blackness of a peripheral skin segment (eg, toes, fingers, earlobes), mottling of one extremity, or absent or greatly diminished pulses in one extremity.

c. Desired outcome
   i. Patient displays normal pink, warm skin, with equal pulses.
   ii. Normal urine output.
3. Altered body image due to bleeding, bruising, or hematoma formation
   a. Problem: Vascular occlusion and tendencies to bleed can cause cyanosis, extensive subcutaneous tissue bleeding, or overt bleeding; purplish bruising in all body areas, edema with purplish discoloration, petechiae, bleeding from every orifice or puncture site, bloody urine, bloody stool, bloody tears. Patients or their families may be very distressed regarding these changes in body image.
   b. Intervention
      i. Provide patient and/or family with an idea of expected changes that may occur with these disorders.
      ii. Be sensitive to nursing interventions that may worsen these symptoms. Avoid the following:
         - Automatic BP cuff.
         - Trendelenburg positioning.
         - Use of nonelectric razors.
         - Intramuscular (IM) or subcutaneous injections.
         - Rectal procedures (eg, temperatures) and medications.
         - Constipation or straining during defecation.
         - Dry mucous membranes of the nose and mouth.
         - Hard-bristled toothbrush.
      iii. Reassure patient and family that the blood in the subcutaneous tissue will be reabsorbed as the patient gets better.
      iv. Encourage family to participate in providing comfort measures and pressure on bleeding sites.
   c. Desired outcome
      i. Patient prepared for the body image changes that may occur with bleeding disorders.
      ii. Ecchymoses resolve.
4. Potential fluid volume deficit due to hemorrhage
   a. Problem: Blood lost through micro- and macrovascular bleeding will deplete blood volume as well as produce a deficit of coagulation components.
   b. Interventions
      i. Monitor fluid status through intake and output measurements.
      ii. Monitor vascular volume through central venous pressures, orthostatic vital signs, and jugular venous pulsations.
      iii. Obtain daily weights to compare to intake and output records.
      iv. Administer isotonic IV fluids (eg, Ringer's solution, normal saline) or blood products to replenish lost vascular volume.
   c. Desired outcome
      i. Normal blood pressure, central venous pressure, and stable weights.
5. Altered sensory perception (eg, vision) due to bleeding
   a. Problem: Thrombosis (in DIC) and bleeding occur in the microvasculature of the retina, particularly if accompanied by hypertension. These

hemorrhages alter visual acuity and may cause temporary or permanent visual deficits.

b. Interventions

    i. Assess visual sensation every shift in awake patients.

    ii. Presume visual deficits in the disoriented patient, and provide verbal descriptions of all nursing care behaviors and personnel who enter the room.

    iii. Note ophthalmic findings and communicate with peers regarding the patient's status.

    iv. Explain to family why the patient may be unable to focus his or her vision when spoken to.

c. Desired outcome

    i. Normal visual acuity.

References

1. Shelton, B. K. Life-threatening coagulopathies and thrombolytic disease. In J. E. Wright and B. K. Shelton (eds.), *Desk Reference for Critical Care Nursing*. Boston: Jones & Bartlett, 1993. P. 1181.
2. Shelton, B. K. Disorders of hemostasis in sepsis. *Critical Care Nurs Clin North Am* 6:378, 1994.

CHAPTER 9

Immunologic Disorders

Brenda Shelton

The immune system is the body system responsible for recognizing and destroying invading pathogens (bacteria, fungi, viruses, parasites) and mutant cells (cancer). When both specific and nonspecific immunity is intact, there are three major levels of immune response. The first level of defense is barrier immunity, which includes physical, microbial, and chemical deterrents to pathogen entry. When barrier immunity is breached, the second line of defense is activated and includes nonspecific granulocyte reactions called phagocytosis and complement immunity. The third defensive weapon of the body is specific immunity conferred by antibodies produced by B lymphocytes (humoral immunity) or cytokines (cell killer substances) secreted by T lymphocytes (cellular immunity). Immunologic disorders include those of hyperactivity of the immune system or suppression of its function. A more complete listing of immune disorders and their clinical manifestations are outlined in Table 9.1 [1].

Immune hyperactivity may be the result of uncontrolled nonspecific inflammatory disease or of excess stimulation of antibodies or cytokines. The two most common disorders of hyperactivity, which are described in this chapter, are anaphylaxis and autoimmune disease. Anaphylaxis involves abnormal antibody production to a naturally occurring substance such as pollen, which does not generally cause immune activity. Anaphylactic reactions may be true antibody production (IgE type) or may have similar symptoms without a clear etiology (anaphylactoid). Anaphylaxis has an acute onset, but it has rapid resolution if the etiologic factor is removed. Patients are often treated effectively without requiring intensive care unit (ICU) admission. Autoimmune diseases are syndromes in which the body detects normal body tissue as foreign and creates autoantibodies that destroy the normal tissue. Examples of autoimmune diseases include glomerulonephritis, idiopathic autoimmune thrombocytopenia purpura, immune hemolytic anemia, systemic lupus erythematosus (SLE), and rheumatoid arthritis. The clinical manifestations of autoimmune disease vary according to the target tissue involved, although progression of many of these syndromes affects other body tissues. This chapter provides detail on the nursing care of patients with anaphylaxis and "immune complex diseases." Because immunosuppressive medications are used in the management of these diseases, there are some similar nursing problems in the care of patients with either hyperactive immune system disorders or immunosuppression.

Table 9.1 Overview of Clinical Immunodeficiencies

Disease	Clinical Manifestations	Defect	Therapy
Humoral			
Bruton's hypogammaglobulinemia	Recurrent pyogenic infections, especially pneumonia, sinusitis, otitis, furunculosis, meningitis, sepsis, panhypogammaglobulinemia, arthritis of the large joints	Decreased IgA, IgG, IgM; no plasma cells; low number of B cells; pre-B cells present	Aggressive, appropriate, and judicious use of antibiotics
Selective IgA deficiency	Bacterial infections of respiratory tract, GI tract, and GU tract; diarrhea; malabsorption; increased autoimmune disease	Synthesis but no secretion of IgA, high circulating anti-IgA antibody	Immune serum globulin (except in IgA deficiency)
Common variable immunodeficiency (acquired)	Recurrent pyogenic infections similar to Bruton's but less severe; malabsorption, diarrhea, giardiasis, increased lymphoreticular malignancies	Normal number of circulating B cells; low immunoglobulin levels, no plasma cells	Plasma transfusions
Cellular			
DiGeorge's syndrome	Thymic hypoplasia, hypocalcemia, parathyroid hypoplasia, otitis, tuberculosis, *Candida*, abnormal facies, congenital cardiac anomalies, chronic diarrhea, failure to thrive, esophageal atresia	Deficient T cells; thymic and parathyroid hypoplasia; often increase in B cells	Treatment of infections, tumors, and symptoms Immunologic reconstitution: bone marrow transplant, fetal thymus transplant, lymphocyte transfusion Immunologic enhancement: thymosin, transfer factor, interleukin 2
Chronic mucocutaneous candidiasis	Chronic, resistant C. *albicans* infection of skin, nails, and mucous membranes; some endocrine abnormalities	Normal number of T cells, but failure of T cells to respond to antigen by production of lymphokine	Same as above
AIDS (acquired)	Kaposi's sarcoma, opportunistic infections (*Pneumocystis carinii, Candida*, toxoplasmosis, mycobacteria)	Decrease in number and/or function of T4 subset; reverse T4/T8 ratio; abnormalities in B cell function, NK cell function, and monocyte function	Same as above

Combined			
Severe combined immunodeficiency	Multiple severe infections of many kinds (bacterial, fungal, and viral); graft-vs-host disease; diarrhea; extreme wasting	Low T cells; low B cells; no antibody	Careful, early treatment of infections Protective isolation ISG, bone marrow, and fetal thymus transplants
Wiskott-Aldrich syndrome	Thrombocytopenia with hemorrhagic tendency, eczema, recurrent infection, herpes, and high increase in lymphoreticular malignancy	Hypercatabolism of immunoglobulins; low IgM and IgG with high IgA and E; decreased T cells	Fetal liver transplants
Phagocytic			
Chronic granulomatous disease	Marked lymphadenopathy with draining lymph nodes, hepatosplenomegaly, recurrent pneumonias, abscesses, dermatitis, conjunctivitis, osteomyelitis, usually with unusual organisms of low virulence (*Staphylococcus aureus*, *S. epidermidis*, *Escherichia coli*, *Candida*, *Aspergillus*)	Abnormal neutrophil function with decreased intracellular killing because of enzyme deficiency (NADH or NADPH oxidase)	Surgical drainage or excision Broad-spectrum antibiotics Amphotericin B White cell transfusions
Job's (hyper-IgE) syndrome	Recurrent "cold" abscesses of skin, lymph nodes, and subcutaneous tissue; eczema; otitis media	Abnormal chemotaxis, increased eosinophils, increased IgE, abnormal antibody synthesis	Same as above
Chediak-Higashi syndrome	Recurrent cutaneous bacterial infections; hepatosplenomegaly; partial albinism; progressive CNS abnormality; increased lymphoreticular malignancy	Defective neutrophil and monocyte chemotaxis and delayed neutrophil killing time	Same as above

Table 9.1 Overview of Clinical Immunodeficiencies (*Continued*)

Disease	Clinical Manifestations	Defect	Therapy
Complement			
Selective complement deficiencies	Multiple, serious pyogenic infections; immune complex disease (ie, glomerulonephritis)	Decreased ability to opsonize bacteria; decreased chemotaxis; decreased cytolysis; decreased ability to clear immune complexes	Aggressive, appropriate antibiotic therapy Fresh frozen plasma
Hereditary angioedema	Episodic edema of throat, abdomen, face	Decreased C1 esterase inhibitor	Anabolic steroids and fibrinolytic agents
Secondary immunodeficiency			
Due to disease, injury, or treatment	Increased susceptibility to infection, malignancy, autoimmune phenomena	Variable—most commonly, decrease in number of neutrophils	Protection from infection Treatment of cause, if possible Early detection and appropriate treatment of infections

From Allen, M. A. The Immune System. In J. E. Wright and B. K. Shelton (eds.). *Desk Reference for Critical Care Nursing*. Boston: Jones & Bartlett, 1993. Pp. 1092–1094.

Suppression of the immune systems of the body is a common problem in the intensive care setting. The clinical consequences of inadequate immune function depends on the immune activity being altered. For example, compromised nonspecific function is more likely to result in bacterial infections. Abnormalities in specific immunity result in abnormal antibody protection, viral or opportunistic infections, and cancer. Many physiologic states alter one or several of these immunologic processes. This chapter describes in detail the key characteristics of neutropenia, T-lymphocyte suppression (as with immunosuppression after transplantation or human immunodeficiency virus [HIV] infection), and cancer.

Anaphylaxis

I. Definition: This is an acute generalized hypersensitivity reaction in which the immunologic cells and mediator substances that normally respond to foreign proteins are uncontrolled and disproportionate to the antigen presented. Anaphylaxis presents as one of four patterns: immediate onset, delayed onset (hours to days after antigen exposure), biphasic (immediate symptoms followed by improvement before subsequent worsening), and protracted anaphylaxis (not resolved with initial interventions). The resulting cardiopulmonary effects of distributive shock occur due to an excess inflammatory response.

II. Etiology: Excess inflammatory mediators are often triggered by production of an antigen-specific immunoglobulin of the IgE subtype. The widespread inflammatory mediators are triggered by stimulation of specialized immunologic cells such as basophils and mast cells. Cell reactivity may be activated by presence of IgE or by immune complex formation. It is important to note that since the disorder is chiefly stimulated by preexisting antibody, the first exposure may not in fact produce the most severe symptoms; instead, symptoms tend to worsen with each subsequent exposure.

The majority of life-threatening episodes of anaphylaxis are related to insect venom, penicillin-derivative antimicrobials, and food substances; however, there are as many other possible etiologies as there are items to which one might be allergic. Any substance that produces allergy can result in anaphylactic reactions with some individuals. In fact, some individuals develop anaphylaxis to exercise or unidentified self-substances. The most likely etiologies of anaphylactic reactions are listed in Table 9.2.

When inflammatory mediator substances are released intravascularly, the consequence is widespread large vessel vasodilation, pulmonary vasoconstriction and bronchoconstriction, and capillary permeability.

III. Nursing process

  A. Assessment

    1. Signs and symptoms

      a. Anxiety, restlessness, and agitation occur due to intense air hunger and the uncomfortable sensation of breathing through spastic airways.

      b. Dyspnea, wheezing, cough with or without sputum, and chest tightness are reflections of the bronchospasm and stimulation of mucus production that occurs due to inflammatory mediators.

Table 9.2 Etiologies of Anaphylaxis

Environmental
   Exercise
   Seminal fluid
Venom
   Ant bites
   Bee stings
   Mosquito bites
   Scorpion bites
   Spider bites
Food
   Egg whites
   Peanuts
   Shellfish
   Tree nuts
   Grains
   Seeds
   Cottonseed oil
   Preservatives
Medications/Diagnostic agents
   Anesthetics
   Antimicrobials
   Cytotoxic agents
   Dextran
   Nonsteroidal anti-inflammatory agents
   Opiates
   Vitamins
Biologic agents
   Biotherapy
   Blood products
   Hormones

c. Hypotension, particularly with low diastolic BP, occurs as a result of the inflammatory mediators' effect on the vasculature. They cause vasodilation, which lowers the diastolic BP and expands the vascular pool, causing a decrease in mean arterial pressure (MAP) or perfusion pressure.

d. Dysrhythmias, especially sinus or supraventricular tachycardia, are the result of excess sympathetic nervous system stimulation that occurs from the stress response.

e. Erythema, warmth, and hyperthermia, followed by cool, clammy extremities reflect the vasodilatory phase of increased blood flow that is caused by inflammatory mediators and followed by cool, poorly perfused and oxygenated extremities as the oxygen deficit worsens.

f. Urticaria, pruritus, and angioedema occur due to histamine and other inflammatory mediator release. Angioedema is particularly prominent in the face, but it may occur throughout the body due to a capillary permeability syndrome seen in inflammatory responses.

g. Nausea, vomiting, abdominal cramping, and diarrhea occur because of smooth muscle contraction.

2. Diagnostic parameters
   a. Serum tests
      i. IgE antibody.
   b. Urine tests
      i. None.
   c. Other tests
      i. Arterial blood gases initially show respiratory alkalosis with mild to moderate hypoxemia as the patient compensates with tachypnea to achieve oxygenation. This becomes respiratory acidosis with moderate to severe hypoxemia as the condition worsens and the patient is unable to effectively inhale or exhale through bronchospastic airways.

B. Patient management
   1. Altered gas exchange related to pulmonary vasoconstriction and bronchoconstriction
      a. Problem: Bronchoconstriction and vasoconstriction in the lungs decrease the ability to ventilate effectively, to exchange oxygen at the tissue level, and to exhale carbon dioxide.
      b. Interventions
         i. Administer oxygen therapy as ordered to achieve a PaO_2 greater than 60 mm Hg and oxygen saturation greater than 90%.
         ii. Position patient in high Fowler or reverse Trendelenburg position to permit maximal chest excursion with breathing.
         iii. Auscultate breath sounds frequently and within 10–15 minutes after every intervention to determine effectiveness in alleviation of symptoms.
         iv. Administer bronchodilator therapy via nebulizer for immediate bronchodilation.
         v. Administer ordered sympathomimetics (eg, subcutaneous epinephrine 1:1000 concentration 0.4–1.0 mg) to bronchodilate and block mediators.
         vi. Administer rapid-acting corticosteroid (eg, hydrocortisone 100 mg or dexamethasone 2–10 mg) to counteract pulmonary inflammation.
         vii. Remove restraining clothing to permit maximum ventilation.
         viii. Provide emotional support and/or sedation to decrease oxygen consumption and enhance efficacy of breathing pattern.
      c. Desired outcomes
         i. PaO_2 greater than 60 mm Hg on arterial blood gas analysis (ABG).
         ii. PcO_2 less than 45 mm Hg on ABG.
         iii. Clear breath sounds on auscultation.
         iv. No difficulty breathing.
   2. Altered tissue perfusion related to cardiovascular collapse and mediator activity
      a. Problem: Mediators released during the inflammatory process cause severe vasodilation and perfusion deficit. Dysrhythmia or congestive heart failure occurs due to sympathetic stimulation.

    b. Interventions

        i. Administer fluids to dilute toxins causing reaction and to expand vascular volume to increase BP in dilated vessels.

        ii. Administer sympathomimetics (epinephrine) subcutaneously to counteract mast cell degranulation and generation of mediators. Monitor for increased dysrhythmias or chest discomfort due to myocardial ischemia.

        iii. Provide cardiac monitoring to detect dysrhythmias and invasive or noninvasive blood pressure monitoring to note early symptoms of response to interventions or worsening of condition.

        iv. Administer vasopressor agents as ordered for refractory hypotension. Dopamine (see Table 5.1) may be used, but if tachycardia is present, phenylephrine (Neosynephrine), a pure alpha stimulant, may be used to decrease the adverse effects on heart rate.

    c. Desired outcome

        i. BP within normal limits for patient

        ii. Skin warm and dry

        iii. Peripheral pulses strong and equal bilaterally

3. Anxiety related to difficulty breathing, possible chest discomfort

    a. Problem: Severe air hunger, chest tightness, and oxygen deprivation in a patient leads to anxiety that worsens the condition.

    b. Interventions

        i. Position patient comfortably.

        ii. Permit visitors to stay and comfort patient if they are emotionally stable.

        iii. Reassure patient that although symptoms are severe, there are medications that will relieve them.

        iv. Prepare the patient for expected adverse effects of therapy, such as palpitations or headache.

        v. Administer oxygen if patient feels subjective relief of symptoms, even if oxygenation does not improve.

        vi. Administer ordered sedatives or antianxiety agents to calm patient. While opiates bronchodilate, they also enhance histamine (a mediator) release and, thus, should be avoided if possible.

    c. Desired outcome

        i. Patient verbalizes relief of discomfort.

        ii. Patient appears to be physiologically and emotionally coping with anaphylactic reaction.

        iii. Patient is visibly less anxious and agitated.

4. Altered comfort from rash, itching, edema, difficulty breathing, tachycardia, abdominal discomfort

    a. Problem: There are multiple symptoms that negatively affect coping because the patient is uncomfortable. Symptomatic support reduces the anxiety-related component of the patient's oxygen deficit.

    b. Interventions

        i. Provide cool environment to enhance breathing and decrease feeling of warmth.

        ii. Administer cool compresses as needed to promote comfort.

    iii. Administer H_1 blockers such as diphenhydramine, as ordered, to counteract itching, rash, and the mast cell degranulation that perpetuates reaction.

    iv. Administer H_2 blockers (eg, cimetidine, ranitidine) to halt mast cell degranulation and release of histamine. (Theoretical benefits of these agents are not proven.)

    v. Administer mentholated or corticosteroid creams to decrease itching and inflammation.

    vi. Position patient in high Fowler or reverse Trendelenburg position to permit maximal chest excursion with breathing.

    vii. Apply warm pad to abdomen for relief of cramping.

  c. Desired outcome

    i. Patient verbalizes comfort.

    ii. Absence of edema, redness, and pruritus

5. Altered elimination related to GI distress

  a. Problem: Smooth muscle contraction leads to increased bowel motility, with cramping and diarrhea.

  b. Interventions

    i. Provide bedside commode during acute event.

    ii. Reassure patient that this is an expected effect of the reaction and will subside as the condition improves.

    iii. Measure intake and output and ensure fluid replacement for lost fluids.

    iv. Monitor electrolyte values for losses and replace as ordered.

  c. Desired outcome

    i. Normal fluid and electrolyte balance

    ii. Absence of abdominal discomfort

    iii. Normal stool pattern

6. Altered health maintenance

  a. Problem: Patients who experience anaphylaxis, especially to normal environmental substances, must alter their lifestyles to avoid these stimuli. In addition, for 24–72 hours after the event, patients must alter their physical activity to prevent recurrence of symptoms.

  b. Interventions

    i. Ensure that patient obtains and can administer self-care with an anaphylaxis kit.

    ii. Advise patient on how to avoid antigens that trigger anaphylaxis.

    iii. Refer patient to vendor for Medic Alert bracelets and cards.

    iv. Inform patient of need for the next 72 hours to avoid warm showers, saunas or whirlpools, exercise, or other activities that cause vasodilation.

    v. Be certain a follow-up appointment is made with medical staff and/or visiting nurses for within 1–3 days of anaphylaxis episode.

    vi. Assist patient in obtaining prescriptions for H_1 and H_2 blockers and steroids to last about 24 hours after anaphylaxis episode.

    vii. Advise patients who have had reactions to contrast media to obtain premedication as needed for future radiologic and nuclear studies.

      c. Desired outcomes

          i. Patient vocalizes understanding of allergens, reaction(s) to them, and appropriate emergency measures to be instituted if exposed.

          ii. Patient wears identification regarding allergic reactions.

Autoimmune Disease

I. Definition: The term *autoimmune disease* is derived from the antigen-antibody reactions that occur when the body's humoral defense system (B-lymphocyte production of antibodies) determines that normal self-proteins are foreign and a rejection phenomenon occurs. "Auto" and "immune" are joined to describe the immune reaction against self.

Autoimmune disorders are classified by the organ specificity of the reaction and the exact mechanisms of immunologic rejection. Autoimmune diseases are categorized as organ specific if their tissue destruction is confined to the target organ; major disease manifestations occur when body tissue is rejected. For example, interstitial nephritis causes destruction of the glomerular basement membrane and results in renal failure. Other examples of these disorders include Graves' disease, type I diabetes mellitus, autoimmune hemolytic anemia, and Goodpasture's syndrome. Non–organ-specific disorders have antigen-antibody immune complexes that circulate freely in the serum and lodge in a variety of tissues before causing immunologic tissue destruction. The clinical manifestations of organ nonspecific disorders such as SLE, rheumatoid arthritis, and sarcoidosis are multisystem organ dysfunction.

II. Etiology: The exact etiologic mechanisms of autoimmune disease are unclear, but many of these disorders are linked to recent viral infection, immune stimulation such as pregnancy, or a genetic predisposition for immune disease. The consequence of immune stimulation is development of inappropriate antibody. Tissue damage occurs by one of five mechanisms: (1) direct blocking of an activity by the antibody (eg, hemophilia, myasthenia gravis); (2) antibody causes cell lysis by combining with receptor site on cell surface (eg, autoimmune hemolytic anemia); (3) antibodies fix to mediator-containing cells, and mediator release causes cell damage (eg, allergy); (4) specific autoantibodies bind to specific tissue (eg, autoimmune thyroid disease); and (5) immune complexes of antibody and antigen circulate and by their own immunocompetence damage tissue (eg, SLE).

III. Nursing process

  A. Assessment

    1. Signs and symptoms: The signs and symptoms of immune complex disease vary widely, according to the specific disorder. The most common autoimmune diseases and their clinical manifestations are noted in Table 9.3.

    2. Diagnostic parameters: depends on disorder (see Table 9.3).

      a. Serum tests (see Table 9.3).

      b. Urine tests (see Table 9.3).

      c. Other tests

         i. Tensilon test: diagnostic for myasthenia gravis

Table 9.3 Autoimmune Disorders

Autoimmune Disorder	Diagnostic Tests (Autoantigen)	Clinical Manifestations
Diabetes (type I)	Autoantibody to B-islet cells	Abnormal glucose metabolism with hyperglycemia, increased risk of atherosclerosis, poor wound healing, neuropathies (peripheral and autonomic)
Goodpasture syndrome	Autoantibody to glomerular basement membrane and tubulobasement membrane	Pulmonary hemorrhage and glomerulonephritis
Guillain-Barré syndrome	Autoantibody to peripheral nerve myelin	Progressive weakness and flaccidity of voluntary and involuntary muscles that develop in an ascending pattern; the earliest manifestations may be heaviness or numbness and tingling of the lower extremities
Hashimoto's thyroiditis, Graves' disease, primary myxedema	Thyroglobulin autoantigen against TSH, thyroid microsomes	Patients present with either hyperthyroid or hypothyroid manifestations
Hemolytic anemia	Autoantibody to erythrocyte surface antigen	Lysis of RBCs in the circulation rather than by normal splenic or hepatic means causes increased bilirubin and blood urea nitrogen; increased reticulocytes reflect rapid RBC turnover, although refractory anemia is common in severe disease
Idiopathic neutropenia	Neutrophil autoantigen	Leukopenia with increased risk of bacterial infection and decreased inflammatory response
Idiopathic thrombocytopenic purpura	Platelet autoantigen	Thrombocytopenia with a bleeding tendency
Interstitial nephritis	Autoantibody to glomerular basement membrane and tubulobasement membrane	Proteinuria, fluid retention, and renal failure
Multiple sclerosis	Unknown	Central nervous system and spinal cord lesions leading to diffuse neurologic deficits; common complaints include blurred vision, unsteadiness, focal weakness, headaches, profound fatigue, and weakness

Table 9.3 Autoimmune Disorders (*Continued*)

Autoimmune Disorder	Diagnostic Tests (Autoantigen)	Clinical Manifestations
Myasthenia gravis	Autoantibody binds at acetylcholine receptor site of voluntary and involuntary muscles	Diffuse weakness, decreased muscle strength
Rheumatoid arthritis	IgG (rheumatoid factor)	Chronic systemic symmetrical inflammation of joints and the surrounding muscles, tendons, ligaments, and blood vessels
Scleroderma	SCL-70 centromere	Systemic sclerosis of skin, blood vessels, synovial membranes, skeletal muscle, and internal organs (especially esophagus, GI tract, thyroid, heart, lungs, kidneys); localized disease more common
Sjögren's syndrome	Antinuclear antibody, IgG (rheumatoid factor), Ro (SS-A/ La(SS-B)	Chronic exocrine gland dysfunction; causes decreased lacrimation and salivary secretion; Raynaud's syndrome may also be manifested
Systemic lupus erythematosis	Antinuclear antibody Small nuclear ribonucleoprotein (SmRNP) Ro (SS-AO) La (SS-B) Cardiolipin Histone Ribosome	No one clear pattern of manifestations due to unpredictable nature of immune reactivity against a variety of organ structures; common clinical findings include arthritis, fatigue, anemia, inflammation of heart and lungs, fever, rashes, sun sensitivity, kidney inflammation (nephritis), and central nervous system disease

TSH, thyroid-stimulating hormone.

   B. Patient management. (Autoimmune disease-specific nursing implications are included in Table 9.3, and universal nursing problems for all disorders of immune compromise are described in the final section of this chapter.)

      1. Altered protection due to autoantibody or immune-complex–induced tissue destruction

         a. Problem: Autoantibodies or immune complexes produce tissue destruction or blocking of normal activity from a variety of mechanisms. The treatment must be aimed at counterblocking, suppressing, or removing these immune complexes.

         b. Interventions

            i. Administer corticosteroids and immunosuppressive agents as ordered (see Chap. 14).

ii. Assist in plasmapheresis therapy as needed. Plasmapheresis removes blood and selectively filters the plasma, which contains autoantibodies or immune complexes, then reinfuses other blood components. Specialized protein-coated filter columns (eg, staphylococcal protein A) capture the antibodies so that the patient has fewer disease symptoms. Donor plasma is frequently infused to replace coagulation proteins lost in this process. This therapy works best in disorders where known autoantibodies exist.

iii. Prepare patient for large-bore access device insertion (similar to dialysis catheter).

iv. Plan care so that patient can remain immobile approximately 3–5 hours for the daily pheresis procedure. These procedures may be done for 3 days or up to 2 weeks while the patient is acutely symptomatic.

v. Assist patient in diversional activity during pheresis procedure.

vi. Immediately after setup on pheresis, check vital signs for hypovolemic symptoms.

vii. Monitor for lower ionized calcium levels during pheresis procedure, as the pheresis solution binds with serum calcium.

viii. Maintain catheter patency between treatments—the same as institutional protocols for temporary dialysis devices.

c. Desired patient outcomes

i. Pheresis procedure is well tolerated hemodynamically and metabolically by the patient.

ii. Clinical improvement in symptoms is apparent within 2 days of therapy's conclusion.

2. Altered skin integrity related to edema common to many autoimmune disorders

a. Problem: Most immune complex diseases stimulate inflammatory mediators that produce capillary permeability and result in edema.

b. Interventions

i. Passive or active range of motion to all joints to maintain integrity and enhance venous blood return.

ii. Apply skin lotions at least daily to prevent drying, which can alter skin integrity.

iii. Apply skin protectant (eg, skin barrier or benzoine) to areas exposed to pressure or abrasion (eg, heels, elbows, sacrum) to prevent breakdown.

iv. Elevate edematous extremities when possible.

v. Check splints, stockings, and straps periodically for excess induration and risk for breakdown on edematous areas.

vi. Limit fluid intake.

vii. Monitor albumin levels and administer albumin replacement therapy as ordered.

c. Desired outcome

i. Skin smooth, clean, dry, and free of lesions or wounds.

ii. Edema in extremities is alleviated.

3. Altered health maintenance due to chronic illness and possible progressive organ failure.
   a. Problem: The chronic, progressive nature of tissue destruction in immune complex diseases requires lifestyle adjustments, limitations on activities or diet, and taking of multiple medications. Immunosuppressant treatments place patient at risk for infection, which further restricts their social activities.
   b. Interventions
      i. Encourage family-centered activities and development of special activities that are within the patient's limitations.
      ii. Refer to social worker, psychotherapist, or clergy as needed to assist with coping strategies.
      iii. Refer to durable medical equipment company for home use as needed to accommodate for physical limitations.
      iv. Assess abilities of family and friends to provide necessary physical and emotional support after discharge.
   c. Desired outcome
      i. Patient displays effective coping mechanisms.
      ii. Family and patient demonstrate adaptability to physical limitations.
      iii. Patient has adequate financial resources to obtain needed equipment, supplies, and medications.
4. Potential for ineffective coping due to chronic illness and possible progressive organ failure
   a. Problem: Many of these diseases lead to life-threatening progressive disease and require healthy family communication patterns to meet resulting demands. The longevity and chronicity of health problems are taxing to family relationships and may eventually result in patient being unable to work, thereby increasing stress.
   b. Interventions
      i. Provide open communication and encourage discussion of issues and concerns regarding both health care and home care.
      ii. Refer to social worker, psychotherapist, or clergy as needed to assist with development of effective coping strategies.
      iii. Teach and facilitate relaxation or guided imagery to assist with coping if the patient is receptive to this therapy plan.
      iv. Refer the patient or family to support groups as needed.
      v. Refer to appropriate agency for financial counseling or assistance with obtaining disability benefits.
   c. Desired outcome
      i. Patient and family express healthy grieving for loss of physical functioning and chronic health problems.
      ii. Patient and family vocalize that coping strategies are meeting their needs.
      iii. Patient and family are able to cope with financial strains of illness.

Neutropenia

I. Definition: Neutropenia occurs when absolute neutrophil count decreases. There is disagreement as to whether it is defined as a level of 2500 cells/mm^3 or less [2] or 500 cells/mm^3 or less [3]. In patients with normal WBC counts, the higher, more conservative number is used to trigger infection precautions. Normally the total WBC count is 5000–10,000 cells/mm^3, and 35–75% of these cells are neutrophils. A diminished number of neutrophils alters the body's defenses against bacterial invaders. The major consequence of neutropenia is infection with bacteria. Common infections in the immunocompromised host are described in Table 9.4 [4], systemic signs and symptoms of infection in Table 9.5, and nursing management of antimicrobial therapy in Table 9.6.

II. Etiology: Neutrophils are decreased in diseases involving bone marrow production (eg, agranulocytosis, aplastic anemia) or when excess destruction occurs. Malnutrition, prolonged infections, increased age, and medications are the most common causes of neutropenia. Even among these likely causes, cancer chemotherapeutic agents that suppress bone marrow activity report the highest incidence of neutropenia. Immune neutropenia is caused by immune complex disease, but it has the same manifestations and general management guidelines as neutropenia from other causes. A more comprehensive listing of these etiologies is included in Table 9.7.

III. Nursing process

A. Assessment

    1. Signs and symptoms

      a. Fatigue alone without overt signs or symptoms of infection has been noted by patients with neutropenia. It may be present with or without infectious complications.

      b. Fever is the cardinal symptom of infection in the neutropenic patient; however, other inflammatory symptoms (eg, swelling, erythema, pus formation) may not occur due to the lack of WBCs.

      c. Reduced symptoms of inflammation are typical, since the WBCs that mount this response are insufficient in number to generate typical pain, erythema, and WBC exudate.

      d. Organ-specific signs and symptoms of infection are the prevalent clinical presentations of neutropenia, since many patients develop infection, and virtually all who are neutropenic for more than 21 days become infected. Organ-specific signs and symptoms of infection are included in Table 9.5.

    2. Diagnostic parameters

      a. Serum tests

        i. Total WBC count is performed to determine whether there is an adequate amount of WBCs to combat infection and mount inflammatory responses to injury. Although not specifically diagnostic for neutropenia, a low WBC count signals the probability of reduced neutrophil efficacy.

Table 9.4 Common Infections in the Immunocompromised Host

Organisms	Source	Likely Infection Site	Signs and Symptoms	Treatment*
Gram-positive bacteria				
Staphylococcus aureus	Normal flora: hand, nasopharynx	Wounds, open lesions, invasive lines, cellulitis, pneumonia, colon, blood	High fever, purulent secretions, septic emboli	Semisynthetic penicillins: nafcillin, methicillin (vancomycin)
Streptococcus: beta-hemolytic, *S. pyogenes*, *S. viridans*, *S. pneumoniae*	Normal flora: nasopharynx, skin, droplet transfer	"Strep" throat, scarlet fever, impetigo, strep gangrene, neonate and postpartum, otitis media, meningitis, pneumococcal pneumonia, endocarditis	Thin serous secretions, sudden onset of fever, maculo-papular rash with vesicle formation, fluffy infiltrates on chest x-ray	Penicillin or erythromycin ± aminoglycoside if severe (ampicillin)
Meningococcus	Normal flora: nasopharynx, droplet transfer	Meningitis, pneumonia, purulent conjunctivitis, sinusitis, endocarditis, genital infections	Arthralgias and myalgias, hypotension, petechial rash, thrombosis and hemorrhage	Penicillin, ampicillin, cephalosporins (chloramphenicol)
Corynebacterium diphtheriae	Skin, GI tract, other persons	Upper respiratory, wound, skin, occasional GI tract in immunocompromised host	Skin disorders, membranous covering on tissues	Penicillin or erythromycin
Actinomyces	Normal flora: mouth, throat, tooth decay	Abscesses head and neck, thorax, abdomen	Painful indurated swelling mouth/neck, fistulas, bowel obstruction	Penicillin or tetracycline
Nocardia	Soil	Pulmonary infection, arthritis, cardiac, abdominal	Mucopurulent sputum, night sweats, fistulae	Trimethoprim/sulfameth-oxazole for 12–18 mo or high-dose sulfonamides

Gram-negative bacteria

Organism	Source	Site	Signs and symptoms	Treatment
Enterobacteriaceae: *Klebsiella*, *Escherichia coli*, *Proteus*, *Serratia*, *Shigella*, *Salmonella*, *Yersinia*	Exogenous sources (others, environment) Endogenous (one part body to another) pathogenic strain of normal flora	Diarrhea, colitis, bacteria	Watery diarrhea with blood/pus and abdominal cramping, blood infections, peritonitis if GI tract connection with abdomen, urinary tract infection with GI contamination	Aminoglycosides and third-generation cephalosporins (trimethoprim/sulfamethoxazole)
Pseudomonas	Standing liquids	Any site—wounds contacted with contaminated water, pneumonia in mechanically ventilated patients, GI and GU	Sickly sweet odor and blue-green drainage	Aminoglycoside and penicillin derivative, eg, ticarcillin

Fungi

Organism	Source	Site	Signs and symptoms	Treatment
Candida albicans, *C. tropicalis*, *C. krusei*	Normal flora: GI and GU tract, vagina, mouth, skin; *C. krusei* is resistant strain not normally in flora	Nails, skin, mucous membranes (oral, esophageal, vaginal, GU) bacteremia	Scaly, erythematous rash of skin, cream/yellow lacelike irregular lesion, white discharge	Topical antifungals (nystatin), ketoconazole (amphotericin B, amphotericin)
Aspergillus	Damp, molding plants or areas, ventilation systems	Corrosive fungal ball in lungs, ear, cornea, sinuses, brain; abscess	Cough, blood tinged sputum, reddened and swollen eye	Amphotericin
Cryptococcus neoformans	Dust contaminated by pigeons (urban areas)	Pulmonary, meningitis	Rare pulmonary symptoms, frontal headache and progressive neurologic decline in meningitis	None; possibly amphotericin B
Blastomyces	North American soil	Bronchopneumonia, bacteremia	Viral pulmonary symptoms, painless skin macules, abscesses	Amphotericin B
Histoplasma	Inhalation in areas where soil is contaminated with bird or bat excrement	Pneumonitis with other inflammatory reactions, pleural effusions, pericarditis, sinusitis	Fever, headache, chills, cough, chest pain, sore throat, GI distress	Amphotericin B

Table 9.4 Common Infections in the Immunocompromised Host (*Continued*)

Organisms	Source	Likely Infection Site	Signs and Symptoms	Treatment*
Viruses				
Herpesvirus causing herpes simplex	Common naturally occurring virus, transmitted via body secretions, contact, or transplantation	Type I: gingivostomatitis, extraoral lesions Type II: genital, extragenital May disseminate; in compromised patients, both types are found in any body location. Herpes simplex viral pneumonia and meningitis are not uncommon in immunocompromised patients	Oral or extraoral ulcers with raised outer border, extraoral/genital vesicles with crusting and clear drainage; occasional erythema; paresthesias and pain in the area	Skin lesions in immunocompetent patients: vidarabine or topical acyclovir; refractory or disseminated infections: intravenous acyclovir, and investigationally ganciclovir or foscarnet
Herpesvirus causing herpes zoster	Reactivation of the varicella virus that has lain dormant in the cerebral ganglia	Unilateral skin eruptions around the thorax or vertically on legs or arms	Fever, malaise, severe deep pain, pruritus, paresthesias in the area involved even before the small red nodular lesions that fill with fluid or pus. Lesions occur vertically.	Acyclovir
Cytomegalovirus	Common naturally occurring virus transmitted by direct contact; however, may be transmitted through blood product transfusion if the patient has had no previous contact	Lungs, liver, GI tract, retina, central nervous system; less commonly may occur as a septicemia	Mild, nonspecific influenza-like symptoms are the usual manifestation of primary disease, although immunocompromised hosts exhibit localized infections. Diffuse infiltrates may be seen on chest x-ray or organ-specific dysfunction	Ganciclovir, cytomegalovirus immunoglobulin, new indication for acyclovir

Parasites/Opportunistic organisms

Pneumocystis carinii	Many sources for airborne protozoa	Primarily alveolar/parenchymal lung infection	Low-grade fever, cough, mild hypoxemia, dyspnea, minimal sputum, progressive infiltrates and respiratory symptoms	Trimethoprim/sulfamethoxazole, or alternatively pentamadine, pyrimethamine sulfamethoxazole, or dapsone; prophylaxis with pentamidine in immunocompromised patients
Legionella	Gram-negative bacteria most common in ventilation systems	Primarily diffuse interstitial pneumonia, possibly GI tract	High spiking fevers, dyspnea, hypoxemia, large amount white sputum, widespread infiltrates on chest x-ray	Erythromycin ± rifampin
Mycoplasma	Naturally occurring in many locations; most resistant to pathogenesis	Primarily cavitating pneumonia, although liver infections or bacteremia have been noted	High fever, cough with large amount of sputum, lobular pneumonia	Tetracycline and/or erythromycin
Toxoplasma	Ingestion through raw or uncooked meat or exposure to cat feces, although other unknown means as well	Generalized infection, encephalitis, myocarditis, hepatitis, and pneumonitis	Fever and mononucleosis-like syndrome, delirium, maculopapular rash (especially palms and soles of feet)	Pyrimethamine + folinic acid + sulfadiazines, with clindamycin added in refractory patients
Cryptosporidium	Present in animals, fish, birds, reptiles; spread by contact or fecal contamination of water supply	GI tract, cholecystitis	Watery diarrhea, cramping abdominal pain, weight loss, anorexia, nausea, vomiting, malaise	No specific antimicrobials are known to be effective antidiarrheal agents

Table 9.4 Common Infections in the Immunocompromised Host (*Continued*)

Organisms	Source	Likely Infection Site	Signs and Symptoms	Treatment*
Mycobacterium tuberculosis	Airborne spread through close proximity to infected person	Cavitating lung lesions with apical localization most common, skin, liver, or renal TB	Persistent cough, lymph-adenopathy, pleural effusions, inter-mittent fevers, night sweats, increased liver enzymes	Isoniazid ± rifampicin + pyrazinamide or ethambutol and streptomycin
Mycobacterium avium-intracellulare	Soil, water, animals, birds, foodstuffs; can be aerosolized but is usually contracted via ingestion	Milder pneumonitis than with *Mycobacterium tuberculosis*; lymphadenitis	Gradual onset fever, night sweats, anorexia, weight loss, diarrhea, weakness	Isoniazid, rifampicin, and ethambutol (strepto-mycin, esthionamide, or kanamycin)

*Second-line therapy in parentheses.

Adapted from Shelton, B. K. Infections and Immune Disorders. In *Advanced Management of Clinical Emergencies*. Baltimore: The Johns Hopkins Staff Development Program, 1990.

Table 9.5 Signs and Symptoms of Infection

Body System	Complication	Signs and Symptoms*
Neurologic	Encephalitis	Confusion, lethargy, difficulty arousing, headache, visual difficulty/photosensitivity, nausea, hypertension
	Meningitis	Lethargy and somnolence, confusion, nuchal rigidity
Head/neck	Conjunctivitis	Reddened conjunctiva, excess tearing of eye, pus-like exudate from eye, blurred vision, swelling of eyelid, eye itching
	Otitis media	Earache, difficulty hearing, itching inner ear, ear drainage
	Sinusitis	Discolored nasal mucus, nasal congestion, face pain, eye pain, blurred vision
	Oropharyngeal infection	Oral ulcerations or plaques, halitosis, reddened gums, abnormal papillae of the tongue, sore throat, difficulty swallowing
	Lymphadenitis	Swollen neck lymph glands, tender lymph glands, a lump felt when swallowing
Pulmonary	Bronchitis	Persistent cough, sputum production, gurgles in upper airways, wheezes in upper airways, hypoxemia and/or hypercapnea
	Pneumonia	Chest discomfort pronounced with inspiration, persistent cough, sputum production, diminished breath sounds, crackles or gurgles, asymmetrical chest wall movement, labored breathing, nasal flaring with breathing, hypoxemia
	Pleurisy	Chest discomfort pronounced with inspiration, sides of chest more painful, usually unilateral discomfort, splinting with deep breaths
Cardiovascular	Myocarditis	Dysrhythmias, murmurs or gallops, elevated jugular venous pulsations, weak thready pulses, hypotension, point of maximal impulse shifted laterally
	Pericarditis	Aching constant chest discomfort unrelieved by rest or nitrates, pericardial rub, muffled heart sounds
Gastrointestinal	Gastritis	Nausea, vomiting within 30 minutes of eating, heme-positive emesis, aching stomach (initially improved by eating)
	Infectious diarrhea	More than six loose stools per day, clay-colored stools, foul-smelling stools, abdominal cramping, abdominal distention
	Pancreatitis	Epigastric discomfort, intolerance to high-fat meal, clay-colored stools, nausea and vomiting, hyperglycemia, hypocalcemia, hypoalbuminemia, increased lipase and amylase
	Hepatitis	Jaundice, right-upper–quadrant discomfort, hepatomegaly, elevated transaminases and bilirubin, fatty-food intolerances, nausea and vomiting, diarrhea

Table 9.5 Signs and Symptoms of Infection (*Continued*)

Body System	Complication	Signs and Symptoms*
Genitourinary	Urethritis	Painful urination, difficulty urinating, itching of GU orifice
	Cystitis	Small frequent urination (urinary urgency), feeling of fullness of the bladder
	Nephritis	Flank discomfort, oliguria, protein in urine
	Vaginitis	Itching of vaginal area, vaginal discharge
Musculoskeletal	Arthritis	Joint discomfort, swollen and warm joints
	Myositis	Aching muscles, weakness
Dermatologic	Superficial skin infection	Rashes, itching, raised and/or discolored skin lesions, open and draining skin lesions; patterns unique to specific microorganisms
	Cellulitis	Redness, warmth and swelling of subcutaneous tissue area, radiating pain from area toward middle of body
Hematologic-immunologic	Bacteremia	Low diastolic BP, headache, confusion, oliguria, decreased bowel sounds, warmth, flushing, positive blood cultures

*Signs and symptoms presented in this table are unique features of each process and do not include the constitutional signs and symptoms seen with all infections such as fever, chills, malaise, leukocytosis, positive tissue culture for microorganisms, or increased erythrocyte sedimentation rate.

      ii. Absolute neutrophil count (ANC) is calculated with the WBC differential count:

$$\text{total WBC count} \times \text{neutrophils (\%)} = \text{ANC}$$

For example,

$$5000 \text{ cells/mm}^3 \times 0.25 \text{ (25\%)} = 1250 \text{ cells/mm}^3$$

    b. Urine tests
      i. None.
    c. Other tests
      i. None.
  B. Patient management (universal nursing problems for all immune compromise disorders are described in the final section of this chapter).

T-Lymphocyte Suppression

    The suppression of T-lymphocyte function results in reduced ability to recognize foreign tissue, malignant cells, and viruses. T-lymphocyte suppression may be therapeutically induced as when suppression of rejection of an engrafted organ transplant is desired, or it may be an acquired phenomenon from other physical disorders. Congenital T-lymphocyte suppression is relatively rare, but it occurs in the form of severe combined immunodeficiency syndrome, neonatal HIV infection, thymic dysfunction, and other deficiencies manifested as pediatric cancers.

Table 9.6 Antimicrobial Therapy

Antibiotic	Coverage	Nursing Implications
Aminoglycosides Gentamicin Amikacin Tobramycin Kanamycin	Most gram-negative *Enterobacter (Serratia, Proteus, Klebsiella, E. coli)*, *Pseudomonas, Erwinia*	1. Assess urine output for oliguria and signs of decline in kidney function 2. Monitor blood urea nitrogen (BUN) and creatinine for evidence of renal failure 3. Assess hearing for vestibular and auditory damage 4. Provide skin lotions and antipruritic medications for rash 5. Obtain peak and trough blood levels to monitor for toxicity 6. Administer dose over at least 30 minutes
Penicillins Penicillin G Penicillin V Ampicillin Amoxicillin Ticarcillin Piperacillin Carbenicillin Imipenem	*Actinomyces, Clostridium,* meningococcemia, *Proteus* (ampicillin), *Salmonella* (ampicillin/amoxicillin), *Streptococcus, Staphylococcus* (2nd line)	1. Observe frequently during initial infusions—signs/symptoms of hypersensitivity may include dyspnea, stridor, itching, rash (especially ampicillin and amoxicillin), hypotension 2. Administer oral doses with food or milk to reduce risk of GI intolerance 3. Antidiarrheal medications as needed for diarrhea (especially ampicillin) 4. Assess for bruises and petechiae signaling abnormal platelet activity (especially carbenicillin and ticarcillin) 5. Monitor for neuromuscular twitching 6. Monitor urine output for renal insufficiency 7. Monitor BUN and creatinine for evidence of renal failure 8. Replenish potassium as needed; drugs cause potassium depletion
Quinolones Norfloxacin Ciprofloxacin	Resistant *Enterobacter*	GI intolerance Headache with/without dizziness Malaise Insomnia Rare visual disturbances Hepatic dysfunction
Gram-positive coverage Nafcillin Oxacillin Vancomycin	*Staphylococcus, Clostridium difficile, Corynebacterium diphtheriae*	"Red man syndrome" (vancomycin) Fever Rash, allergic reactions Neutropenia Hypotension with rapid infusion

Table 9.6 Antimicrobial Therapy (*Continued*)

Antibiotic	Coverage	Nursing Implications
Cephalosporins		
Cefamandole	General *Enterobacter*	Phlebitis
Cefazolin	coverage (*E. coli,*	Diarrhea
Cephalothin	*Klebsiella, Proteus,*	Allergic reactions
Ceftazidime	*Serratia*), *Staphylo-*	Platelet dysfunction
Cefuroxime	*coccus aureus,*	Rare hepatic dysfunction
Moxalactam	*Haemophilus*	
	influenzae	
Tetracyclines		
Tetracycline	Tick fever, *Clamydiae,*	GI intolerance
Demeclocycline	*Klebsiella,* urinary tract	Vertigo
Monocycline	infection (UTI), *Myco-*	Vaginitis
	plasma pneumoniae	Hepatotoxicity
	(2nd line)	Teeth staining
		Photosensitivity
Other antibacterials		
Clindamycin	Gastrointestinal bacilli	GI intolerance
		Diarrhea
		Colitis
		Rash
Erythromycin	*Campylobacter, Chlamy-*	Phlebitis
	dia conjunctivitis,	Diarrhea
	Corynebacterium	Stomatitis
	diphtheriae,	Cholestatic hepatitis
	Legionella, Myco-	Rash
	plasma pneumoniae	Dose-related ototoxicity
Metronidazole	*Bacteroides,* various	Metallic taste
	normal flora,	Headache
	Clostridium difficile	Phlebitis
		Reversible peripheral neuropathies
		Antabuse-like reaction
Sulfa-trimethoprim	*E. coli* UTI, *Haemophilus*	Hypersensitivity
	influenzae, Shigella,	Rash
	Pneumocystis carinii,	Anaphylaxis
	some strains of	GI intolerance
	Pseudomonas,	Bone marrow aplasia (platelets, WBCs)
	Salmonella, Yersinia	
Sulfonamides (Gantricin)	Nocardia	Allergic reactions—rash, pruritus
		Fever
		Crystalluria
		GI intolerance
		Photosensitivity
Antifungals		
Ketoconazole	Widely spread localized	GI intolerance
	fungal infections,	Hepatotoxicity
	oral/mucocutaneous	Decreased testosterone levels (gyneco-mastia, dysmenorrhea)
	Candida	

Table 9.6 Antimicrobial Therapy (*Continued*)

Antibiotic	Coverage	Nursing Implications
Amphotericin B	Topical—mucocutaneous fungal infection IV—disseminated fungal infections (*Candida, Aspergillus, Cryptococcus*)	Fever, rigors, headache Hypokalemia Renal failure Anemia Phlebitis Metallic taste
Flucytosine	Disseminated or septicemic *Candida, Coccidioides, Cryptococcus*	Nausea and vomiting Rash Hepatotoxicity Bone marrow suppression Confusion
Antivirals		
Acyclovir	Herpes simplex I and II, varicella-zoster	Irritation at injection site Renal insufficiency Hepatotoxicity Rash Bone marrow suppression (platelets and WBCs) Metabolic encephalopathy
Ganciclovir	Cytomegalovirus	Neutropenia Thrombocytopenia Rash Hepatotoxicity Headache, fever Psychosis Myopathy

Table 9.7 Etiologies of Neutropenia

Malnutrition
  Protein deficiency
  Calorie deficiency
  B vitamin deficiency
Health states
  Chronic fever
  Chronic illness
  Diabetes mellitus
  Elderly
Medications
  Alkylating agents (antineoplastic and immunosuppressive), eg, cyclophosphamide
  Antidysrhythmics, eg, procainamide, quinidine
  Antimetabolites, eg, methotrexate, azathioprine
  Antiretroviral agents, eg, zidovudine
  Antitumor antibiotics, eg, bleomycin, adriamycin
  Plant alkaloids, eg, vincristine, vinblastine, paclitaxel
  Trimethoprim-sulfamethoxazole
  Zyloprim (allopurinol)

In adults, most T-lymphocyte lymphomas are of the Hodgkin's subtype and have been linked to familial tendencies, history of retroviral infection, or unknown causes thought to be congenital. The patient with acquired specific immune system dysfunction may have HIV infection with acquired immunodeficiency syndrome (AIDS) or receive medications, such as corticosteroids, that suppress T-lymphocyte function. T-lymphocyte suppression in the setting of transplantation is addressed in Chapter 14 and is comparable to cases of patients receiving corticosteroids, such as for autoimmune disease. The patient problems and goals of care likewise are similar.

Acquired Immunodeficiency Syndrome

   I. Definition: Acquired immunodeficiency syndrome (AIDS) is a specific acquired immune deficient state due to retroviral infection with HIV. The virus insinuates itself into the human T4 helper lymphocyte RNA, causing viral replication rather than normal cell multiplication. The consequences include destruction of T4 helper lymphocytes with an increased propensity for opportunistic infections, lymphoreticular cancers, and neurologic involvement.

   II. Etiology: AIDS was first identified in 1979, when an otherwise healthy man developed an opportunistic infection (*Pneumocystis carinii*), which was believed to occur only in immunocompromised patients. We now know that HIV is the etiology of this selective destruction of T4 helper lymphocytes (cells with CD4 receptor sites) and monocytes having CD4 molecules on their surface. HIV is primarily a bloodborne pathogen, and the proposed transmission occurs when there are breaks in barrier integrity or when there is direct access to blood and mucous membranes. Currently the most common methods of disease transmission are through blood exposure with IV drug use, anal intercourse, fetal exposure to maternal blood, or sexual contact with a member of a high-risk group.

   III. Nursing process

   A. Assessment

   1. Signs and symptoms: The major clinical manifestations of HIV infection are grouped into five categories: (1) acute retroviral illness, (2) constitutional disease, (3) neurologic disease, (4) opportunistic infection, or (5) cancer. Low T4 helper cell counts associated with one of the defined indicator diseases are considered definable as AIDS. The Centers for Disease Control (CDC) classifications and indicator diseases correlated to helper counts are listed in Table 9.8 [5]. Symptoms vary widely, depending on the indicator condition involved. Key signs and symptoms of opportunistic infections are listed in Table 9.4, and other AIDS-related signs and symptoms are included in this discussion.

   a. Constitutional symptoms including generalized lymphadenopathy, fever, chills, night sweats, unexplained weight loss (more than 10% of body weight), and malaise are clinical manifestations of both acute retroviral illness and constitutional disease. Acute retroviral illness occurs 3–6 weeks after the initial exposure to HIV. Patients may have

Table 9.8 1993 Revised Classification System for HIV Infection and Expanded AIDS Surveillance Case Definition for Adolescents and Adults*

	Clinical Categories		
CD4 + T-cell Categories	(A) Asymptomatic, acute (primary) HIV, or PGL	(B) Symptomatic, not (A) or (C) conditions	(C) AIDS-indicator conditions
(1) ≥500/μL	A1	B1	C1
(2) 200–499/μL	A2	B2	C2
(3) <200/μL	A3	B3	C3

PGL = persistent generalized lymphadenopathy. Clinical category A includes acute (primary) HIV infection.
*Categories A3, B3, C1, C2, and C3 represent the expanded AIDS surveillance case definition. Persons with AIDS-indicator conditions (category C) as well as those with CD4 + T-lymphocyte counts <200/μL (categories A3 or B3) became reportable as AIDS cases in the United States and territories effective January 1, 1993.
Adapted from Centers for Disease Control. 1993 Revised Classification System for HIV infection and expanded surveillance case definition for AIDS among adolescents and adults. *MMWR* 41(RR-17):2, 1992.

these symptoms and not progress to other forms of the disease, or these symptoms may be a prodrome to more serious symptoms.

b. In the early phase of disease, neurologic manifestations include short-term memory deficit, impaired concentration, emotional lability, or numbness of the extremities. As neurologic impairment advances, symptoms become more pronounced, and the patient may display disorientation, agitation, combativeness, acute paranoia, severe memory deficits, impaired judgment, and paresthesias that affect the patient's ability to care for him- or herself.

c. Patients with indicator cancers usually exhibit a more aggressive metastatic disease that is refractory to traditional treatment modalities. The most common cancer is Kaposi's sarcoma, tumors that cause hemorrhaging of the microvasculature. The characteristic lesions are raised; purplish, reddish, or black; and irregularly shaped. They usually appear first in the extremities or on the face, but in advanced disease they can spread to the GI tract or lungs. Lymphoreticular cancers (especially non-Hodgkin's lymphoma or lymphocytic leukemia) may present with lymphadenopathy, infection, or organ dysfunction. The tumors often involve extranodal sites (eg, brain, lung) and metastasize quickly. Invasive cervical carcinoma has also been identified as an indicator disease of HIV infection. Usually a slow-growing tumor with mild dysmenorrhea is the major symptom, and these patients exhibit severe bleeding, fungating growth of tumors, and anemia.

2. Diagnostic parameters

   a. Serum tests

      i. Enzyme-linked immunosorbent assay (ELISA) is the diagnostic test of choice for identifying the presence of antibody to viral proteins (particularly HIV). After staining, the presence of highlighted antibody indicates that exposure to the virus occurred at least 8–12 weeks prior to testing. This test has false-positive results and is often repeated twice to reduce the risk of incorrect diagnosis. ELISA is also used to test donated blood for possible HIV contamination.

   ii. Western blot test is a protein electrophoresis test that selectively identifies one of the key envelope proteins found in HIV: gp160/120, gp41, or p24.

   iii. Viral cultures involve growth in culture of patient monocytes and lymphocytes, with periodic evaluation of the cultured cells' reverse transcriptase. Clumped helper T cells are indicative of HIV infection.

   iv. Polymerase chain reaction involves removal of patient monocytes and lymphocytes, with growth and replication several times, and subsequent testing for HIV DNA.

   v. Absolute lymphocyte count is a test that quantifies the number of lymphocytes. The total lymphocyte count is normally 600–1200 cells/mm^3. When the lymphocyte count is below 500 cells/mm^3, immune compromise occurs, and when there are less than 200 cells/mm^3, opportunistic infections occur.

   b. Urine tests
      i. None
   c. Other tests
      i. None.

B. Patient management. (Universal plan of care for the immunocompromised patient is applicable for patients with AIDS, and unique problems are outlined in this section.)

   1. Potential for infection with progression to sepsis or new onset of opportunistic infections

   a. Problem: Depression of the immune system combined with malnutrition, and in the presence of multi-infectious processes or microorganisms, potentiates the patient's risk of developing life-threatening sepsis or additional opportunistic infections. The use of antimicrobial therapy also alters normal body flora, which further potentiates the risk of infection.

   b. Interventions (see p. 260, "Universal Nursing Problems in the Immunocompromised Patient" for additional guidelines).

      i. Maintain universal precautions, and instruct patient and visitors in these precautions so that they can comply both in the hospital and when the patient is discharged.

      ii. Monitor temperature (may be hyperthermic or severely hypothermic) and laboratory studies (more severe leukocytosis, left shift toward granulocytosis) for evidence of infection.

      iii. Examine skin and mucous membranes (eg, oral cavity) for redness, white patches, open lesions, and sore areas. Provide appropriate cleansing and dressing measures, as well as topical antimicrobials for open lesions, as ordered.

      iv. Encourage good personal hygiene to decrease risk of infection. Measures include bathing daily, perineal care twice daily, and brushing teeth with a soft toothbrush three times daily. Avoid products that dry the skin (wet areas) and oral agents (commercial mouthwashes with high alcohol content) that further disrupt barrier integrity.

v. Inspect wounds and catheter insertion sites for signs of local inflammation, infection, abnormal drainage, redness, pain, and swelling.

vi. Note increased respiratory distress exhibited by cough, production of thick odorous sputum, congested lungs on auscultation.

c. Desired outcomes

i. No new opportunistic infections.

ii. Signs and symptoms of progressing infection recognized early with appropriate interventions implemented in a timely fashion.

iii. Maintained skin and mucous membrane integrity.

2. Altered thought processes related to HIV neurologic disease, malignant brain involvement, or infection

a. Problem: Neurologic disease in HIV may produce increased intracranial pressure, seizures, and cognitive dysfunction.

b. Interventions

i. Assess orientation, motor activity, central reflexes (eg, pupils), and cognitive function frequently. Report focal deficits and changes from baseline.

ii. Assess need for safety precautions (eg, restraints) due to altered cognitive function.

iii. Maintain seizure precautions.

iv. Keep head of bed elevated to reduce risk of increased intracranial pressure.

v. Provide orientation cues in the room whenever possible (eg, calendars, clocks, open curtains).

vi. Refer to home care agency to provide follow-up for patients with known or suspected neurologic disease. Be certain the patient has a support network in place and that visits are frequent and regular.

vii. Administer sedation cautiously.

viii. Administer antiretroviral agents as ordered, since they seem to improve the clinical symptoms of neurologic disease. Nursing care of the patient receiving retroviral medications is summarized in Table 9.9.

c. Desired outcome

i. Alert; well-oriented to person, place, and time; appropriate in verbal responses

ii. Safe environment

3. Altered gas exchange due to opportunistic infections of the lung

a. Problem: The pulmonary system is often the target of microbial invasion that develops into life-threatening pneumonia in the AIDS patient.

b. Interventions

i. Administer oxygen as ordered and for oxygen saturation less than 90% or PaO_2 less than 60 mm Hg.

ii. Assess oxygen saturation frequently or continually.

Table 9.9 Antiretroviral Agents

Drug	Dosage and Administration	Nursing Implications
Zidovudine (previously known as azidothymidine [AZT])	Symptomatic/asymptomatic HIV infection with CD4 count <500 cells: 100 mg PO 5–6 times per day. Some current studies using 200 mg tid appear to be equally effective Pregnant women after 14th week of pregnancy: 100 mg PO 5 times daily throughout pregnancy and optional intrapartum intravenous retrovir 2 mg/kg loading dose followed by 1 mg/kg/h until delivery Newborns of HIV-positive women: 2 mg/kg oral elixir q6h beginning 8–12 h postpartum and continuing for 6 wk. Children with confirmed HIV infection: 90–240 mg/m^2 PO q6h or 80–160 mg/m^2 IV q6h	Use cautiously in hepatic and renal disease—metabolism occurs in the liver and is renally excreted Monitor hematologic tests for anemia, leukopenia (especially neutropenia) Implement infection prevention precautions Administer blood products as ordered Discuss with health care team plans to provide therapy breaks in bone marrow toxicity Administer bone marrow stimulants such as erythropoietin or granulocyte colony-stimulating factor as ordered to eliminate bone marrow toxicity Administer mild analgesics as ordered for headache or myalgias Administer with meals to reduce incidence of nausea Assist patient in relaxation procedures Report and develop a plan to address insomnia if present Apply warmth to muscle aches as needed
Didanosine (commonly known as dideoxycytidine [ddC])	Each dose should be at least two tablets of specialized buffered powder to make oral solutions to ensure adequate buffering Chewable tablets: 25, 50, 100, 150 mg Pediatric solution: 10 mg/mL Buffered powder for solution: 100, 167, 250, 375 mg Dosage is reduced in renal or hepatic impairment Dose is based on weight: <60 kg, 25–100 mg tablet increments bid (average dose approximately 100 mg bid); >60 kg, 200 mg tablet increments bid (average dose approximately 200 mg bid)	Half-life in children is reduced (adult half-life 1.3–1.6 h, child half-life 0.8 h) Bioavailability greatly variable (average 20–25%) based on dose form, gastric pH, food in GI tract Administer cautiously to renally impaired patients; drug and its metabolites thought to be cleared renally Monitor for paresthesias or altered sensation in periphery, discuss possible therapy break with health care team Encourage patient to avoid clothing with small buttons that require manipulation if peripheral neuropathies are present Provide safety measures in patients with peripheral neuropathies Evaluate abdominal discomfort for severity and location, then check amylase and lipase levels for evidence of pancreatitis

Zalcitabine (commonly known as dideoxyinosine [ddI])	0.750 mg (one tablet) PO alone or concomitantly with zidovudine 200 mg q8h 0.375 mg PO with zidovudine 200 mg q8h is given after therapy break for peripheral neuropathies No dose reduction is required for children and infants	Administer between meals; bioavailability reduced when taken with food Administer with caution in hepatic or renal disease Monitor for paresthesias or altered sensation in periphery; discuss possible therapy break with health care team Encourage patient to avoid clothing with small buttons that require manipulation if peripheral neuropathies are present Evaluate abdominal discomfort for severity and location, then check amylase and lipase levels for evidence of pancreatitis Administer mild analgesics as ordered for headache Provide oral anesthetics if ulcerations are present Discuss need for oral antimicrobials (eg, nystatin as prophylaxis against thrush) if ulcerations are present Assess airway when there is oral or esophageal ulceration that may cause difficulty breathing Monitor carefully for several hours after the first few doses of medication due to the risk of anaphylactoid reactions Provide frequent rest periods and assist patient in planning activities of daily living to allow rest and reduce severity of drug-induced fatigue Weigh patient daily to assess for weight gain Monitor urine output for oliguria that signals fluid retention If used long term, check breath sounds, peripheral edema, and jugular venous pulse every shift to detect heart failure If used long term, monitor chest x-rays for heart enlargement

       iii. Ensure obtainment of daily chest x-rays as ordered during times of respiratory impairment.

       iv. Assess frequently breath sounds for diminished sounds, adventitious sounds, or egophony.

       v. Administer prophylaxis against pulmonary infection as ordered (see "Pneumonia" in Chap. 13 for specific nursing implications of these medications and additional management strategies): against tuberculosis—isoniazid (INH) 5 mg/kg every day; against *P. carinii*—pentamidine 300 mg via nebulizer every 4 weeks.

  c. Desired outcome

      i. Pa_{O_2} is greater than 60 mm Hg on ABG.

      ii. Pc_{O_2} is less than 45 mm Hg on ABG.

      iii. Clear breath sounds on auscultation.

      iv. The patient reports no difficulty breathing.

      v. Compliance with prophylactic antimicrobial regimens.

4. Altered body image due to weight loss, Kaposi's sarcoma lesions, permanent indwelling IV access devices

  a. Problem: Certain clinical manifestations of HIV and their treatment cause several changes in physical appearance that may alter the patient's perception of self. Patients with HIV infection also receive multiple prophylactic and therapeutic medications to prevent or treat opportunistic infections that require IV access.

  b. Interventions

      i. Assist the patient in devising methods of masking physical changes related to therapy (eg, use of scarves, pouches for IV lines).

      ii. Refer patient to support programs that explore use of makeup or props to mask effects of treatment.

      iii. Encourage patient to wear stylish clothes when possible.

      iv. Provide a mirror and other supplies and encourage patient to take care with appearance.

  c. Desired outcome

      i. Patient vocalizes satisfaction with appearance.

      ii. Patient has improved feelings of self-worth.

5. Altered elimination, diarrhea

  a. Problem: Several opportunistic infections common in HIV infection cause diarrhea.

  b. Interventions

      i. Measure intake and output, and monitor for dehydration or electrolyte imbalances.

      ii. Encourage fluids, if needed, to prevent fluid volume deficit.

      iii. Provide bedside commode or other rapidly accessible means of toileting. Be certain antiseptic cleansing supplies are accessible for use afterward.

      iv. Provide incontinent pads or adult diapers to reduce embarrassment, especially if patient must go to other departments for tests.

      v. Provide rectal skin care with petroleum-based ointments to protect the skin from breakdown.

    vi. If the patient's condition permits, provide sitz baths or witch hazel compresses for soreness of the rectum.

    vii. Send stool samples for culture (daily for 3 days) with new onset or worsening of diarrhea. Be certain testing for opportunistic infections is done.

    viii. Apply occlusive dressings on all broken skin surfaces that might come into contact with stool.

    ix. Provide clean linens as needed.

    x. Encourage consumption of foods that may decrease diarrhea and normally cause constipation—bananas, cheese, yogurt, carbohydrates.

    xi. Have patient avoid additional stimulants of rapid GI motility—caffeine, fatty foods, leafy vegetables.

    xii. Administer antidiarrheals as ordered; no clearly preferred agent has been identified, so choices should be based on patient preference (eg, anticholinergics, bulking agents, opiate derivatives).

  c. Desired outcome

    i. Patient has fewer than six stools per day, and stool is less than 500 cc/d.

    ii. Skin integrity of rectal area is maintained.

    iii. Absence of fluid volume deficit.

6. Altered sensory perception or vision related to possible cytomegalovirus (CMV) infection.

  a. Problem: In HIV patients, CMV is a common opportunistic infection that can damage the retina and cause blindness.

  b. Interventions

    i. Assess visual acuity periodically: Ask the patient to read items at a distance and note changes from baseline.

    ii. Administer ganciclovir 2.5–5.0 mg/kg daily 5–7 times per week as ordered when the CD_4 counts are less than 100 cells/mm^3.

  c. Desired outcome

    i. Patient will not have deterioration of visual acuity.

    ii. Compliance with prophylactic antimicrobial regimen.

7. Potential for injury related to altered clotting factors

  a. Problem: The risk of abnormal bleeding occurs due to decreased vitamin K absorption, altered hepatic function, presence of autoimmune platelet antibodies, malignancies (Kaposi's sarcoma), adverse effects of antineoplastic therapy, circulating endotoxins from sepsis, and as an adverse effect of antiretroviral therapy.

  b. Interventions

    i. Avoid intramuscular injections, rectal temperatures, and rectal tubes, which may increase bleeding tendency.

    ii. Apply pressure over venipuncture (venous or arterial) sites and locations of removed catheters for at least 5 minutes and longer if oozing persists. A sandbag or topical hemostatic agents (eg, topical thrombin) may be used to prevent or stop bleeding from these sites.

    iii. Maintain a safe environment to prevent patient bumps and falls, which can precipitate bleeding episodes.

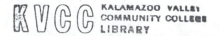

    iv. Use Trendelenburg position with caution, because the increased intracranial pressure it causes may precipitate an intracranial hemorrhage.

    v. Avoid use of salicylates or nonsteroidal anti-inflammatory drugs (NSAIDs), which have an anticoagulant effect. Instruct the patient and family to consult a physician before using any medications after discharge.

    vi. Monitor blood counts (hematocrit [HCT], hemoglobin [Hgb], RBC count), platelet count, and coagulation studies (prothrombin time [PT], partial thromboplastin time [PTT], fibrinogen level) and administer blood products as ordered and indicated.

    vii. Heme test body fluids (urine, stool, sputum, emesis).

    viii. Monitor for changes in vital signs (orthostasis, tachycardia), skin color (increased paleness, cyanosis), and cool extremities, which signal occult bleeding.

    ix. Assess the patient every shift for petechiae and ecchymoses, which may precede overt bleeding.

    x. Observe for epistaxis, frank hematuria, hemoptysis, nonmenstrual vaginal bleeding, oozing around catheters, and gum bleeding, which signals overt coagulation problems with bleeding.

  c. Desired outcomes

    i. No evidence of occult or overt bleeding.

    ii. No injury is incurred.

    iii. Patient and family verbalize methods of monitoring and preventing bleeding problems after discharge.

8. Anticipatory grieving

  a. Problem: The experience of a critical illness such as AIDS forces patient and family to recognize the loss of a normal way of life. They must learn to handle the uncertainty of the illness and its possible outcomes or losses. The patient could lose a body part or function, the ability to work, and possibly his or her life. How the patient's life is affected by this illness, as well as the patient's coping strategies, is influenced by past methods of dealing with stress, anxiety, and loss, in addition to the presence of supportive relationships with others.

  b. Interventions

    i. Identify how the patient and family are coping with the stresses of illness and provide them with opportunities to verbalize their needs.

    ii. Acknowledge appropriate feelings of grief and loss. Help the patient and family work through grief stages as appropriate.

    iii. Assist individuals to identify their strengths and areas in which they can master their feelings of powerlessness.

    iv. Provide, as needed, appropriate referrals to social worker, community agencies, clergy, mental health professionals, and support groups.

    v. Provide privacy as needed, for patient to conduct personal matters such as legal paperwork.

  c. Desired outcomes

    i. Patient and significant others demonstrate appropriate coping measures and begin to identify methods of handling the stress of loss.

ii. Patient shows acceptance of loss.

9. Potential for social isolation

   a. Problem: Patients with HIV infection are still perceived by many as being contagious with a life-threatening illness. There is significant risk that the fear of contracting HIV infection will affect interactions with the patient. Because of unfounded fears, friends, family, and volunteers may provide less social support to a patient with HIV. For other HIV-infected patients, the risk of contracting an opportunistic infection from a friend also may decrease their interactions with this person.

   b. Interventions

      i. Assess perceptions of family and friends regarding their risk of contracting HIV from the patient.

      ii. Provide education to these individuals as needed to reduce their anxiety about this risk.

      iii. Practice universal precautions in all patient encounters.

- Use protective barriers when in contact with blood, urine, stool, semen, or blood-contaminated excretions.
- Use needleless systems whenever possible.
- Clean all multipatient devices (eg, thermometers, noninvasive BP cuffs, pulse oximeter probes) between patient use.
- Wear goggles for procedures that risk splashing contaminated secretions (eg, line insertions, bronchoscopy).
- Bag all specimens in impermeable plastic bags before transport.
- Place all patient waste and excrement-contaminated linen in biohazard containers.

      iv. Provide social support for patients whenever possible, through diversional activity such as television, telephone access, and volunteer or clergy visits.

      v. Refer to support groups depending on patient's condition.

   c. Desired patient outcomes

      i. Patient verbalizes feelings of being supported by family, friends, or health care providers.

      ii. All in contact with the patient or their specimens/linen have minimal concerns about contracting HIV infection.

Cancer

I. **Definition:** Cancer comprises a group of diseases in which mutant cells escape the immune surveillance system that normally detects and removes mutant cells from the body. Neoplasms (new growths) may be benign (non-cancerous) or malignant (cancerous). The malignant status of the growth will determine its local invasiveness, ability to grow out of control, and ability to spread to other parts of the body. Cancers are named according to the cell type from which they originate: Carcinomas are from squamous or epithelial tissues, sarcomas arise from connective tissue, and hematologic cancers develop from the blood cells or lymphoid organs. Cancers characteristically have irregular borders, are immovable, and involve a complex blood supply. Cancers spread from one area of the body to another (metastasis) via lymphatics, direct extension, or hematogenous connections. The location of the primary tumor, degree of tissue differentiation, and severity of metastases are predictive of prognosis for patients with cancer. While cancer may arise from an immune deficit, the clinical complications of cancer are more often related to tumor location and characteristics.

II. **Etiology:** Theories of cancer development have ranged from failure of immune surveillance (T-lymphocyte function), to abnormal and excessive responses to inflammatory foci, and even include genetic abnormalities (oncogenes) or retroviral infection (link of cancer to HIV infection). The exact mechanisms of cancer development are unknown, but the most supported theories describe cancer initiators and promoters. Cancer initiators are carcinogens (eg, toxic chemicals, radiation, or medications), genetic defects, viral infection, or other stimuli known to produce mutations of normal cells. Under normal circumstances, these mutant cells should be removed from the circulation before they can establish "a home." Cancer promoters are those variables that cannot produce cancer alone but, in the presence of an initiator, have been shown to enhance the possibility of cancer development. Diet (eg, high-fat diet is associated with breast and colon cancers; high alcohol intake with esophageal, pancreas, stomach, and liver cancers), hormones (eg, estrogens are associated with uterine and vaginal cancers), dysplastic tissue (eg, cervical dysplasia, dysplastic nevi of the skin), immune suppression (eg, AIDS-related lymphomas), and other diseases are known promoters of cancer growth. Despite this knowledge of the behavior of malignancies, unexplained malignant growth and tumors refractory to antineoplastic therapy claim many lives yearly. In the United States, cancer is the second most common cause of death [6]. The critical care nurse is likely to encounter patients with many different kinds of cancer and must be familiar with the typical clinical presentations, diagnostic tests, and usual management strategies. These are reviewed in Table 9.10.

The phase of the cancer illness continuum predicts cancer-related complications and guides the clinician in determining the best course of therapy. Cancer is divided into chronologic and physiologic stages in which complications are likely to occur: (1) at diagnosis, (2) as an adverse effect of antineoplastic treatment, (3) during progressive disease, and (4) as a late effect of cancer or its therapy. Complications are categorized as related to compression or invasion of normal body processes, or as a metabolic consequence of the cancer or its treatment. The most common crises and their malignant associations are discussed in Table 9.11.

III. **Nursing process**

A. Assessment

1. Signs and symptoms (vary with type of cancer and location of tumor; see Table 9.10). The primary tumor and metastatic disease are both considered when symptomatology is defined. The seven warning signals of cancer as defined by the American Cancer Society are outlined here:

   a. *C*hange in bowel or bladder habits.
   b. *A* sore that does not heal.
   c. *U*nusual bleeding or discharge.
   d. *T*hickening or lump in the breast or elsewhere.

Table 9.10 Cancer Overview

Cancer	Presenting Symptoms	Diagnostic Tools	Metastatic Patterns	Treatment
Brain	Headache Altered mental status Motor deficits	CT scan MRI scan Positron-emission tomographic scan	Direct extension most common	1. Surgical excision or debulking 2. External beam radiotherapy 3. Implanted radioactive seeds 4. Chemotherapy: cisplatin regimens
Breast	Nontender, immovable breast lump Nipple discharge Nipple dimpling Peau d'orange	Mammogram Dye-enhanced mammography Breast lump biopsy Thermography Zerogram	Regional lymph nodes first Liver common Lung common Bone (especially spine and pelvis) common Pericardium Pleural space	1. Surgical excision (ranges from lumpectomy to mastectomy with lymph node dissection) 2. External beam radiation 3. Implanted radioactive seeds 4. Chemotherapy given even as adjuvant therapy to postoperative disease-free patient with high risk of recurrence (more than two positive nodes); regimens consist of cyclophosphamide and an antitumor antibiotic (eg, doxorubicin); some patients also receive methotrexate, 5-fluorouracil, or thiotepa 5. Hormonal manipulation (eg, tamoxifen) used in older women with estrogen or progesterone receptor positive status 6. Autologous bone marrow transplant
Colon	Altered bowel habits Rectal bleeding Thin, ribbon-like stools Back pain	Colonoscopy guided colon biopsy p54 gene CT scan	Regional lymph nodes most common Early hematologic spread to liver Extensive disease often involves omentum and peritoneal cavity, causing significant ascites Bone Occasionally to lung	1. Surgical excision with re-anastomosis or colostomy/ileostomy 2. External beam radiation 3. Chemotherapy: 5-fluorouracil containing regimen; many regimens add leukovorin or levamisole because it enhances the effects of 5-fluorouracil 4. Chemotherapy may also be given via hepatic artery for isolated liver metastases

Table 9.10 Cancer Overview (*Continued*)

Cancer	Presenting Symptoms	Diagnostic Tools	Metastatic Patterns	Treatment
Head/Neck	Dysphagia Hoarseness Oral lump Head and neck lymphadenopathy	CT scan Lesion biopsy	Direct extension occurs first Regional lymph nodes Oral/sinus cavities Carotid artery erosion by tumor Brain metastases (late) Lung metastases	1. Radical surgical excision with or without tracheostomy and feeding tube 2. External beam radiation 3. Chemotherapy: cisplatin-containing regimen is most common

Leukemia	Infection
	Bleeding
	Bruising
	Gum hyperplasia
		Complete blood count shows blasts
		Bone marrow aspirate and biopsy
			Disseminated disease to start	1. Always requires systemic chemotherapy
				2. Chemotherapy agents chosen depend on cell type; common drugs include
				  a. Acute nonlymphocytic: cyclophosphamide (acute severe symptoms), cytosine, arabinoside, daunorubicin, etoposide
				  b. Acute lymphocytic: l-asparaginase, methotrexate, prednisone, vincristine, intrathecal medication, or radiation
				  c. Chronic nonlymphocytic: oral alkylating agents if symptoms are not severe, systemic alkylating agents (eg, cyclophosphamide, busulfan) as disease progresses; in acute phase conversion is treated like other acute nonlymphocytic leukemias
				  d. Chronic lymphocytic: treated with oral alkylating agents
				3. Bone marrow transplant

Lung	Cough Hemoptysis Hoarseness Dyspnea Unexplained weight loss	Chest x-ray offers strong suspicion CT scan Bronchoscopy biopsy	Superior vena cava Hilar lymph nodes Brain metastases common Spinal cord involvement with spinal cord compression	1. Surgical excision 2. External beam radiation 3. Chemotherapy: cisplatin-containing regimen

Cancer	Signs/Symptoms	Metastatic Sites	Diagnostic Tests	Treatment
Lymphoma	Lymphadenopathy Bowel obstruction or abdominal distention common Difficulty breathing common with pulmonary tumor	Any organ Rare brain metastases except with HIV lymphoma Bone marrow (common with certain subtypes)	Lymph node biopsy MRI Lymphangiogram	1. Systemic chemotherapy: multidrug regimen; common regimens include alkylating agent (eg, cyclophosphamide), antitumor antibiotic (eg, doxorubicin), plant alkaloid (eg, oncovin), and steroids (eg, prednisone) 2. Local radiation therapy used for large lesions, usually palliative therapy unless only one node group is involved in disease
Multiple myeloma	Unresolvable infection Anemia Neurologic changes (usually from hyperviscosity caused by excess M protein) Bone demineralization with possible pathologic fractures Renal dysfunction	Renal involvement Bone disease	Protein M levels Urine for Bence Jones protein Protein electrophoresis Bone scan (nonspecific) Plasma viscosity levels (usually to monitor disease status)	1. Systemic chemotherapy: most common agent is melphalan 2. Plasmapheresis may abate symptoms of excess M protein 3. Bone marrow transplant reserved for resistant disease
Ovary	Irregular menses Dysmenorrhea Bleeding between menses Abdominal pain Abdominal distention	Bowel metastases with or without obstruction Omentum Pleura Bone Liver Lung (unusual or late in disease)	CT scan Surgical pathology of ovary CA-125 (used more often to monitor disease status)	1. Surgical excision desirable but not usually possible 2. External beam radiation 3. Chemotherapy may be given intraperitoneally or systemically or both; most regimens contain cisplatin or similar drug
Pancreas	Jaundice Dyspepsia Fullness of abdomen Ascites	Liver Pleura Lung	CT scan Endoscopic retrograde pancreatotomy with biopsy	1. Surgical excision offers short-term, disease-free state for a small percentage of patients 2. Systemic chemotherapy is offered, but no clear superior agent is available

Table 9.10 Cancer Overview (Continued)

Cancer	Presenting Symptoms	Diagnostic Tools	Metastatic Patterns	Treatment
Prostate	Dysuria Urinary frequency Urinary urgency Hematuria	Digital examination findings of enlarged prostate is suspicious in older male Cystoscopy biopsy	Direct extension occurs first Bone involvement of the sacrum or pelvic girdle is common Bladder Bowel Liver and/or lung involvement is late	1. Surgical resection performed if able, but debulking for unresectable tumors is not usually the chosen treatment 2. Hormonal manipulation (estrogens) are common first-line therapy in nonresectable or resistant disease 3. External beam radiation or radiation seeds implanted in the prostate used in progressive or nonresectable disease 4. Systemic chemotherapy rarely used
Renal	Hematuria Back/flank pain	CT scan Renal biopsy	Adrenals usually involved with large tumor Inferior vena cava often involved at diagnosis Bone (especially spine) Bowel/omentum Pleura and lungs Brain metastases occur with moderate frequency	1. Surgical excision or debulking usually performed first. Surgical procedure may include ureterostomy in severe disease 2. Biologic therapy common early treatment 3. External beam radiation therapy given in refractory disease or with brain metastases 4. Few chemotherapeutic agents have proven effective
Sarcoma	Painless tissue masses that may be regular or irregular in shape, usually fixed, usually firm About half are in lower extremities Tissue masses may be internal (eg, GI tract) for some subtypes Peripheral neuralgias Constitutional symptoms such as fatigue, malaise, fever	Tissue biopsy CT scan determines extent of primary and metastatic disease	Lung is common Liver	1. Surgical excision most common therapy 2. External beam radiation used postoperatively for patients at high risk for recurrence and in residual disease 3. Chemotherapy given in unresectable or metastatic disease; most effective agent is doxorubicin; other drugs added may include dacarbazine, cyclophosphamide, vincristine

Table 9.11 Tumor-Specific Oncologic Emergencies

Emergency	Description	Brain	Breast	Colon	Head/Neck	Leukemia	Lung	Lymphoma	Multiple myeloma	Ovarian	Pancreatic	Prostate	Renal	Sarcoma
Anaphylaxis	Acute severe allergic reaction that occurs secondary to a major ABO incompatibility. Usually associated with respiratory distress	X	X	X	X	X	X	X	X	X	X	X	X	X
Bowel obstruction	Primary or metastatic cancers involving the GI tract and occluding a section of bowel. Mechanism may be inflammatory fibrosis or direct compression		X	X		X		X	X	X	X	X	X	X
Chemotherapy induced cardiomyopathy	Characterized by a dilated and hypertrophied myocardium with poor contractility; caused by a direct toxicity of chemotherapy; may be acute and idiosyncratic or dose related		X			X		X						X
Coagulation abnormalities	Qualitative or quantitative deficit in platelets or coagulation factors leading to increased risk of bleeding. Abnormalities may arise from platelet abnormalities, liver-produced coagulation factors, or disorders of fibrinolysis	X	X	X	X	X	X	X	X	X	X	X		X
Disseminated intravascular coagulation	Excessive and accelerated clotting in the microvasculature; trigger mechanisms are the same as for the normal clotting cascade, but the response becomes uncontrolled; syndrome results in depletion of clotting factors, thrombotic events, and rupturing of thrombotic vessels, leading to hemorrhage	X				X	X	X		X	X			

Table 9.11 Tumor-Specific Oncologic Emergencies (*Continued*)

Emergency	Description	Brain	Breast	Colon	Head/Neck	Leukemia	Lung	Lymphoma	Multiple myeloma	Ovarian	Pancreatic	Prostate	Renal	Sarcoma
Hemorrhagic cystitis	Chemotherapy metabolite irritation and damage to the endothelial lining of the bladder leading to "mucosites of the bladder"	X	X			X		X						X
Hyperammonemia	Sudden and unprecipitated rise in ammonia levels during the aplastic period that does not correlate to a rise in hepatic enzymes such as SGOT or SGPT. Cause is uncertain but believed to be a metabolite of leukemic cell destruction					X		X						
Hypercalcemia	Serum calcium concentration exceeding 11 mg/dL; the abnormal release of calcium is caused by bone destruction from metastases, prolonged immobilization, high concentrations of parathyroid hormone found in some tumors, and presence of prostaglandins or osteoclast activating factor		X			X	X	X	X		X	X	X	
Hyperviscosity	Increase in solute or cell concentration in the blood, leading to prolonged circulatory time, venous stasis, and tendency for thromboembolic complications	X				X			X					
Increased intracranial pressure	Caused by tumors, edema, or bleeding in the brain; characterized by altered level of consciousness, irregular breathing patterns, bradycardia, nausea and vomiting, and papilledema	X	X		X	X	X	X			X		X	X

Infections and sepsis	Development of bacterial, fungal, viral, or opportunistic infections, leading to a systemic response and stimulation of the inflammatory-immune response; the inflammatory-immune response causes further cell damage from an excessive response by inflammatory mediators such as histamine, bradykinin, complement, and thromboxane	X	X	X	X	X	X	X	X	X
Malignant effusions	Development of effusions from tumor-, infection-, or inflammation-stimulated production of fluid in body compartments normally containing small amounts of lubricating fluid; excessive fluid accumulation leads to organ compression with dysfunction; common effusions occur in the abdomen (peritoneal), pericardium, and pleural areas	X	X	X	X		X	X	X	X
Meningeal carcinomatous	Infiltration of tumor cells to the arachnoid and pia mater, causing diffuse or multifocal involvement of the leptomeninges (arachnoid, pia, dura mater surrounding brain)	X	X	X	X	X				
Metabolic encephalopathy	Electrolyte and osmolarity changes resulting in brain edema or irritability; mimics several specific brain disorders with altered level of consciousness, seizures, and diminished central brain reflexes	X	X	X	X	X	X	X	X	X
Pathologic fractures	Results from bone metastases or bone resorption in chronic illness; tumor infiltration or bony matrix collapse leads to fractures without related injury; long bones are most susceptible	X	X	X	X	X	X	X	X	X
Pneumonitis	Inflammation of pulmonary endothelium with resultant capillary permeability and excessive lung water May be induced by bacteria, fungi, viruses, medications, or radiation or may be idiopathic	X	X	X	X	X	X	X	X	X

Table 9.11 Tumor-Specific Oncologic Emergencies (Continued)

Emergency	Description	Brain	Breast	Colon	Head/Neck	Leukemia	Lung	Lymphoma	Multiple myeloma	Ovarian	Pancreatic	Prostate	Renal	Sarcoma
Pulmonary capillary leak syndrome	Noncardiogenic pulmonary edema occurs after chemotherapy or with lung infections, probably because of endothelial lung injury; typical symptoms are those of diffuse lung infiltrates, respiratory distress, and hypoxemia		X			X		X						X
Scalded skin syndrome	Group of disorders with clinical presentation of surface skin burns; it is caused by drugs or staphylococcal infection or may be idiopathic		X		X	X		X						
Syndrome of inappropriate secretion of ADH	Certain cancers stimulate ADH receptors in the brain or lungs or make ectopic ADH; the excess ADH produces a water intoxication syndrome with hypo-osmolarity, hyponatremia, and primarily neurologic disturbances	X	X	X	X	X	X	X			X			
Spinal cord compression	Malignancies originating in or near the spinal column and resulting in compression and damage to the spinal cord	X	X	X	X	X	X	X	X	X	X	X	X	X
	Extravertebral lesions originate through the vertebral foramen and partially involve the cord; extradural tumors develop between the bone structures, causing destruction of the bone surrounding the spinal cord													

Superior vena cava syndrome	Occurs when the superior vena cava is occluded by external pressure, invasion by neoplasm, or intraluminal obstruction with tumor or thrombosis; leads to impaired venous return from the head and upper extremities with facial, right shoulder, chest, and arm edema
Thromboembolic complications	Development of clots in venous, arterial, or intra-organ as a result of a hypercoagulable state; clots dislodge and then travel to the lung and produce pulmonary emboli or to the brain and cause a cerebrovascular accident
	Hypercoagulability may be caused by large numbers of hyperactive circulating coagulation factors or by viscosity due to proportionately higher numbers of cells per plasma volume
Tumor lysis syndrome	Rapid and bulky destruction of tumor cells resulting in intravascular spilling of intracellular contents; leads to hyperkalemia, hyperphosphatemia, hypocalcemia, hyperuricemia, and acidosis
Urate nephropathy	Excessive amounts of uric acids crystallize within the renal tubules, cause obstruction to the outflow of filtrate, and lead to obstructive renal failure or hydronephrosis
Veno-occlusive disease of the liver	High-dose chemotherapy (especially alkylating agents) and radiation therapy cause damage to the hepatic vessels, which leads to inflammatory occlusion of hepatic circulation
	Characterized by weight gain, ascites, hyperbilirubinemia, and eventually hepatic failure

  e. *I*ndigestion or difficulty swallowing.

  f. *O*bvious change in a wart or mole.

  g. *N*agging cough or hoarseness.

 2. Diagnostic parameters

  a. Serum tests (Table 9.12) like the carcinoembryonic antigen, prostate-specific antigen, or alkaline phosphatase level. While not exclusively diagnostic in cancer, they may be used to monitor persons at risk for disease or its recurrence. Tumor markers may also be used to monitor response to therapy [7].

  b. Urine tests

   i. Cytology for malignant cells may be seen when the cancer involves the urinary tract, especially the bladder or urethra, but these are not considered diagnostic without other confirmatory tests.

  c. Other tests

   i. CT scans, magnetic resonance imaging, or positron-emission tomographic scans will detect masses that are likely to be cancerous in many circumstances. The probability of malignancy may depend on the shape, density, specific location, vascularity, and other systemic symptoms or signs that are present.

   ii. Tissue biopsy is the definitive diagnostic tool for any type of cancer. This permits characterization of cells and invasion of normal tissue by the tumor. The site of biopsy corresponds to the primary tumor or suspected metastatic lesions. The method of obtaining biopsy will depend on how the tumor can be accessed by "scopic" procedures such as endoscopy, by percutaneous aspiration, excision, or operative procedure.

B. Patient management: Problems depend on the type of cancer, site of metastasis, and treatment-related complications. Organ failure due to tumor involvement can be deduced from outlines of organ failure in other chapters. The universal care plan for the immunocompromised patient is appropriate for patients with cancer. Certain therapies are unique to cancer; thus, this care plan is based on the common problems of patients undergoing these therapies.

 1. Altered protection related to cancer development

  a. Problem: Cancer is a disease in which mutant cells bypass normal immune surveillance and proliferate uncontrollably, defining it as an alteration in protective mechanisms. If unchecked by therapy, the tumor's replacement of normal cells eventually causes widespread tissue destruction, organ dysfunction, and death.

  b. Interventions

   i. Assess family risks for cancer (eg, immediate family members with any cancer; familial tendencies for leukemia, breast, colon, and prostate cancers are supported by the scientific literature). Provide referrals and educational materials for other family members.

   ii. Assess personal risks for cancer (or second cancers) (eg, high-fat diets place patient at risk for breast or colon cancer; cigarette smoking for lung and oral cancer; sun exposure for skin cancer; more than moderate alcohol intake increases risk of larynx, esophageal, pancreas, liver, and stomach cancers). Assist patients and families in identifying methods of reducing risks for another malignancy.

Table 9.12 Select Laboratory Values from Blood Samples and Their Clinical Significance in the Diagnosis and Monitoring of Malignant Disease

Laboratory Test	Normal Reference Range	Oncologic Clinical Significance
Biochemical tests		
Acid phosphatase	M: 2.5–11.7 U/L F: 0.3–9.2 U/L	↑ Acute leukemia, multiple myeloma, metastatic prostate and breast cancer (bone)
Alkaline phosphatase	30–150 IU/L	↑ Cancer of bone, liver, leukemia, lymphoma, tumors causing extrahepatic biliary obstruction
Calcium	8.5–10.5 mg/dL	↑ Leukemia, lymphoma, multiple myeloma, bone metastasis, cancer of lung (squamous), kidney, esophagus, pancreas, bladder, liver, parathyroid
Immunoglobulins		
IgG	650–1600 mg/dL	↑ IgG myeloma
IgA	50–400 mg/dL	↑ IgA myeloma
IgM	18–280 mg/dL	↑ Waldenström's macroglobulinemia
IgD	0.5–3.0 mg/dL	↑ IgD myeloma
IgE	0.1–0.04 mg/dL	↑ IgE myeloma
		↓ Advanced neoplasms
Lactic dehydrogenase	70–250 IU/L	↑ Lymphoma, liver cancer, acute leukemia, metastatic carcinoma
Lysozyme	4.0–13.0 mg/L	↑ Acute leukemia (monocytic or myelomonocytic), chronic myeloid leukemia
Parathyroid hormone	430–1860 ng/L (C-terminal fragment) 230–630 ng/L (N-terminal fragment)	↑ Ectopic hyperparathyroidism from cancer of the kidney, lung (squamous), pancreas, ovary
Progesterone	M: 0.12–0.3 ng/mL F: 0.02–30 ng/mL	↑ Luteinizing tumors, adrenocortical tumors
Serum alanine aminotransferase (SGPT)	6–24 U/mL	↑ Metastatic liver cancer
Serum aspartate aminotransferase (SGOT)	10–30 U/mL	↑ Metastatic liver cancer

Table 9.12 Select Laboratory Values from Blood Samples and Their Clinical Significance in the Diagnosis and Monitoring of Malignant Disease (*Continued*)

Laboratory Test	Normal Reference Range	Oncologic Clinical Significance
Biochemical tests (*cont.*)		
Serum gamma glutamyl transferase (SGGT)	1–70 U/mL	↑ Metastatic liver cancer, pancreas cancer
Testosterone	M: 300–1200 ng/dL F: 10–100 ng/dL	↑ Cancer of adrenals, ovary, extragonadal tumors producing ectopic gonadotropin
Uric acid	M: 4.0–8.0 mg/dL F: 2.5–7.5 mg/dL	↑ Leukemia, multiple myeloma, disseminated cancer ↓ Hodgkin's disease, multiple myeloma, lung cancer
Tumor markers		
Alpha-fetoprotein	0–30 ng/mL	↑ Nonseminomatous germ cell testicular cancer, choriocarcinoma, gonadal teratoblastoma in children, cancer of the pancreas, colon, lung, stomach, biliary system
Carcinoembryonic antigen	Nonsmokers: 0–2.5 ng/mL Smokers: 0–3 ng/mL	↑ Cancer of the colon, rectum, stomach, pancreas, prostate, lungs, breast
Human chorionic gonado-tropin, beta subunit	0–5 IU/L	↑ Choriocarcinoma, germ cell testicular cancer, ectopic production in cancer of stomach, pancreas, lung, colon, liver
Prostate acid phosphatase	<4.0 ng/mL	↑ Metastatic cancer of prostate
Calcitonin	<100 pg/mL	↑ Cancer of thyroid (medullary), lung (small cell), breast, carcinoid
CA-125	<35 U/mL	↑ Cancer of ovary (epithelial)
Prostatic specific antigen	0–4 ng/mL	↑ Prostate cancer
Hematology		
Hematocrit	M: 41–53% F: 36–46%	↓ Anemia, nonspecific
Hemoglobin	M: 13.5–17.5 g/dL F: 12.0–16.0 g/dL	↓ Anemia, nonspecific
Leukocyte count (WBC)	M: 3.9–10.6/mm^3 F: 3.5–11.0/mm^3	↑↓ Leukemia, lymphomas, tumors involving peripheral blood marrow ↓ Leukemia, ↓ metastatic disease to bone

Leukocyte differential		
Neutrophils	54–75%	↑ Acute myeloblastic leukemia, chronic myelocytic leukemia, lymphoma ↓ Carcinoma, leukemia, sarcoma, myeloma
Lymphocytes	29–40%	↑ Leukosarcoma, lymphocytic leukemia, multiple myeloma, lymphoma, carcinoma ↓ Hodgkin's disease, leukemias (chronic, granulocytic, monocytic), lymphosarcoma, terminal carcinoma
Monocytes	2–8%	↑ Hodgkin's disease, lymphoma, monocytic leukemia, chronic myelogenous leukemia, multiple myeloma ↓ Hairy cell leukemia
Eosinophils	1–4%	↓ Chronic myelogenous leukemia, Hodgkin's disease, metastatic carcinoma, eosinophilic leukemia
Basophils	0–1%	↑ Chronic myelogenous leukemia, Hodgkin's disease
Platelet count	150,000–400,000/mm^3	↑ Myeloproliferative disorders, chronic myelogenous leukemia, carcinoma, Hodgkin's disease, lymphoma ↓ Acute leukemia, myelogenous or lymphocytic, monocytic leukemia, multiple myeloma

From O'Mary S. S. Diagnostic Evaluation, Classification, and Staging. In S. L. Groenwald et al. (eds.), *Cancer Nursing Principles and Practice* (2nd ed.). Boston: Jones & Bartlett, 1993. Pp 164–165.

      iii. Teach patient lifestyle changes that can enhance normal immunologic eradication of cancer cells (eg, adequate rest, balanced diet, relaxation, guided imagery).

      iv. Support patient through the treatment plans directed at destroying cancer. The major treatment modalities for cancer include (1) surgery, (2) radiotherapy, (3) antineoplastic chemotherapy, (4) biotherapy, and (5) bone marrow transplantation. (Tables 9.13 and 9.14 [8] describe the most common antineoplastic chemotherapy and biotherapy agents.)

   c. Desired patient outcome

      i. No clinical or pathologic evidence of cancer after therapy completion.

      ii. Control of disease symptoms; stabilization of disease progress.

      iii. Assist patient and significant others in coping with terminal disease when cure or remission is not possible.

      iv. Family or significant others are able to identify unhealthy behaviors or genetic predispositions that increase their risk of cancer.

2. Altered nutrition due to anorexia, nausea, and vomiting from therapy

   a. Problem: All therapies for cancer may alter the patient's ability or desire to eat a well-balanced diet. The mere diagnosis of cancer may cause depression and decreased appetite. After surgery, patients may be unable to tolerate oral intake until the GI tract returns to function. Radiation therapy in the abdominal region and chemotherapeutic agents alter the villi of the GI tract and increase serotonin secretion, which is thought to be one of the major stimulants of nausea and vomiting in these therapies. Radiation to the head affects proprioception centers and may cause nausea. Abdominal radiation causes increased cell death of GI tissues, resulting in impairment of digestion, intolerances to certain foods, increased irritation with increased bowel motility, and diarrhea. These effects can last months or years. Certain chemotherapeutic agents such as cisplatin have a direct effect on the chemoreceptor trigger zone in the brain and produce an almost instant severe nausea and vomiting effect.

   b. Interventions

      i. Provide premedication and postmedication with antiemetics for at least 24 hours for patients receiving therapy with known emetogenic potential. Antiemetics are of three major classes: phenothiazines (eg, chlorpromazine), cholinergic agents (eg, metoclopramide), and serotonin-blocking agents (eg, ondansetron). Adjuvant medications such as steroids, diphenhydramine, and benzodiazepines are used to enhance antiemetic effects.

      ii. Control strong odors (eg, food trays, perfume, cleaning solutions), which cause nausea for many patients.

      iii. Encourage small, frequent meals, which do not cause overfilling of the stomach.

      iv. Monitor intake and output every shift and weigh daily to assess for GI losses. Provide replacement as ordered.

      v. Monitor electrolytes daily and replace as ordered. Vomiting causes

Table 9.13 Commonly Used Chemotherapy Agents

Classification	Effects	Nursing Implications
Alkylating agents Nitrogen mustard Chlorambucil Busulfan Thiotepa	Cell cycle phase–nonspecific; destroy resting and dividing cells; cause inability of DNA to replicate	Major side effects are related to rapidly dividing normal cells: hematopoietic, gastrointestinal, and reproductive Nausea and vomiting are common Leukopenia reaches nadir in 7–14 days; recovery in about 30 days
Nitrosoureas Carmustine (BCNU) Semustine Lomustine (CCNU) Streptozocin	Cell cycle phase–nonspecific; affect DNA formation by inhibiting several enzymatic steps	Cross the blood-brain barrier; cause bone marrow suppression and gastrointestinal toxicities; delayed nadir at 3–5 weeks Severe nausea and vomiting; thrombocytopenia common
Antibiotics Actinomycin D Mitomycin C Adriamycin Daunorubicin Bleomycin Mithramycin	Cell cycle phase–nonspecific; interfere with nucleic acid synthesis and block DNA-directed RNA and DNA transcription	Bone marrow suppression common, especially leukopenia and thrombocytopenia; nadir occurs at 10–14 days with recovery in 21 days; stomatitis and alopecia can be anticipated Dose-related cardiotoxicity may be seen with doxorubicin and daunorubicin; bleomycin may cause severe pulmonary toxicity
Antimetabolites Methotrexate 5-Fluorouracil 6-Mercaptopurine Cytosine arabinoside 6-Thioguanine	Cell cycle phase–specific; inhibit DNA synthesis	Bone marrow suppression common; nadir in 1–2 weeks Alopecia, mucositis, nausea, vomiting, and diarrhea common Methotrexate can be lethal in high doses without leucovorin "rescue" of normal cells; treatment with 6-mercaptopurine and 6-thioguanine can cause liver damage
Plant alkaloids (vinca alkaloids) Vinblastine Vincristine	Cell cycle phase–specific; destroy cells by crystallizing spindle proteins during metaphase, arresting mitosis	Vinblastine causes myelosuppression with nadir in 4–10 days and recovery in 10–21 days Vincristine may cause neurotoxicity often evidenced by peripheral neuropathy, cranial nerve palsies, vocal cord paralysis, and autonomic nervous system dysfunctional constipation
Hormones Estrogens Androgens Progestins Corticosteroids	Presence of specific receptor proteins inside cytoplasm of cell allows binding of the hormone; receptor proteins facilitate synthesis of messenger RNA; using hormones antagonistic to process causes antitumor effects	Side effects are directly related to the normal action of the hormone Sexual hormones: fluid retention and changes in secondary sexual characteristics can occur Corticosteroids: cushingoid state, peptic ulcer, hypertension, diabetes, and osteoporosis

From Majiewski, A., McCoy-Adabodi, A. Oncologic Emergencies. In S. Dunbar (ed.), *AACN Clinical Reference Manual* (3rd ed.). St. Louis: Mosby–Year Book, 1993.

Table 9.14 Biotherapy agents

Agent	Action	Side Effects
Interferons Alpha Beta Gamma	Proteins that enhance antiviral immunity; capable of modifying immune responses and enhance natural killer cell activity	Influenzalike syndrome: fever, chills, malaise, fatigue, myalgias CNS: mild confusion and somnolence to seizure activity GI: nausea, vomiting, diarrhea, anorexia, weight loss Hematologic: leukopenia, thrombocytopenia, anemia Cardiovascular: hypotension, tachycardia, dysrhythmias, myocardial ischemia
Interleukins Interleukin-2	Peptides that signal between cells in the immune system; mediate expansion of T-lymphocytes	Influenzalike syndrome: fever, chills, headache Cardiovascular/pulmonary: capillary leak syndrome with resultant hypotension, decreased central venous pressure, oliguria, peripheral edema Renal: proteinuria, hematuria, increased blood urea nitrogen and creatinine, azotemia Neurologic: mental changes ranging from lethargy to psychosis GI: nausea, vomiting, diarrhea, mucositis Hepatic: increased liver function studies Integumentary: erythematous rash to dry desquamation
Monoclonal antibodies	Antibodies produced by B-lymphocytes targeted against tumor-cell antigen	Potential for severe allergic reactions, fever, rigors, chills Pulmonary: dyspnea, respiratory stridor Renal: potential renal failure from tumor lysis
Tumor necrosis factor	Soluble factor, produced by macrophages, cytotoxic for some tumor cells and some parasites	Influenzalike syndrome: fever, chills, headache, fatigue Hematologic: leukopenia, thrombocytopenia Hepatic: trglyceride elevation, decreased cholesterol Cardiovascular: hypotension Pulmonary: dyspnea
Colony-stimulating factors Granulocyte colony-stimulating factor Granulocyte macrophage colony-stimulating factor	Naturally occurring glycoproteins that stimulate the growth of colonies of maturing blood cells from their hematopoietic precursors	Influenzalike syndrome: fever, chills, rigors, myalgias, headache (usually granulocyte macrophage colony-stimulating factor)

From Majiewski, A., McCoy-Adabodi, A. Oncologic Emergencies. In S. Dunbar (ed.), *AACN Clinical Reference Manual* (3rd ed.). St. Louis: Mosby–Year Book, 1993.

hypokalemia, hypocalcemia, hypochloremia, alkalosis, and hypo-magnesemia.

    vi. After each episode of vomiting, hold all intake for 2–3 hours and medicate the patient prior to trying food again.

    vii. Heme test the emesis every shift to monitor for occult GI bleeding.

    viii. If possible, schedule administration of nausea-producing drugs for 2–3 hours after mealtime or before bedtime to reduce anorexic effect.

  c. Desired patient outcomes

    i. Patient denies the sensation of nausea or verbalizes control adequate to permit some oral intake.

    ii. Absence of vomiting.

3. Altered elimination due to diarrhea

  a. Problem: Radiation therapy to the GI tract and many chemotherapeutic agents (most all except plant alkaloids) destroy the mucosal lining of the GI tract, enhancing GI motility and causing diarrhea. The loose stools may be worsened by administration of broad-spectrum antimicrobial agents that kill the normal bacterial flora.

  b. Interventions

    i. Provide antidiarrheals as ordered. Major classes of agents include anticholinergics (eg, atropine-containing agent) and opiate derivatives (eg, tincture of opium).

    ii. Encourage food intake with fluids to provide bulk for fluid.

    iii. Provide readily available bathroom facilities (eg, bedside commode, bedpan).

    iv. Use skin barrier or protectant cream on the rectal area to prevent skin breakdown.

    v. Consider use of fecal incontinent bag if patient is unable to anticipate when he or she needs to stool or if patient has frequent incontinent stools.

    vi. Administer sources of GI-fermenting bacilli if ordered (eg, yogurt, acidophilus milk).

    vii. Offer sitz baths, warm compresses, or witch hazel compresses if hemorrhoids are aggravated by diarrhea.

    viii. Avoid taking rectal temperatures, because this action stimulates bowel movement and can injur or irritate the rectal mucosa.

    ix. Heme test all stools.

    x. Rule out infectious etiologies of diarrhea with stool cultures. Use contact precautions until negative stool cultures are confirmed.

    xi. If a patient has an ileostomy or colostomy, use appropriate skin care measures to prevent stoma irritation or skin breakdown. Teach the patient and family these measures so that they can be continued at home.

  c. Desired patient outcomes

    i. Fewer than three stools per day.

    ii. Stool less than 500 cc/d.

    iii. Prevention of fluid deficit.

    iv. Patient states he or she is comfortable.

4. Altered oral mucous membranes related to treatment induced stomatitis
   a. Problem: Rapidly dividing cells are destroyed by radiation and chemotherapy, so the mucosal cells of the entire GI tract are damaged. The clinical manifestation of this tissue damage in the oral cavity includes erythema, soreness, ulcerations, bleeding, xerostomia (dry mouth), and altered taste sensations.
   b. Interventions
      i. Inspect the oral cavity and assess at least every shift for oropharyngeal pain.
      ii. Provide oral rinsing and light toothbrushing with an oxidizing solution (one-quarter strength peroxide or weak bicarbonate solution) every 2–4 hours while awake if there is visible debris in mouth.
      iii. Culture first oral lesions or slow-to-heal lesions as ordered (bacteriology, mycology, virology).
      iv. Provide antifungal prophylaxis (eg, nystatin) as ordered for patients with stomatitis.
      v. Administer oral anesthetic agents (eg, viscous xylocaine) cautiously as ordered for painful stomatitis. Be careful to assess gag reflex after administration and use less than what compromises this reflex.
      vi. Position head of bed upright to reduce risk of aspiration from severe edema and inability to handle secretions.
      vii. Provide readily available oral suction device.
      viii. Instruct patient and caregivers about oral care measures.
   c. Desired patient outcomes
      i. Patient denies oral or pharyngeal discomfort.
      ii. Pink, moist, intact oral mucosa.
      iii. Oral symptoms do not impair normal eating and fluid intake patterns.
      iv. Patient verbalizes comfort.
5. Altered skin integrity due to rashes, burns, desquamation, immobility
   a. Problem: Rapidly dividing cells are destroyed by radiation and chemotherapy, making the skin susceptible to injury during therapy. The symptomatic sites in radiation therapy are in the area directly over the radiation treatment port. Radiated skin may show "tattoo" or sunburn effect, and these areas are more prone to injury. Chemotherapy produces a wide range of symptoms from blisters on hands and feet or total body rashes, to breakdown in skin folds. Radiotherapy and some antineoplastic drugs cause photosensitivity as well.
   b. Interventions
      i. Gently massage and cleanse skin daily to prevent infections.
      ii. Apply skin protectant/barrier to areas that are reddened, on bony prominences, and other areas prone to breakdown.
      iii. Administer antihistamines (eg, diphenhydramine) as ordered to relieve pruritus, so patients do not break skin integrity with their nails.

     iv. Perform passive range of motion or encourage active range of motion every shift.

     v. Turn immobile patients every 2–4 hours.

     vi. Provide pads (eg, heel pads) or pillows to cushion pressure on skin sites that are susceptible to breakdown.

     vii. Consult skin care experts (enterostomal therapist, wound care specialist, dermatologist) for specialty skin products with severe burns or desquamation. Dead tissue may need debridement or application of enzymatic debriding ointment to promote healing and prevent infection. Antimicrobial creams (eg, silver sulfadiazine) may be indicated in some circumstances.

     viii. Apply antifungal powder as ordered in moist, dark, skin folds where *Candida* is most likely to grow.

     ix. Culture suspicious open skin areas as ordered for bacteriology, mycology, virology.

     x. Rotate endotracheal tube from one side of the mouth to the other to prevent lip breakdown.

     xi. Limit additional invasions of barrier integrity whenever possible, because healing may be impaired after cancer therapy.

  c. Desired patient outcomes

     i. Skin is clean, dry, intact, with normal color and texture.

     ii. Patient denies skin discomfort.

     iii. Patient and caregivers learn proper techniques for maintaining skin integrity.

6. Sensory impairment due to peripheral neuropathies

  a. Problem: Plant alkaloid antineoplastic agents selectively destroy cells in the mitotic phase, the same phase in which many peripheral nerve cells exist. Patients receiving these agents are more susceptible to selective neuropathies. Peripheral neuropathies are most common, but autonomic neuropathies (eg, gastroparesis or tachycardia–bradycardia syndromes) may also occur.

  b. Interventions

     i. Monitor patients receiving long-term therapy for decreased sensation of fingertips (eg, have patient button dress shirt; as neuropathies develop, this task becomes difficult to perform).

     ii. Protect extremities from injury (eg, use a foot cradle) since altered sensation makes the patient less likely to note injury.

     iii. Assist patient when out of bed, and note ability to walk with altered sensation of bottom of feet. Sturdy shoes decrease this risk. Assistive devices (eg, cane, walker) may be obtained from physical therapy.

     iv. Obtain physical therapy and occupational therapy consults.

     v. Report intermittent tachycardia or bradycardia.

     vi. Report gradual onset of intolerance to large meals.

     vii. Monitor for constipation, because these nerves are frequently affected.

  c. Desired patient outcomes

     i. Patient develops alternative systems to detect injury to extremities and demonstrates appropriate safety measures.

     ii. Patient develops methods of accommodation for defects.

     iii. Patient is made aware of early signs of chemotherapy-induced neuropathy (constipation) and understands the need to report it promptly.

7. Potential for bleeding (see Chap. 8, "Hematologic Disorders," for more detailed guidelines in caring for patients with bleeding problems).

  a. Problem: Bone marrow cells divide rapidly and are susceptible to injury from direct beam radiation or antineoplastic chemotherapy. Suppression of platelet growth leads to thrombocytopenia and a bleeding tendency. Suppression of WBCs increases patient risk of infection.

  b. Interventions

     i. Administer coagulation products (platelets, fresh frozen plasma, cryoprecipitate) as ordered (see Chap. 8).

     ii. Elevate head of bed to decrease intracranial pressure, which can cause bleeding in susceptible patients.

     iii. Minimize breaks in barrier (eg, venous laboratory tests) by inserting long-term lines or by using noninvasive monitoring devices.

     iv. Avoid intramuscular (IM) and subcutaneous injections.

     v. Use topical hemostatics to prevent bleeding from unavoidable skin alterations.

  c. Desired patient outcomes

     i. No overt or occult bleeding.

8. Altered body image due to alopecia (hair loss), skin changes, edema, weight loss, surgical intervention (eg, colostomy, urostomy, implanted vascular access devices).

  a. Problem: Rapidly dividing cells such as hair follicles and epithelial cells are prone to damage from antineoplastic therapy. The subsequent alopecia and changes in skin may greatly alter the patient's appearance and self-image. Surgery to treat the patient's cancer may cause drastic changes in body appearance (eg, radical neck dissection, mastectomy, colostomy) that may contribute to the patient's loss of self-esteem.

  b. Interventions

     i. Advise patient that hair loss is temporary (begins 2 weeks into treatment and ends about 2 months after last treatment) and that hair often returns a different color or texture.

     ii. Encourage haircut or style changes as loss begins, so that hair does not come out in large clumps and so that thinning hair is disguised by the new hairstyle. Haircuts also shield sterile dressings from loose hair.

     iii. Provide scarves, hats, turbans, or other head coverings to cover baldness.

     iv. Offer a mirror for the patient to see changes and assist with methods to enhance appearance. Encourage patient to join a support group to learn how other patients cope with similar problems.

    v. Advise patient and family of likely darkening of skin color and texture changes. Suggest purchase of makeup with a broader color palette to accommodate changes. Encourage use of makeup to improve appearance and improve self-image.

    vi. Provide moisturizing creams to maintain smooth skin.

    vii. For patients with major changes in body appearance or functional changes, provide appropriate instruction on care and function. If desired and appropriate, arrange for a visit from a cancer survivor with similar problems. Refer to support group on discharge.

  c. Desired patient outcomes

    i. Patient uses techniques to optimize his or her appearance.

    ii. Patient verbalizes satisfaction with appearance.

    iii. Patient adjusts to changes in body structure or function and seems to accept loss without loss of personal self-esteem.

9. Altered perception of sexuality

  a. Problem: Radiation therapy to the pelvic region and most antineoplastic therapies reduce gonadal function, and some are known to be teratogenic. In addition, fatigue, anemia, and other metabolic imbalances often cause impotence in men and decreased libido in women. Patients receiving opposite-sex hormonal therapy may be upset about the effects of these drugs: women receiving androgens experience masculinizing effects, and men receiving estrogens exhibit feminization effects. Hormonal therapy is usually temporary, and these effects cease after therapy ends.

  b. Interventions

    i. Inform patient of possible sterility associated with therapy. Patients of child-bearing age must practice nonhormonal birth control while on teratogenic therapy (antineoplastic drugs and radiation). Patient and partner may need to consult a fertility specialist should parenthood be desired after therapy.

    ii. Refer patient and significant other to sperm banking facilities as indicated.

    iii. Monitor other physiologic disorders that alter sexual function (eg, hyperglycemia, anemia, hyperthyroidism, hypothyroidism, adrenal insufficiency).

    iv. Inform patient with sexual or reproductive concerns that a specialist can be consulted. Refer to a mental health professional if sexual counseling is not provided in the care setting. Provide privacy and encourage patient and partner to maintain intimacy through close physical contact.

  c. Desired patient outcomes

    i. Patient decides whether sperm banking or birth control measures are appropriate interventions for his or her family situation.

    ii. Patient is able to verbalize anticipated changes in sexuality during and after therapy and plans adaptive measures.

    iii. Patient and significant other explore alternative methods of intimacy during hospitalization.

        iv. Patient suffers no loss of self-esteem or feelings of rejection. Patient and partner are able to express their love despite problems of illness.

10. Anticipatory grieving

    a. Problem: The experience of cancer, especially if accompanied by critical illness, forces the patient and family to recognize their loss of a normal way of life. They must learn to handle the uncertainty of the illness and its possible outcomes or losses. The patient could lose a body part or function, lose ability to work, and possibly his or her life. How the patient's life is affected by this illness and his or her coping strategies are influenced by past methods of dealing with stress, anxiety, and loss, as well as supportive relationships with others.

    b. Interventions

        i. Identify how the patient and family are coping with the stresses of illness and provide them with opportunities to verbalize their needs.

        ii. Acknowledge appropriate feelings of grief and loss. Help the patient and family work through grief stages as appropriate.

        iii. Assist individuals to identify their strengths and areas in which they can control their feelings of powerlessness.

        iv. Provide appropriate referrals to social worker, community agencies, clergy, mental health professionals, and support groups as needed.

        v. Provide privacy, as needed, for patient to conduct personal matters such as legal paperwork.

        vi. Maintain an open and honest relationship in which the patient and family feel comfortable asking for prognostic information.

    c. Desired outcomes

        i. Patient and significant others demonstrate appropriate coping measures and begin to identify methods of handling the stress of loss.

        ii. Patient shows acceptance of loss.

11. Potential for altered gas exchange due to pulmonary fibrosis from radiation and chemotherapy

    a. Problem: Unshielded radiation to the lung fields and certain chemotherapy agents cause pulmonary injury. The two types of lung damage are fibrosis of the alveolar interstitium (especially antitumor antibiotics and radiation) and acute inflammatory or hypersensitivity reactions (especially antimetabolites and certain alkylating agents). Either type of lung injury eventually reduces pulmonary compliance and gas exchange.

    b. Interventions

        i. Check total life dose of bleomycin; consult physician as it nears 400–500 U (considered the maximum dose before pulmonary toxicity).

        ii. Administer supplemental oxygen cautiously after radiation or chemotherapy—oxygen toxicity occurs at lower levels for these patients (possibly as low as 30%).

iii. Assess respiratory rate, pattern, and breath sounds every shift. Report tachypnea, dyspnea, labored breathing, use of accessory muscles to breathe, diminished or adventitious sounds.

iv. Monitor chest x-rays as ordered.

v. Check oxygen saturation periodically and with every acute respiratory distress episode.

vi. Monitor arterial blood gases as ordered; note respiratory acidosis.

vii. Monitor peak airway pressures and compliance (peak pressure minus static pressure) for decreasing compliance (a cardinal sign of pulmonary toxicity).

viii. Note presence and qualities of sputum.

ix. Be certain ventilator provides adequate humidification. Patients with pulmonary toxic therapy have thicker, more tenacious secretions and are prone to mucous plugging.

x. Administer corticosteroids as ordered for suspected acute pulmonary toxicity or radiation pneumonitis.

xi. Note increases in pulmonary artery pressures that may signal the increased thoracic pressure seen with pulmonary fibrosis.

xii. Note physical activity tolerance and whether symptoms reflect restrictive pulmonary disease.

c. Desired patient outcomes

i. Patient denies dyspnea.

ii. PaO_2 greater than 60 mm Hg on arterial blood gas analysis.

iii. Oxygen saturation greater than 90% by oximeter.

iv. Functional residual capacity (FRC) greater than 2 liters.

12. Potential for altered cardiac output due to cardiomyopathies from radiation and chemotherapy

a. Problem: Unshielded radiation to the heart and certain chemotherapy agents (especially antitumor antibiotics, biotherapy, cyclophosphamide) cause hypertrophy of myocardial cells with subsequent symptoms and signs of heart failure. This may be idiosyncratic or dose dependent.

b. Interventions

i. Assess heart sounds, jugular venous pulsations (JVP), pulses, and ECG rhythm every shift. Report murmurs, gallops, increased JVP, irregular rhythms, tachycardia.

ii. Assess for peripheral edema every shift.

iii. Compare intake and output with weight to determine whether fluid is improperly excreted and may be interstitially retained.

iv. Monitor pulmonary artery or central venous pressures for elevations indicating heart failure.

v. Monitor chest x-ray for enlargement of cardiac silhouette (greater than one-half chest width).

vi. Administer fluids and colloidal products carefully, assessing for heart failure symptoms as given. Many patients require slow infusions, split blood units, or diuretics with colloids.

vii. Monitor Adriamycin or daunomycin doses; report if nearing total life dose of 500 mg/m^2.

       viii. Note physical activity tolerance and whether symptoms reflect heart failure.
    c. Desired patient outcomes
       i. Normal heart sounds
       ii. Normal heart size on chest x-ray
       iii. Absence of symptoms of heart failure

Universal Nursing Problems in the Immunocompromised Patient

I. Potential for infection

A. Problem: Patients with reduced numbers or activity of WBCs are at risk for the development of life-threatening infections. The type of infecting organism will depend on which WBC activities are altered and other host risk factors for infection. The signs and symptoms of infection in the immunocompromised host are greatly subdued because there is insufficient WBC activity to produce the usual inflammatory symptoms.

B. Interventions

    1. General interventions to control environmental risks of infection include the following:
       a. Hand washing between patients and all procedures is one of the most effective methods of reducing nosocomial infection.
       b. Follow universal precautions (see Chap. 1).
       c. Plan nurses' assignments to reduce the possibility of spread of infection between patients.
       d. Be particularly careful handling secretions/excretions that are known to be infected so that cross-contamination does not occur (eg, use different washcloth for rectum and urinary areas).
       e. Monitor visitors for any recent history of communicable diseases.
       f. Clean all multipurpose equipment (eg, oximeter probes, noninvasive BP cuffs, bedscale slings, infusion pumps, electronic thermometers) between patient use.
       g. Do not permit live flowers or standing water (eg, in vases) in the patient's room.
    2. Assessment standards
       a. Monitor temperature every 2–4 hours. Rectal temperatures are not advised due to the possibility of breaking mucosal integrity.
       b. Observe all dressings daily for signs and symptoms of infection.
       c. Inspect all orifices (oral cavity, rectal area, urethra) every shift for evidence of localized infection.
       d. Inspect all excrement every shift for cloudiness, altered color, or odors that may signify infection.
       e. Assess for any localized pain: Inspect painful areas for erythema, swelling, exudate, or rebound tenderness of abdomen that may signal pocketed infection.
       f. Auscultate breath sounds at least every shift, and report new adventitious sounds or diminished breath sounds that may herald pulmonary infection.

g. Monitor WBC elevations for evidence of infections and response to interventions. If the WBC count is low, assess WBC total count and ANC daily (see formula on p. 222). Interpret these findings by applying the following guidelines: ANC count less than 2000 cells/mm^3, risk of infection mild; less than 1000 cells/mm^3, risk moderate; less than 500 cells/mm^3, risk severe.

3. Patient care routines
   a. Bath and linen change daily, oral care three to four times daily, perineal care twice daily.
   b. Ensure that nutritional needs are being met to enhance resistance to infection and aid in healing.
   c. Protect the patient from consuming possibly contaminated foods by noting that all foods brought from home should be discarded in 1–2 days; avoid commercial foods with meat, eggs, or mayonnaise; and clean fresh fruits and vegetables before giving them to the patient. Some institutions require a "cooked-food diet," in which only foods previously cooked are permitted, with no fresh fruits or nuts, pepper, or other raw or possibly contaminated foods.
   d. Ensure that sleep needs are being met to enhance resistance to infection and aid in healing.
   e. Control glucose levels, so that unintentional hyperglycemia does not occur. (Hyperglycemia compromises phagocytic activities that fight infection.)
   f. Consider noninvasive monitoring methods whenever possible.
   g. Report characteristics of excrement or wound drainage.
   h. Use sterile technique for inserting and dressing IV catheters. Sites should be changed at least every 72 hours when possible.
   i. Invasive lines exposed to contaminating secretions (eg, jugular or femoral lines) may require antimicrobial ointment, occlusive dressings, and more frequent dressing changes.
   j. Cover all open wounds with sterile dressing. Skin abrasions may be treated with antimicrobial ointment and dressings, or left open to air provided frequent cleansing is performed.
   k. Encourage incentive spirometry or deep breathing and coughing.
   l. Apply skin protectant to sites at risk for skin breakdown.
   m. If construction is occurring, consider applying a mask on the patient during intrahospital transport. If hepa filtration or other airflow protection is provided to the patient while in the unit, and building air systems are old, masks may be considered for transport as well.
   n. Avoid stopcocks in IV systems; use closed injection site systems.
   o. IV tubing is changed every 72 hours if a closed system is maintained. More frequent changes are advocated if the line is open or if open (semipermeable membrane) transducer systems are used.
   p. Consider closed endotracheal tube suction systems provided there is an in-line flush port to clean the catheter after each use.
   q. Change oxygen setups with standing water (eg, nasal cannula, ventilator tubing) every 24 hours.
   r. For first fever or new fever, perform routine culture and assessment

functions as indicated or ordered prior to initiation of antimicrobial therapy. (New fever is defined as one that exceeds 38.3°C after 72 hours on an antibiotic regimen.)

    i. Blood cultures from two sites.

    ii. Blood cultures from existing venous/arterial access devices.

    iii. Urine culture.

    iv. Stool culture (if diarrhea is present cultures are performed daily for 3 consecutive days).

    v. Sputum culture.

    vi. Chest x-ray.

    vii. Orifices cultured—nose, mouth, rectum. Some institutions advocate culture of skin where darkness and moistness are a problem such as skin folds in groin or under arm.

    viii. Assess breath sounds and report adventitious or diminished sounds.

s. Administer antimicrobial therapy as ordered. (Common agents and their nursing implications are included in Table 9.6.) Administration of these agents should be changed to IV form if the patient is unable to take medication orally.

t. Perform antimicrobial peak and trough levels as ordered. Be certain that the exact time of last medication is listed in order to calculate levels accurately.

u. Be alert to superinfection with fungal flora at any time 7–10 days after initiation of broad-spectrum antibiotics. Prophylaxis (eg, oral nystatin or topical nystatin powder) may be started in some individuals.

v. Enhance immune system functioning.

    i. Ensure that nutritional needs are being met to enhance resistance to infection and aid in healing.

    ii. Ensure that sleep needs are being met to enhance resistance to infection and aid in healing.

    iii. Control glucose levels, so that unintentional hyperglycemia does not occur. (Hyperglycemia compromises phagocytic activities that fight infection.)

    iv. If neutropenia is a problem, discuss with multidisciplinary team; consider use of granulocyte-stimulating factor.

> **granulocyte colony-stimulating factor (Filgrastim)**
> *Administration Guidelines* Single daily IV dose of 5 μg/kg every day for up to 2 weeks based on postchemotherapy nadir. When given outside of planned nadir ANC, as with antineoplastic therapy, may be given for up to 2 weeks. Should not be used 24 hours before or 24 hours after the administration of antineoplastic chemotherapy. Therapy should be continued within this 2-week time frame until the WBC count reaches 10,000 cells/mm^3. Administer single dose over 1 minute or less.
> *Nursing Considerations* IV administration of the single dose over 1 minute or less. Use extreme caution in any myeloid malignancy; can act as growth factor for any tumor. Use caution in patients with preexisting cardiac disease; cardiac events (eg, myocardial infarction) have occurred, but relationship to filgrastim is unclear. Discontinue therapy and notify physician immediately if allergic reactions (itching, redness, swelling at the injection site) occur. Discontinue therapy after ANC surpasses 10,000 cells/mm^3, and chemotherapy nadir has occurred.

    w. If total bone marrow suppression is a problem or fungal infection is a high risk, discuss with multidisciplinary team considering use of granulocyte-macrophage colon-stimulating factor or erythropoietin replacement.

> **granulocyte-macrophage colony-stimulating factor**
> *Administration Guidelines* Daily infusion of 250 μg/m^2 for 21 days. Initiate 2–4 hours after autologous bone marrow infusion and not less than 24 hours after the last dose of chemotherapy or 12 hours after the last dose of radiation. Reduce dose in impaired renal or hepatic function. Each 250- or 500-μg vial must be diluted with 1 mL preservative-free sterile water for injection.
> *Nursing Considerations* Administer each single dose over 2 hours. Reduce rate or discontinue therapy if allergic reactions occur. Should be clear and colorless. If the final concentration will be below 10 μg/mL, add albumin to normal saline (1 mL of 5% albumin to each 50 mL normal saline) before addition of medication. Use caution when administering for any malignancy with myeloid characteristics. Monitor CBC and differential before and twice weekly thereafter to detect any leukocytosis (WBC > 50,000 cells/mm^3; or ANC > 20,000 cells/mm^3). Reduce dose or discontinue therapy if leukocytosis is detected. Observe for fluid retention (peripheral edema, pleural effusion, and/or pericardial effusion). Use caution in individuals with a history of renal or hepatic dysfunction.

    x. Check IgG levels, and if low discuss with the multidisciplinary team considering IV administration of immune globulin infusions.

> **immune globulin**
>
> *Administration Guidelines* Single IV dose of 100–200 mg/kg
> and retest IgG levels: level should be > 300 mg/dL after infusion
> therapy. Dilute in large volume of fluid (approximately 1 liter) and
> administer over at least 2 hours.
> *Nursing Considerations* Hypersensitivity may occur. Administer
> slowly, observing frequent vital signs (about every 15 minutes) and
> signs and symptoms of respiratory distress for the first 30–60
> minutes of infusion. High-volume infusion may precipitate
> congestive heart failure in susceptible patients—monitor to detect
> signs and symptoms early. Administer through central venous
> access only—produces severe phlebitis. Dose may be repeated
> monthly if levels decrease or clinical improvement is not evident.

    y. Granulocyte transfusions are reserved for individuals with overwhelming sepsis and little hope of return of their white cell function during the crisis. Nursing care of patients receiving granulocyte transfusion includes the following:

      i. Premedicate with acetaminophen 625 mg and benadryl 25–50 mg

      ii. Take baseline vital signs.

      iii. Hang on blood infusion set, but without microaggregate filter Have normal saline available for flushing.

      iv. Be certain that patient has an additional patent IV access for possible emergency medication administration.

      v. Administer slowly, approximately 5 mL/min for first 5 minutes then increase rate as ordered by blood bank, because WBC should be transfused at a certain number of cells per minute, and the blood bank has determined how much diluent is in cells.

      vi. Monitor for anaphylaxis or severe allergic reactions: respiratory distress, wheezing, hypotension, pain at IV site, chest pain.

      vii. Agitate bottom of bag every 15 minutes to ensure mixing of cells in solution. (Cells will settle to bottom of bag and infuse rapidly if not agitated.)

      viii. Draw postinfusion WBC count 2–4 hours after infusion.

      ix. Observe for inflammatory symptoms at site of suspected infection

C. Desired patient outcome

  1. Afebrile.

  2. No exudative signs of infection.

  3. Negative cultures for microbes.

II. Hyperthermia

A. Problem: Infections that commonly occur in the immunocompromised patient produce an elevated body temperature that increases metabolic demands and causes discomfort and physical decompensation.

B. Interventions

  1. Administer acetaminophen every 4 hours as tolerated and as ordered Drug is given with caution for individuals with compromised liver function, or before broad-spectrum antimicrobial therapy has been implemented.

2. Administer warmed blankets as needed for chills experienced by the patient as the temperature increases.

3. Chills can be diminished or broken by administration of small doses of IV meperidine (12–25 mg initially, may be repeated two to three times) or morphine sulfate (0.5 mg every 3–5 minutes until relief).

4. Monitor respiratory status during hyperthermia; oxygenation often goes down, but the effects of increased temperature may make oxygen saturation remain the same.

5. Monitor platelet count, since it may decrease due to the hypermetabolism of hyperthermia.

6. Avoid feeding patient when febrile, since nausea and vomiting are common problems at that time.

7. Avoid additional causes of fever while trying to resolve (eg, try not to give blood products until fever is resolved).

C. Desired outcome

  1. Body temperature less than 38°C

III. Alteration in comfort related to fever, vasodilation (headache), diffuse myalgias and arthralgias, sweating after temperature returns to normal

A. Problem: Immunosuppressed patients who develop infections have uncomfortable constitutional symptoms that require intervention. Vasodilation produces warm feeling, headache, dizziness, and orthostasis. Vague multisystem aches signal infection.

B. Interventions

  1. Acetaminophen 650 mg q4h, as needed, as ordered for minor flulike symptoms

  2. Darken room and promote rest when patient is symptomatic.

  3. Apply cool compresses to head as needed for comfort.

  4. Perform orthostatic blood pressure checks and supervise activity when out of bed.

  5. Bathe patient and change linen after fever breaks.

C. Desired outcome

  1. Patient verbalizes relief of uncomfortable symptoms.

IV. Impaired wound healing

A. Problem: Suppression of immune function impairs the body's ability to provide an appropriate WBC response to injury with inflammation and subsequent healing. Wounds are slow to heal when the patient has a suppressed immune system.

B. Interventions

  1. Assess the skin every shift for breaks in integrity that must be monitored for infection.

  2. Apply antimicrobial ointments to open skin lesions or other therapies as ordered for incisions or surgical wounds.

  3. Perform wound care with sterile technique.

  4. Limit invasive procedures when possible (eg, insert a saline lock for blood drawing to minimize venipunctures).
  5. Enhance nutrition to offset some immune dysfunction.
C. Desired outcome
  1. Patient is without open wounds, lesions.

V. Social isolation

A. Problem: Individuals with immune compromise must always limit activities and social interactions. Exposure to crowds or communicable diseases can cause life-threatening infections, so patients often must alter their lifestyles and family structures to accommodate this need.
B. Interventions
  1. Teach patient situations to be avoided (eg, day care centers in which communicable diseases are common).
  2. Encourage alternative methods of socializing (eg, videotaping events, video telephones).
  3. Refer patient and family to mental health professional for assessment of the impact of this problem on relationship with significant other and family.
C. Desired outcome
  1. Patient and significant others verbalize satisfying relationships.

References

1. Allen, M. A. The Immune System. In J. E. Wright and B. K. Shelton (eds.), *Desk Reference for Critical Care Nursing*. Boston: Jones & Bartlett, 1993. Pp. 1092–1094.

2. Allen, M.A., Shelton, B. K. Neutropenia. In J. E. Wright and B. K. Shelton (eds.), *Desk Reference for Critical Care Nursing*. Boston: Jones & Bartlett, 1993. Pp. 1128–1130.

3. Maguire-Eisen, M., Edmonds, K. S. Leukemias. In J. C. Clark and R. F. McGee (eds.), *Core Curriculum for Oncology Nursing* (2nd ed.). Philadelphia: Saunders, 1992. P. 486.

4. Shelton, B. K. Infection and Immune Disorders. In *Advanced Management of Clinical Emergencies*. Baltimore: The Johns Hopkins Staff Development Program, 1990.

5. Centers for Disease Control. 1993 Revised classification system for HIV infection and expanded surveillance case definition for AIDS among adolescents and adults. *MMWR* 41(RR-17):2, 1992.

6. Wingo, P. A., Tong, T., Bolden, S. Cancer Statistics, 1995. *CA* 45(1):8, 1995.

7. O'Mary, S. S. Diagnostic Evaluation, Classification, and Staging. In S. L. Groenwald et al. (eds.), *Cancer Nursing Principles and Practice* (2nd ed.). Boston: Jones & Bartlett, 1993. Pp. 164–165.

8. Majiewski, A., McCoy-Adabodi, A. Oncologic Emergencies. In S. Dunbar (ed.), *AACN Clinical Reference Manual* (3rd ed.). St. Louis: Mosby-Year Book, 1993. Pp. 1077–1100.

CHAPTER 10

Burns

Jennifer Hebra

I. Definition: Burn injuries are estimated to affect approximately 2 million individuals each year, with 80% of the victims having less than 20% total body surface area (TBSA) involvement. A burn injury is defined as damage to the skin from a thermal, electrical, or chemical agent. The severity or depth of the injury depends on the temperature, intensity, and duration of contact with the causative agent.

A. Extent of burn injury: Either the Lund and Browder method (Table 10.1) [1] or the "Rule of Nines" (Fig. 10.1) can be used to estimate percentage of TBSA burned. Although the Rule of Nines is not as accurate as the Lund and Browder method, it can provide the practitioner with a quick estimation of the surface area involved. Burns that involve greater than 2% TBSA of full-thickness injury or greater than 10% TBSA of deep partial-thickness injury usually require inpatient treatment. Major burns should be evaluated for possible transfer to a burn center. See Table 10.2 [2] for the evaluation criteria for transfer to a specialized burn center. Patients with partial- or full-thickness injuries that extend greater than 20% TBSA should receive intravenous (IV) fluid resuscitation.

B. Depth of injury: Correct determination of the depth of injury is vital and will assist the health care team in planning treatment, estimating prognosis, and calculating fluid and nutritional requirements. A superficial partial-thickness (first-degree) injury involves only the outer layer of skin, while deep partial-thickness (second-degree) and full-thickness (third-degree) injuries involve the epidermis and varying degrees of the dermis and possibly the subcutaneous tissue. Table 10.3 describes the skin layer involved and provides an assessment description of the various injury depths.

C. Location of injury: Inpatient treatment is required for all partial- and full-thickness burns of the face, hands, feet, or genitalia. Burns of major flexor joints should be hospitalized for treatment to minimize contracture formation.

II. Etiology: When skin integrity is challenged by environmental hazards, the skin responds immediately. Heat, chemical, and electrical injuries may cause protein coagulation and cell death, depending on the intensity and time of exposure. Cold-temperature injuries (eg., frostbite) result in vascular spasm. All exposures result in temporary or permanent interruption in blood flow to

268 ▼ 10. Burns

Table 10.1 Estimation of Percentage Total Body Surface Area Burned
(Lund and Browder)

Location	Burn Age (yr)					Percent (%)		
	0–1	2–4	5–9	10–15	Adult	Second Degree	Third Degree	Total
Head	19	17	13	10	7			
Neck	2	2	2	2	2			
Anterior trunk	13	13	13	13	13			
Posterior trunk	13	13	13	13	13			
R buttock	2½	2½	2½	2½	2½			
L buttock	2½	2½	2½	2½	2½			
Genitalia	1	1	1	1	1			
R upper arm	4	4	4	4	4			
L upper arm	4	4	4	4	4			
R lower arm	3	3	3	3	3			
L lower arm	3	3	3	3	3			
R hand	2½	2½	2½	2½	2½			
L hand	2½	2½	2½	2½	2½			
R thigh	5½	6½	8½	8½	9½			
L thigh	5½	6½	8½	8½	9½			
R leg	5	5	5½	6	7			
L leg	5	5	5½	6	7			
R foot	3½	3½	3½	3½	3½			
L foot	3½	3½	3½	3½	3½			
								Total

R, right; L, left.
Note: Numbers in table body equal percentage of BSA affected at each burn location.
Adapted from Harvey, J. S., Watkins, G. M., and Sherman, R. T. Emergent burn care. *South Med J* 77:204, 1984.

Table 10.2 Criteria for Transfer to a Specialized Burn Center

- 20% or greater TBSA of deep, partial-, or full-thickness burns
- 10% or greater TBSA full-thickness burn
- Elderly or children (< 10 years) with greater than 10% TBSA burn
- Pulmonary or inhalation injury
- Circumferential burns
- Deep, partial-, or full-thickness burns to the face, hands, feet, genitalia, or joints
- Electrical or chemical burns
- Burns associated with significant trauma or preexistng illness

TBSA, total body surface area.
Adapted from the American Burn Association. Hospital and prehospital resources for optimal care of patients with burn injury: Guidelines for development and operation of burn centers. *J Burn Care Rehabil* 11:97, 1990.

Figure 10.1 Estimate the percentage of the TBSA burned using the Rule of Nines. Shade the burned areas on the diagram using different colored markers to correlate with burn depth. Each area is divided by factors of nine. A. Anterior. B. Posterior.

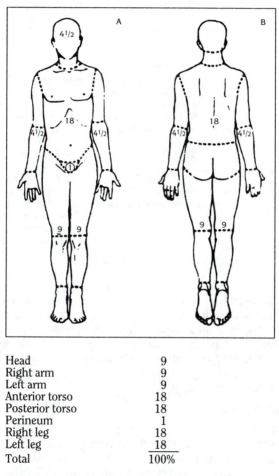

Head	9
Right arm	9
Left arm	9
Anterior torso	18
Posterior torso	18
Perineum	1
Right leg	18
Left leg	18
Total	100%

(Adapted from *Intensive Care Medicine* (2nd ed.). Edited by J. M. Rippe, R. S. Irwin, J. S. Alpert, and M. P. Fink. Published by Little, Brown and Company. 1991. P. 1509.)

the area and increased capillary permeability. Cellular enzymes, histamine, serotonin, prostaglandins, and interleukin-1 are just a few of the substances that are deployed in response to the injury. Burns are always associated with some degree of protein, fluid, and electrolyte shift among the intravascular, interstitial, and intracellular spaces. Generalized edema is commonly seen with injuries that exceed 25% TBSA. This process begins with massive fluid loss from the injured site and is worsened by increased capillary permeability.

Table 10.3 Skin Layer Involvement of Burn Injuries

Burn Injury	Skin Layer Involvement	Assessment Description
Superficial partial-thickness (first-degree burn)	Epidermis, or outer layer of skin that contains melano-cytes (protects from ultra-violet radiation) and Langer-hans' cells (defends against foreign body invasion)	Minor inflammation, erythema (redness); pain and burning sensation; no blisters
Deep partial-thickness (second-degree burn)	The entire epidermis and part of the dermis layer; contains collagen and elastin (sup-portive structure for the hair follicles, blood vessels, nerve endings, sebaceous glands, and the sweat glands)	Major inflammation, mobilizes fluid to the area in an attempt to repair the damage; leaves nerve endings exposed; blis-ters; swelling, moist surface; extremely painful; hypersen-sitive to touch and movement of air
Full-thickness (third-degree burn)	Damage of the entire epidermis and dermis layers and some portion of the subcutaneous tissue	Blood vessels thrombosed, skin completely necrosed causes permanent cell death; no pain (nerve endings destroyed; white, gray, or charred color; waxy and dry appearance; leathery texture)

Tissue edema and cellular swelling occur early as a result of a shift of water and sodium to the intracellular space. This causes further decrease of tissue perfusion related to the increase in interstitial pressure, obstruction to lymphatic flow, and depletion of intravascular volume. Multisystem failure is a constant threat throughout the initial phase of burn recovery due to the systemic inflammatory response combined with the decrease in tissue perfusion to various organs.

III. Nursing process

A. Assessment

1. Signs and symptoms: Although the burn wounds may appear dramatic and life-threatening, the basics of life support must be the priority. Quickly assess and treat airway, breathing, and circulation concerns before addressing the burn injuries. However, the patient should be covered with warm, sterile sheets and blankets to avoid rapid heat loss through the burn wounds.

   a. Burn injury assessment: Hypothermia and large evaporative water losses may occur if the burn wounds are not assessed and covered quickly. Estimate the percentage TBSA burned and determine the depth of injury of each wound using Table 10.1 and Figure 10.1. The estimated TBSA burned is used for determining the fluid requirements of the patient.

      i. Airway obstruction may develop immediately if substantial inhalation injury has occurred or may be delayed with progressive swelling of the airway and can continue for as long as 48 hours after the initial insult. Suspect airway obstruction if burn injury occurred in an enclosed space or in the presence of facial or neck burns or singed nasal hairs, carbon noted in mouth/oropharynx, carbonaceous sputum, circumferential burns to torso or neck, stridor, deteriorating arterial blood gases, hoarseness, rhonchi, dyspnea, or a change in voice. In addition, by-products of the combustion of chemicals may cause pneumonitis that can lead to the development of pneumonia, acute respiratory distress syndrome (ARDS), and even irreversible respiratory failure.

ii. Massive intravascular fluid loss occurs with burns greater than 20% TBSA, and signs of hypoperfusion and hypovolemia may appear if fluid resuscitation is not immediate. Sequelae include marked increase in capillary permeability, partially due to histamine release; loss of plasma and albumin that readily pass through capillary membranes taking fluid along out of the vasculature; drop in blood volume that leads to decreased venous return and blood pressure; and possibly irreversible hypovolemic shock. Symptoms of intravascular hypovolemia include hypotension, weak or absent peripheral pulses, edema, tachycardia, pale mucosal membranes, and decreased filling pressures (pulmonary artery pressure [PAP], pulmonary artery wedge pressure [PAWP], and central venous pressure [CVP]).

iii. Kidney damage may result due to decreased renal perfusion from hypovolemia as capillary leak progresses; associated injury trauma; sepsis; or drug therapy resulting in oliguria, anuria, or renal failure. Also, in very deep integument injuries or in electrical burns, muscle breakdown occurs resulting in the release of myoglobin in the blood contributing to renal damage. Symptoms include urine output less than 30 mL/h, increased specific gravity, urine a very dark amber color, hemoglobinuria, or myoglobinuria.

iv. Most GI disturbances can be attributed to the stress of the burn injury and shunting of blood away from the gut during the hypovolemic state. This combination may cause hypersecretion of acid in the stomach, ischemia to the gastric mucosa, or decreased mucosal production. Signs and symptoms include nausea and vomiting, decreased or absent bowel sounds from altered peristaltic function, paralytic ileus, peptic ulcers, Curling's ulcers (acute peptic ulcers usually associated with burn injuries—a form of stress ulcer), or deep ulcerations in the duodenum.

v. Hypermetabolism secondary to elevated catecholamine levels causes an increase in body temperature by 1–2°F, an increase in heart rate, shivering, protein wasting, an increase in oxygen consumption, and an alteration in glucose balance resulting from evaporative water losses through the burn wounds and catabolic processes.

vi. Associated injuries: It should be kept in mind that burn injuries are a traumatic occurrence, and, therefore, other major injuries may be present. A complete physical assessment and history of related events are crucial. Refer to Chapter 3 for a review of the assessment guidelines and treatment of the trauma patient.

2. Diagnostic tests
   a. Serum tests: Most alterations in electrolyte balances occur because massive intravascular volume is escaping to the interstitium as part of the inflammatory response mechanism.
      i. Hemoglobin/Hematocrit: elevated due to hemoconcentration and intravascular fluid volume loss or decreased as a result of bleeding from associated traumatic injuries; hemoglobin may also be decreased due to hemolysis; hematocrit should decrease as fluid is replaced (24–48 hours).
      ii. Urea nitrogen: increased due to hemoconcentration and intravascular fluid volume loss; acute renal failure.
      iii. Alterations in potassium, sodium, and chloride: increased levels of the electrolytes result from osmotic pressure changes that draw water into the cells, sending potassium out; cell destruction and the hemolysis of red blood cells; overriding hemoconcentration; chloride reabsorption from urine causes increased serum levels and acidosis; however, as rehydration occurs, these electrolytes are decreased as they move back into the cells or lost through diuresis; sodium may also be initially decreased as it is lost in wound exudate.
      iv. Creatine kinase (CK): elevated if skeletal muscle damage has occurred from very deep full-thickness burns or from electrical injuries.
      v. Albumin: reduced due to loss of protein through wounds and increased capillary permeability.
      vi. Arterial blood gases: Metabolic acidosis results from renal failure, poor peripheral perfusion that causes anaerobic metabolism and lactic acid buildup, or from the application of mafenide acetate.
      vii. Carboxyhemoglobin (carbon monoxide bound with hemoglobin): may be present if inhalation injury has occurred (normally less than 5%–10%, depending on area pollution or smoking habits).
   b. Urine tests
      i. Specific gravity: greater than 1.030 indicates a concentrated urine as a result of inadequate fluid replacement, protein wasting, or glucose spillage.
      ii. Protein: positive if in negative nitrogen balance and body burns protein rather than food.
      iii. Glucose: positive; stress response causes the body to underutilize ingested glucose and excess is excreted in the urine.
      iv. Myoglobinuria: myoglobin in the urine due to muscle destruction in severe thermal burns or electrical injuries resulting in potential renal destruction.
   c. Other tests
      i. Bronchoscopy will assist in determining the extent of inhalation injury; there may be mucosal damage or carbon noted in the tracheobronchial tree.
      ii. Chest radiography: A chest x-ray should be done for a baseline

reading and will assist in diagnosing smoke inhalation, respiratory distress, or traumatic injuries.

    iii. ECG: Obtain an ECG for a baseline reading and to assess if ischemic myocardial changes have occurred from electrical injuries or electrolyte imbalances.

B. Patient management

   1. Alteration in gas exchange related to inhalation injury, airway obstruction, carbon monoxide poisoning (inhalation of smoke if burn occurred in enclosed space), and pulmonary edema formation

    a. Problem: decrease in oxygenation (hypoxia), carbon dioxide retention, carboxyhemoglobin (carbon monoxide bound with hemoglobin decreasing oxygen-carrying capacity).

    b. Intervention

      i. Assess every hour for the development of airway obstruction from tracheal edema or secretions; note hoarseness, stridor, change in voice, or carbonaceous sputum.

      ii. Provide supplemental humidified oxygen as required.

      iii. May need intubation or tracheostomy secondary to edema and inhalation injury (tracheostomies through burn injuries are avoided due to increased risk of sepsis).

      iv. Keep airway clear of secretions. (Assess ability of patient to mobilize secretions; be prepared for pharyngeal or endotracheal suctioning; provide humidification.)

      v. Encourage patient to cough, deep breathe, and use incentive spirometer every hour while awake.

      vi. Assist patient to change positions every 1–2 hours to mobilize secretions and use chest wall muscles.

      vii. Perform chest physiotherapy to mobilize secretions.

      viii. Assess level of consciousness every 1–4 hours.

      ix. Monitor pulse oximetry closely, maintain greater than 95%.

      x. Obtain arterial blood gases and monitor results closely.

      xi. To support adequate chest expansion, assess need for escharotomies (incision through eschar to release pressure caused by edema accumulation) if chest or neck have circumferential burns.

      xii. Provide continued ventilatory support or oxygen therapy as needed to maintain adequate blood gases and prevent acid base disturbances.

      xiii. Administer diuretics as needed to maintain optimal fluid volume (only after complete fluid resuscitation has occurred).

    c. Desired outcome

      i. Respiratory rate within normal limits.

      ii. Oxygen saturation greater than 95%.

      iii. Airway remains patent.

      iv. Absence of adventitious breath sounds.

      v. Absence of obstruction from edema, secretions, stridor.

      vi. Absence of dyspnea and cyanosis.

      vii. Normal arterial blood gases and evidence of lung perfusion.

      viii. Absence of acidosis or alkalosis.

        ix. Carboxyhemoglobin less than 10%.

        x. No evidence of pulmonary edema (rales, frothy sputum)

  2. Decrease in cardiac output related to increased capillary permeability and leak of plasma fluid volume from the intravascular space

     a. Problem: decreased tissue perfusion, tissue hypoxia, and possible organ dysfunction (also worsened by local compression due to edema), hypotension, hypovolemia, decreased venous return, depressed myocardial function, and cell damage.

     b. Intervention

        i. IV fluid therapy is required for burns greater than 20% TBSA.

        ii. Insert two large-bore catheters; do not insert distal to circumferential burns.

        iii. IV formulas are available (Table 10.4) [3] to use as a guide; titrate to maintain a urine output of greater than 30–60 mL/h and adequate BP and CVP (2–6 mm Hg).

        iv. Be prepared for the insertion of a central line or a pulmonary artery (PA) catheter.

        v. Monitor and document PA catheter reading every 4 hours; notify physician if a worsening trend appears.

        vi. Fluid replacement should be tailored to the individual patient

Table 10.4 Formulas to Establish Fluid Requirements

Formula	Electrolyte Solution	Colloid Solution	Glucose in Water
Evans—first 24 h	NS—1.0 mL/kg per percent of burn	1.0 mL/kg per percent of burn	2000 mL
Evans— second 24 h	NS—½ of 1st 24-h requirement	½ of 1st 24-h requirement	2000 mL
Brooke—first 24 h	LR—1.5 mL/kg per percent of burn	0.5 mL/kg per percent of burn	2000 mL
Brooke— second 24 h	LR—½ to ¾ of 1st 24-h requirement	½ to ¾ of 1st 24-h requirement	
Modified Brooke— first 24 h	LR—2.0 mL/kg per percent of burn		
Modified Brooke— second 24 h		0.3–0.5 mL/kg per percent of burn	To maintain urine output >30–60 mL/h
Parkland— first 24 h	LR—4 mL/kg per percent of burn		
Parkland— second 24 h		20%–60% of calculated plasma volume deficit*	2000 mL

NS, normal saline; LR, lactated Ringer's solution.
*Estimated plasma volume deficit:
   0.3 mL/kg/% TBSA burn if burn >30% and <50%.
   0.4 mL/kg/% TBSA burn if burn >50% and <70%.
   0.5 mL/kg/% TBSA burn if burn >70%.
Adapted from Davis, J. H., Drucker, W. R., and Foster, R. S., et al. *Clinical Surgery* (vol 2). St. Louis: C. V. Mosby, 1987. P. 2844.

based on percentage of TBSA of open wounds, past medical history, renal function, and age.

vii. Monitor patient carefully for fluid overload, especially in patients older than 65 years, or with renal disease; symptoms include crackles, dyspnea, weight gain, increased edema, jugular venous distention, or auscultation of third heart sound.

viii. Monitor and track electrolyte values.

ix. Monitor urine specific gravity every 4–6 hours; value will return to normal when patient is rehydrated.

x. After capillary permeability returns to normal and fluid reenters the vascular space (approximately 36–48 hours), IV fluid administration should be greatly reduced, and diuretics may be considered to prevent fluid overload.

xi. Administration of blood products and electrolytes should be determined based on laboratory data; consider hemoconcentration effects when replacing blood and electrolytes.

xii. Insert indwelling urinary catheter; strict input and output data must be maintained.

xiii. Weigh patient daily.

xiv. Ensure that hypovolemia has been corrected before considering vasopressors to maintain BP.

c. Desired outcome

i. Perfusion of all vital organs.

ii. Clear sensorium.

iii. Heart rate within 20 beats/min of baseline.

iv. BP with 10 mm Hg to patient baseline.

v. PAP, PAWP, and CVP within normal limits.

vi. Urine specific gravity normal.

vii. Urine output greater than 30 mL/h.

viii. Brisk capillary refill.

ix. Positive pulses in all extremities.

3. Pain and skin integrity disruption related to burn injury

a. Problem: fluid loss, pain, potential for infection, ineffective thermoregulation, loss of presentable cosmetic appearance.

b. Intervention

i. Emergent period.

- Quickly remove burning agent and apply tepid sterile water towels for no longer than 10–15 minutes (due to possible vasoconstriction); do not expose burns to ice or frigid temperatures; the cold will cause further vasoconstriction and extend the cell injury.

- Rinse burn wounds with water.

- Cover entire body with sterile sheets or blankets to keep patient warm until a complete assessment is done and sterile dressings can be applied.

ii. Acute period: Consider transfer to a specialized burn center for major burns (see Table 10.2).

- Superficial partial-thickness burn

- ○ Wash thoroughly with soap and water and observe aseptic technique.
- ○ Leave wound open; ointments should not be applied.
- ○ Chemical burns should be managed according to the causative agent. Consult with local Occupational Safety and Health Administration or poison control office.
- ○ Elevate extremities to decrease edema formation.
- ○ Monitor wound closely to ensure conversion to second-degree injury has not occurred. (Infection can convert a superficial injury to a partial-thickness injury.)
- ▪ Deep partial- or full-thickness burn
- ○ Wash thoroughly to remove all ointments and debris; depending on institutional policy, sterile or tap water and liquid soap may be used.
- ○ Use sterile scissors to remove necrotic skin and to separate loose eschar (scablike tissue that forms over burn wound).
- ○ The management of blisters that form from deep partial-thickness burns should follow the guidelines provided in Table 10.5 [4].
- ○ After wound has dried, an antimicrobial ointment is applied with sterile gloves to completely cover the burned area.

Antimicrobial agents
Action Prevent and treat wound sepsis.
Special Considerations Specific to agent used (Table 10.6) [5].

- ○ Depending on whether the open or closed method is being used, sterile dressings are applied.
- ○ Wounds must be washed with soap and water at least twice a day and antimicrobial ointment reapplied.
- ○ Elevate extremities to prevent edema formation.
- ○ Apply splints to prevent contractures and support limb function.
- ○ Monitor wound carefully for infection: edema, excessive pain, redness, foul odor, purulent drainage, rapid separation of eschar, or systemic signs of sepsis.

Table 10.5 Management of Blister Formation

- ▪ Burns of greater than 20% TBSA that are being treated in a burn center usually call for the debridement of all blisters
- ▪ Blisters on wounds that involve less than 10% TBSA that are intact, small, and filled with clear fluid may be left intact
- ▪ If there are some blisters with partial or complete rupture, all remaining blisters should be debrided, since partial rupture increases the likelihood of wound infection
- ▪ Blisters of the hands and feet are usually debrided to facilitate early physical activity

---

TBSA, total body surface area.
Adapted from W. L., Garner, C. Zuccaro, and C. Marcelo, et al. The effects of burn blister fluid keratinocyte replication and differentiation. *J Burn Care Rehabil* 14:127, 1993.

○ Provide support through frequent operative procedures for surgical debridement and skin grafting.

—Surgical debridement: Care of patients after surgery should include assessment of bleeding at debrided sites every hour and monitoring for excessive fluid loss; in collaboration with the physician, the wound should be opened on postoperative day 1 and washed and dressed similarly to other open wounds.

—Care of skin grafts: Decrease all friction of the grafted area, maintain immobility, ensure dressings remain intact for at least 3 days unless infection is suspected; after third day carefully open dressing, inspect graft, note graft adherence or collection of serous fluid under graft (fluid should be aspirated with a needle and syringe); clip away any loose or necrotic tissue; rinse with sterile normal saline and redress with sterile gauze.

—Care of donor sites: Donor sites are covered with protective dressing and may be exposed to air after the second postoperative day (may require a heat lamp for short periods to maintain dryness); gentle cleansing can be done with soap and water; infected donor sites should be treated as second- and third-degree burns and require at least twice-a-day dressing changes.

○ Liberally administer analgesics to decrease the severe pain associated with burns and wound management procedures of first- and second-degree burns; possible analgesics include

Table 10.6 Commonly Used Antimicrobial Agents

Topical Ointment and Application Guidelines	Indications	Comments
Silver sulfadiazine—liberally apply to burned areas	2nd- and 3rd-degree burns	Poor eschar penetration, painless and easy application; may cause neutropenia
Mafenide—liberally apply to burned areas	Gram-negative and gram-positive infected 2nd- and 3rd-degree burns or patients with WBC <4000/mm^2	Poor eschar penetration, painful, associated with metabolic acidosis
Silver nitrate—pour over burned areas, must resaturate at least q2h	Gram-negative and gram-positive infected wounds without eschar	Poor eschar penetration, associated with electrolyte imbalances, especially hyponatremia and hypochloremia
Dakin's solution—pour over burned areas, must resaturate at least q2h	Gram-negative and gram-positive infected wounds without eschar	Poor eschar penetration, may damage surrounding healthy skin

Kinney, M. R., Packa, D. R., and Dunbar, S. B. Burns. In *AACN's Clinical Reference for Critical Care Nursing* (3rd ed). St. Louis: Mosby–Year Book, 1993. Pp. 1195–1231.

morphine and meperidine, altered weekly to prevent drug tolerance and decreased bowel motility.

---

morphine, meperidine
Action Decrease pain.
Administration Guidelines Morphine 2–10 mg IV every 1–2 hours; meperidine 25–100 mg IV every 1–2 hours.
Special Considerations Monitor respiratory rate (RR) and BP when administering large doses of IV analgesics.

- Recognize that very large doses of analgesics may be necessary to alleviate the severe pain; base dosage requirements on pain relief and patient assessment rather than standardized guidelines.
  —Assess and document pain relief using a 0–10 pain scale
- Administer diazepam and midazolam as needed.

---

diazepam, midazolam
Action Decrease anxiety.
Administration Guidelines Diazepam 2–10 mg IV every 4–6 hours; midazolam 1–4 mg IV during painful procedures.
Special Considerations Monitor RR and BP frequently; have airway management equipment immediately available.

- Nitrous oxide may be used during dressing changes.

---

nitrous oxide
Action Provides analgesia.
Administration Guidelines Must be administered by physician or anesthesiologist.
Special Considerations Physician must remain at bedside to ensure proper mixture of oxygen and nitrogen; have airway management equipment immediately available.

- Alternatives should be offered such as hypnosis or guided imagery, since analgesic pain control is usually insufficient due to the severe discomfort and risk of respiratory depression.
- Maintain warm temperature in dressing change area.
  c. Desired outcome
    i. Restore skin integrity and prevent further deterioration of skin integrity.
    ii. Prevent infection as evidenced by the presence of granulation tissue, the absence of maceration of skin, the absence of foul-smelling odors from skin, redness, pus or purulent drainage; wound biopsies and cultures are negative, grafted skin remains intact, and WBC count remains normal.

   iii. Fluid loss minimized by applying appropriate dressings to wounds.
   iv. Patient affirms pain has been relieved or sufficiently reduced.
   v. Able to participate in range-of-motion (ROM) activities.
   vi. Able to tolerate painful procedures.
   vii. Increase in sleep and rest periods.
   viii. Absence of crying, moaning, complaining, or facial grimacing.
   ix. Normal RR, heart rate (HR), and BP.
 4. Potential for infection related to loss of integumentary protective barrier
  a. Problem: inability to heal wounds, multisystem organ failure.
  b. Interventions
   i. Wash hands before and after each patient contact.
   ii. Implement skin and wound isolation precautions (see Chap. 1).
   iii. Monitor vital signs (HR, BP, RR, and temperature) every 4 hours and as needed.
   iv. Obtain blood, sputum, and urine cultures if patient spikes a temperature greater than 101.5°F, in collaboration with the physician.
   v. Assist in obtaining burn wound biopsy samples.
   vi. Monitor laboratory values that may indicate infection (WBC, glucose intolerance).
   vii. Administer antibiotics on time to maintain therapeutic blood levels.
   viii. Administer tetanus toxoid on admission.

---

tetanus toxoid
Action Stimulates antibody production to provide passive immunity against tetanus infection.
Administration Guidelines 0.5 mL *IM only*, booster given every 10 years.
Special Considerations Do not give in patients with acute respiratory infection, convulsive disorders, immunosuppression, or active tetanus infection.

---

   ix. Observe aseptic technique when providing burn wound care.
   x. Do not allow live plants or flowers in room; soil and water harbor microorganisms.
   xi. Separate all patient items; clean all equipment thoroughly between patient use if shared.
   xii. Provide daily calorie requirements to promote rapid healing and support defense mechanisms.
   xiii. Monitor carefully for signs of infection; symptoms include WBC count greater than or less than normal, thrombocytopenia, temperature greater than 101.5 or less than 98.6°F, glucose intolerance, confusion.
  c. Desired outcome
   i. HR, BP, RR, and temperature remain within normal limits.
   ii. Patient does not develop a nosocomial infection.

       iii. WBC and platelet count remain within normal limits.
       iv. Blood, sputum, urine, and wound cultures remain negative.
       v. Patient avoids an antibiotic-resistant infection.

5. Nutritional deficit related to increased metabolic rate to facilitate wound healing and defend against infection, potential for gastrointestinal dysfunction

  a. Problem: inability to heal wounds, increased potential for infection, development of ulcers and paralytic ileus.

  b. Intervention

     i. Large energy deficits may occur due to high evaporative water losses and hypermetabolism requirements (40% TBSA burns and greater increase metabolic demands by 100% over normal metabolic rates); consult nutritional services or dietician to calculate daily calorie requirements (see Table 10.7 [6] for daily calorie intake equation).

     ii. Provide a high-calorie/high-protein diet if patient is able to eat.

     iii. Provide daily vitamin supplements either orally or in IV fluids.

     iv. Complete calorie counts with each intake.

     v. Caloric intake must be achieved; realize tremendous caloric needs and support patient in creative ways to achieve caloric goals.

     vi. Encourage family members to prepare meals and bring to patient if hospital food is unappealing.

     vii. Provide additional calories by preparing milk shakes with prepared formulas and ice cream or chocolate syrup.

     viii. Space the intake of prepared formula supplements so that patient is not full at meal time.

     ix. Maintain log of daily weights.

     x. Recognize that depression, pain, and ability to self-feed deter adequate food intake.

     xi. If calorie intake cannot be met through eating, hyperalimentation or tube-feeding adjuncts may be required.

     xii. Insert nasogastric tube (NGT) and verify placement at every shift and prior to administration of medications or feeds.

Table 10.7 Calculation of Daily Calorie Needs in Burned Patients*

Ideal daily calorie intake
  Adults: (25 kcal × kg) + (40 kcal × %TBSA burn)
  Children: ([40–60 kcal] × kg) + (40 kcal × %TBSA burn)
  For example: (25 kcal × 75 kg) + (40 kcal × 20% TBSA) = 1875 + 800 = 2675 kcal/day

Nutrients
  Glucose: 55%–60% of daily calories
  Fat: 20%–30% of daily calories
  Protein: 15%–20% of daily calories

*Calculation based on TBSA of open wounds; daily intake requirements must be updated as healing progresses.
Adapted from Harvey, J. S., Watkins, G. M., and Sherman, R. T. Emergent burn care. *South Med J* 77:204, 1984; and Xi, W., Li, A., and Wang, S. Estimation of the calorie requirements of burned Chinese adults. *Burns* 19(2):146, 1993.

   xiii. Check gastric residual every 4–6 hours if continuous enteral feeds given or before each bolus feed; hold feeding and notify physician if residual is greater than 150 mL.

   xiv. Check NGT aspirate for blood and pH every 4–8 hours.

   xv. Administer aluminum hydroxide or magnesium hydroxide antacids to keep GI pH greater than 5.0.

---

antacids: aluminum hydroxide, magnesium hydroxide
Action Treat hyperacidity.
Administration Guidelines 30 mL every 4 hours for gastric pH less than 5.0.
Special Considerations Monitor for renal failure if prolonged use.

---

   xvi. Administer sucralfate (Carafate) as ordered.

---

sucralfate
Action Forms a covering over an ulcer site to prevent further attack by acids, pepsin, and bile salts.
Administration Guidelines 1 g, 2–4 times/day PO, will dissolve readily in water to give per NGT.
Special Considerations Antacids should not be administered within 0.5 hour before or after sucralfate.

---

   xvii. Administer histamine H_2 blockers as ordered.

---

histamine blockers
Action Inhibit action of histamine, thereby decreasing gastric acid secretion.
Administration Guidelines Ranitidine 150 mg PO bid or 300 mg PO at bedtime; 50 mg IV every 6–8 hours; cimetidine 300 mg PO qid with meals and at bedtime; 300 mg IV every 6 hours.
Special Considerations Use cautiously in patients with liver or renal dysfunction; may cause neutropenia, especially if used concomitantly with silver sulfadiazide.

---

   xviii. Assess bowel sounds every 4 hours.

   xix. Document frequency and consistency of bowel movements; test for occult blood.

   xx. Place NGT to suction during period of absent bowel sounds.

   xxi. Consult with dietician and physician to control diarrhea or constipation (see Chap. 4).

   xxii. Total parenteral nutrition (TPN) may be necessary if paralytic ileus is present or enteral feedings are unable to provide daily calories.

   xxiii. Maintain patency and sterility of IV lines used for hyperalimentation.

   xxiv. Verify the accuracy of each TPN bag before hanging.

      xxv. Complete serum and urine nutritional profiles (albumin, trans-ferrin, urine nitrogen, glucose, acetone) should be done every week on patients with extensive burns.

  c. Desired outcome

    i. Absence of ulcers.

    ii. Gastric pH greater than 5.0.

    iii. Bowel sounds present.

    iv. Patient passes formed stools; patient without diarrhea or consti-pation.

    v. 24-hour urine collection demonstrates a positive nitrogen bal-ance (estimation of the adequacy of protein input).

    vi. Urine negative for glucose and acetone.

    vii. Maintain serum albumin greater than 3.0 g/100 mL, serum trans-ferrin greater than 200 mg/100 mL.

    viii. Weight loss less than 5%–10% of baseline.

    ix. Caloric goals are met on a daily basis.

6. Impaired physical mobility related to burn wounds, pain, and scar and contracture formation

  a. Problem: loss of limb function, restricted activity, inability to complete independent activities of daily living.

  b. Intervention

    i. Consult physical and occupational therapy (PT and OT).

    ii. Follow recommendations of PT and OT about splint application and schedule.

    iii. Proper positioning of all burned joints must be initiated early in the recovery period to avoid the formation of contractures.

    iv. Splinting is used when patients are at rest.

    v. Range-of-motion exercises should be done at least once a day, and the patient must be encouraged to complete as many indepen-dent activities as possible.

    vi. Adequate pain control must be accomplished for the patient to participate in physical mobility activities.

    vii. Encourage patients to participate in all activities to maintain mobility throughout burn wound recovery.

    viii. Teach patient the proper use of pressure garments and stress the importance of wearing them continuously for up to 1 year to avoid overscarring and keloid formation.

  c. Desired outcome

    i. Full range of motion of all involved areas and joints equal to preburn function without verbal or nonverbal indication of pain.

    ii. Completion of activities of daily living and independent ambula-tion.

    iii. Patient able to feed self.

    iv. Contractures and hypertrophic scar formation is prevented.

C. Discharge planning (rehabilitative period)

  1. Prepare patient and family for long and stressful rehabilitative process.

  2. Evaluate family for referral to a rehabilitation facility or home health agency if necessary.

3. Review all discharge instructions and prescriptions, especially pain medications (dose, actions, and precautions).
4. Discuss need to wear pressure garments at all times, except for daily showers, for up to a year; garments may be hot and itchy; only lotions without a petroleum base may be used under garments to ease irritation. (Petroleum will destroy material.)
5. Explain importance of protection from *all* sun exposure.
6. Discuss importance of returning for follow-up appointments.
7. Provide the patient and family with a mechanism for attaining answers to questions and concerns after discharge.
8. Recommend local and national support groups for victims of burn injury.
9. Teach patient to continue a balanced diet with adequate protein intake for optimal wound healing.

References

1. Harvey, J. S., Watkins, G. M., and Sherman, R. T. Emergent burn care. *South Med J* 77:204, 1984.

2. American Burn Association. Hospital and prehospital resources for optimal care of patients with burn injury: Guidelines for development and operation of burn centers. *J Burn Rehabil* 11:97, 1990.

3. Davis, J. H., Drucker, W. R., and Foster, R. S., et al. *Clinical Surgery* (vol 2). St. Louis: C.V. Mosby, 1987. Pp. 2822–2903.

4. Garner, W. L., Zuccaro, C., and Marcelo, C., et al. The effects of burn blister fluid keratinocyte replication and differentiation. *J Burn Care Rehabil* 14:127, 1993.

5. Kinney, M. R., Packa, D. R., and Dunbar, S. B. Burns. In *AACN's Clinical Reference for Critical-Care Nursing* (3rd ed). St. Louis: Mosby–Year Book, 1993. Pp. 1195–1231.

6. Xi, W., Li, A., and Wang, S. Estimation of the calorie requirements of burned Chinese adults. *Burns* 19(2):146, 1993.

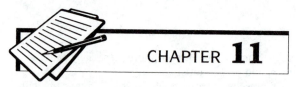

CHAPTER **11**

Neurologic Disorders

Diane Schwenker and Dan Brennan

Arteriovenous Malformations

I. Definition: A tangle of arterial and venous vessels connected by abnormal capillary network causing the vessels to be dilated and high-pressured. The malformation may enlarge progressively over time. Problems associated with this vascular malformation include the following:

A. Hemorrhage.

B. Demand for high volumes of arterial blood leading to shunting of blood away from other areas of the brain with resultant ischemia and atrophy.

C. Pressure on underlying structures causing seizure activity or focal neurologic deficits.

D. Pressure on the ventricular system causing hydrocephalus.

II. Etiology

A. Usually congenital.

B. Usually without familial predisposition.

C. Occur twice as often in men as in women.

D. Most frequently involve middle cerebral artery circulation.

III. Nursing process

A. Assessment

  1. Signs and symptoms: Often develop in or before the third decade of life.
   a. Hemorrhage: The presenting sign in 50–65% of cases resulting from excessive pressure in the malformed vessels.
     i. Decreased level of consciousness (LOC): increased intracranial pressure (ICP) as hemorrhage increases the volume of intracranial contents.
     ii. Risk for vasospasm: Blood in subarachnoid space.
   b. Seizure, also a common presenting sign: Irritation of brain tissue from pressure or ischemia.
   c. Headache: Probably pressure-related.
   d. Bruit depending on the size and location of the malformation: Due to high flow.

    e. Transient episodes of dizziness, syncope, motor or sensory deficits: The effects of vascular steal.

  2. Diagnostic tests

    a. CT scan: Indicates presence of subarachnoid blood and the location of the abnormality.

    b. Arteriogram: Displays the feeding and draining vessels of the arteriovenous malformation (AVM) as well as collateral circulation around the AVM.

    c. Serum laboratory studies: Usual preoperative workup.

B. Patient management

  1. Seizure activity related to ischemia of brain tissue secondary to increased intracranial pressure or vascular steal effects of AVM.

    a. Problem: Seizures may result in permanent injury to the patient from ineffective gas exchange or falls.

    b. Intervention

      i. Protect patient from injury by maintaining side rails of bed in elevated and locked position.

      ii. Position bed height at lowest level.

      iii. Patient should be accompanied by someone when out of bed until anticonvulsant levels are therapeutic and patient is seizure free.

      iv. Oxygen and suction equipment should be at the bedside and ready for use.

      v. See "Seizure Disorders" (p. 322) for management of seizures.

      vi. Administer anticonvulsant drugs and monitor drug levels and side effects.

---

phenytoin (Dilantin)

Action Inhibits the spread of seizure activity; stabilizes electrical threshold of brain cells.

Administration Guidelines 300–400 mg daily in one, two, or three doses. Intravenously mixed in normal saline solution only, delivered at a rate no faster than 50 mg/min to prevent hypotension and respiratory depression.

Nursing Considerations When administered via enteral feeding tube, feedings should be stopped 2 hours before and 2 hours after administration of the drug. Therapeutic and toxic ranges may be relatively close and require monitoring of drug levels and symptoms. May cause drowsiness, GI upset, irritability, rash, anemia, nystagmus, fever, hirsutism, and gingival hyperplasia.

---

    c. Desired outcome: Prevent injury related to seizure activity. Develop a therapeutic regimen for anticonvulsant drugs that controls seizures and minimizes side effects.

  2. Risk for intracranial hemorrhage related to high pressures in abnormal vasculature.

    a. Problem: Ischemia in cerebral vessels may be due to low volume secondary to hemorrhage. Hemorrhage also may result in vasospasm and/or increased intracranial pressure, both of which can result in permanent neurologic disability.

b. Intervention

   i. See "Aneurysms" (p. 287) for management of intracerebral hemorrhage and vasospasm.

   ii. See "Increased Intracranial Pressure" (p. 297).

   iii. Surgical removal or ligation of feeder vessels is done in stages when AVM is extensive.

- The patient is prepared as for craniotomy.
- Following the procedure, patient is monitored for changes in level of consciousness and motor and sensory function. See Table 11.1 (Glasgow Coma Scale).

   iv. Interventional radiology and embolization: May be used before surgical ligation. High pressures in AVM are rapidly diverted during surgical ligation to alternate circulation. This rapid diversion may cause rebound edema and increased intracranial pressure. Embolization allows more gradual diversion of flow.

- The use of embolization preoperatively to occlude feeder vessels will minimize bleeding in subsequent surgical procedures.
- Also used as a primary method of treatment, especially when surgery may not be feasible because of size or location of AVM.
- Patient is fully heparinized during the procedure.

Table 11.1 Glasgow Coma Scale*

Best motor response	
6	Obeys commands
5	Localizes to pain
4	Withdraws to pain
3	Abnormal flexion
2	Abnormal extension
1	No movement
Best verbal response	
5	Oriented and appropriate
4	Confused conversation
3	Inappropriate
2	Incomprehensible sounds
1	No sounds
Eye opening	
4	Spontaneous
3	To speech
2	To pain
1	No eye opening

*Glasgow Coma Scale (GCS) score equals the sum of the scores from each of the three groups.
Source: Trauma. Martuza, R. L., and Proctor, M. R. In *Manual of Neurologic Therapeutics* (5th ed.). M. A. Samuels (ed.). Boston: Little, Brown and Company, 1995. P. 251.

- Procedure is performed with the patient sedated but awake.
- Balloon catheter placed at the feeder vessel(s).
- Balloon inflated and serial neurologic exams performed to evaluate the effect of occluded blood flow.
- If neurologic exams stable, thrombosing material injected to permanently occlude vessel.
- May be done in stages over weeks or months to prevent rebound edema resulting from rapid diversion of high-pressure flow.

    v. Radiosurgery: Stereotactically directed proton beam for destruction of the AVM may be considered for small AVMs in surgically difficult locations.

  c. Desired outcome: Reduction of the risk of hemorrhage by obliterating as much of the AVM as possible while preserving adequate cerebral perfusion.

IV. Discharge planning

A. Anticipate follow-up arteriogram within 6 months.

B. Return to the hospital if a seizure occurs.

C. Report for regularly scheduled checks to evaluate anticonvulsant drug levels and adverse reactions. Abrupt discontinuation of anticonvulsants can result in status epilepticus.

D. Changes in behavior, wakefulness, sensation, or motor ability should be reported immediately.

E. Monitor surgical wounds or arteriogram sites for redness, warmth, or drainage.

F. If postoperative, check temperature on waking and in the evening for the next 5 days; report any elevations above 101°F.

Aneurysms

I. Definition

A. An aneurysm is a localized dilation of the intimal layer of an artery. The media or muscular layer of the vessel stops at the neck of the aneurysm, and the internal elastic layer of the artery continues into the aneurysmal sac. The sac is formed of fibrous tissue; the usual site of rupture is the dome of the sac, where the wall is thinnest. As many as 28,000 cases of subarachnoid hemorrhage caused by aneurysmal rupture occur in North America annually. Subarachnoid hemorrhage has mortality and morbidity rates of 50% and 30%, respectively.

B. Aneurysmal rupture results in bleeding into subarachnoid and/or subdural spaces or into intracerebral tissue. *Rapid* decreases in level of consciousness and/or motor function are indicative of hemorrhage. The risk for rebleeding from a ruptured aneurysm is 35–40% in the first month among those who survive the initial hemorrhage. Blood in the subarachnoid space can result in vasospasm. The incidence of vasospasm is highest at 4 to 14 days after subarachnoid hemorrhage. Symptoms involve *fluctuating* levels of consciousness and motor or sensory deficits. Increased intracranial pressure and ischemia are the etiology of symptoms. Location of the hemorrhage or vasospasm determines specific signs and symptoms.

C. Incidence: Intracranial aneurysmal hemorrhage occurs most often in those 35 to 60 years of age. For those under 40 years old, incidence of hemorrhage is equal among men and women. At 40 years of age, the incidence is higher for women. Overall incidence is higher among cigarette smokers.

II. Etiology: Aneurysms develop in those persons with the following:

A. Arteriosclerotic vessel disease.
B. Hypertension and polycystic kidney disease.
C. History of trauma.
D. Inflammatory or infectious states, ie, vasculitis or sepsis.

III. Nursing process

A. Assessment
   1. Signs and symptoms
      a. Before rupture
         i. Evident in only 50% of cases.
         ii. Related to the size and location of the aneurysm.
         iii. Headache, neck pain, dizziness, or the presence of a bruit on physical exam.
         iv. Significant history
            - Family history.
            - Previous hemorrhage.
            - Hypertension.
            - Cigarette smoking.
      b. After rupture
         i. Sudden onset of headache with a change in level of consciousness or focal neurologic deficit ("the worst headache of my life").
         ii. Symptoms divided into two categories.
            - Those resulting from the irritation of meningeal tissue due to the presence of blood
            - Those related to increased intracranial pressure
         iii. Signs associated with meningeal irritation
            - Headache.
            - Photophobia.
            - Nuchal rigidity.
            - Low-grade temperature elevation.
         iv. Signs associated with increased intracranial pressure
            - Headache.
            - Irritability.
            - Decreased level of consciousness.
            - Cranial nerve deficits: The oculomotor nerve (III), responsible for pupillary constriction and extraocular movement, and facial nerve (VII) are often involved.
            - Papilledema: Optic disk swelling on eyeground exam.
            - Focal motor signs: Weakness contralateral (opposite) to the site of hemorrhage.

    v. Signs specific to the arterial circulation involved (Fig. 11.1)
- Anterior circulation
  - Internal carotid: Visual symptoms may arise from impaired flow to the optic artery, the first bifurcation from the internal carotid.
  - Anterior cerebral artery: Contralateral weakness of the lower extremity, delay in performing commands, decreased initiative, aphasia, decreased level of consciousness
  - Middle cerebral artery: Contralateral weakness of the upper extremity and face (VII), extremity neglect, speech and receptive deficits, decreased level of consciousness, gaze paralysis
- Posterior circulation
  - Vertebral-basilar artery to posterior cerebral arteries: Cerebellar signs, lack of coordination, ataxia due to many perforating vessels to the brainstem; cranial nerve deficits and respiratory and/or cardiovascular signs may occur.

2. Diagnostic tests: Baseline neurologic assessment
- **a.** CT scan: Will demonstrate localized blood within a few hours; may appear normal.
- **b.** Four-vessel cerebral arteriogram: Location, shape, and size of the aneurysm. Vasospasm may occlude the vessel and prevent visualization. Arteriogram may be repeated at a later time if visualization is obscured. All vessels are studied due to 20% incidence of multiple aneurysms.
- **c.** Lumbar puncture: Grossly bloody or xanthochromic due to blood in the subarachnoid space.

3. Laboratory studies
- **a.** Elevated WBC count resulting from irritation of meninges.
- **b.** Electrolyte abnormalities resulting from hypothalamic dysfunction, ie, syndrome of inappropriate secretion of antidiuretic hormone.
- **c.** Electrocardiogram: Nonspecific ST- and T-wave changes, possibly due to hypothalamic dysfunction.

B. Patient management
    1. Potential for bleeding related to disrupted integrity of vessel wall.
- **a.** Problem: Decreased blood supply to brain leads to tissue and cellular injury.
- **b.** Intervention: Institute aneurysm precautions to prevent rebleeding.
  - **i.** Avoid emotional upset.
  - **ii.** Avoid extreme elevations in blood pressure.
  - **iii.** Avoid straining.
  - **iv.** Bed rest.
  - **v.** Low light.
  - **vi.** Low noise level.
  - **vii.** Minimal exertion: Administer complete care.
  - **viii.** Administer antifibrinolytic agents as ordered in specific cases.

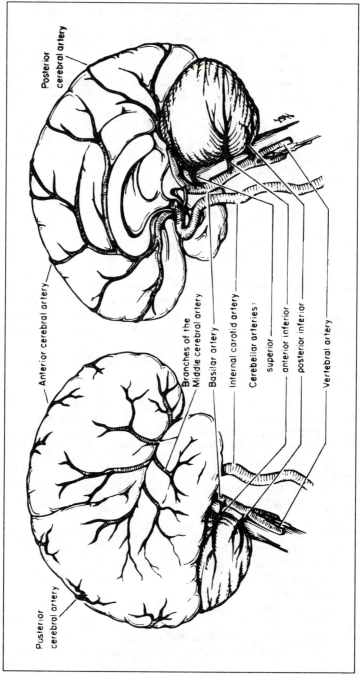

Figure 11.1 Cerebral circulation. (From *Principles of Neurologic Diagnosis*. Montgomery, E. B., Wall, M., and Henderson, V. Boston: Little, Brown and Company, 1985. P. 89.)

> **epsilon-aminocaproic acid**
> *Action* Retards clot lysis.
> *Administration Guidelines* Intravenous (IV) infusion of 1.0–1.5 g/h.
> *Nursing Considerations* Maintain hydration. Monitor closely for signs of neurologic deterioration. Risks associated with cerebral ischemia.

   c. Desired outcome: Prevent rebleeding as evidenced by stable neurologic exam.

2. Impaired cerebral function related to increased intracranial pressure and ischemia.

   a. Problem: Cerebral edema, hematoma formation, ischemia, or vasospasm.

   b. Intervention

      i. Evaluate level of consciousness and motor function.

      ii. Measure level of consciousness using the Glasgow Coma Scale (see Table 11.1) every 15 minutes to 1 hour.

      iii. Perform cranial nerve tests to evaluate neurologic function. Paralysis of a cranial nerve can warn of advancing pressure in the brain.

- Cranial nerve III
  - Eyelid opening: Ask the patient to open eyes; observe for symmetry in the amount of visible eyelid when the eyes are open. In the patient who is unable to follow commands, observe response to noxious stimuli (eg, sternal rub).
  - Pupillary constriction: In response to a bright light beamed directly into the eye; may be more easily observed if the room is darkened and eye is viewed from the side.
  - Eye movement: Up and out; up and in; down and out.
    —Ask the patient to follow an object held 10 inches from the face and moved into the six cardinal positions of gaze.
    —In the patient who is unable to follow commands, observe resting gaze and random movement of eyes when possible.
- Cranial nerve IV: Down-and-in eye movement (see Cranial Nerve III).
- Cranial nerve VI: Lateral eye movement (see Cranial Nerve III).
- Cranial nerve VII: Facial symmetry. Observe the nasolabial fold (line from the nare adjacent to the mouth) and the corners of the mouth for symmetry during a smile or grimace. Weakness is demonstrated by flattening of the fold and droop of the corner of the mouth.
- Cranial nerves IX and X: Swallowing. Be alert for any signs of difficulty in swallowing, such as coughing, choking, or retention of food in mouth after a swallow attempt. If there is suspected dysfunction the patient should receive nothing by

mouth, and formal swallowing evaluations should be performed by qualified personnel.

- Cranial nerve XII: Midline tongue. Ask the patient to stick out tongue. Weakness or paralysis is demonstrated by deviation to the affected side.

iv. Perform motor strength scoring on all extremities. Advancing weakness of paralysis may indicate increasing pressure on the brain or ischemia.

- 5: Normal strength.
- 4: Offers resistance but can be overcome by examiner.
- 3: Able to overcome gravity but offers no resistance to examiner.
- 2: Cannot oppose gravity; moves only in horizontal plane.
- 1: Flicker of muscle movement.

v. Monitor intracranial pressure and institute nursing care protocols to control ICP (see "Increased Intracranial Pressure," p. 297).

c. Desired outcome: Early recognition of neurologic deterioration, which allows early medical or surgical intervention to preserve neurologic function.

3. Potential for vasospasm related to bleeding in subarachnoid space.

a. Problem: Intracerebral arterial vasospasm is a narrowing of the lumen of an artery that results in potential ischemic injury to surrounding brain tissue and areas distal to the site of spasm.

b. Interventions

i. Monitor neurologic function with the Glasgow Coma Scale (see Table 11.1), with cranial nerve testing, and with motor strength scoring.

ii. Administer calcium channel blockers, eg, nimodipine.

---

nimodipine

Action Interferes with calcium movement across cell membrane, which is required for contraction of muscle.

Administration Guidelines 30–60 mg every 4 hours.

Nursing Considerations Must be given at 4-hour intervals. May require puncture of capsule and removal of liquid contents for administration via enteral tube in patients with impaired consciousness.

---

iii. Monitor hemodynamics. Maintain intravascular volume for perfusion of cerebral vessels with infusions of colloids, crystalloids, or whole blood. Therapeutic goals are pulmonary capillary wedge pressure of 18–20 mm Hg or central venous pressure of 10–12 mm Hg.

iv. "Triple H" therapy: hypervolemic, hemodilution, and induced hypertension

- Decrease viscosity of blood by using crystalloid or colloid infusions to adjust hematocrit to 30–35%. Increase central venous pressure (CVP) to 10–12 mm Hg and pulmonary artery diastolic (PAD) pressure to 15–18 mm Hg.

- Maintain mean arterial pressure to perfuse vessels at 160 mm Hg by using vasoactive infusions, ie, phenylephrine or dopamine.

v. Plan for embolization and/or surgical clipping of the aneurysm: Early surgery may be performed for patients with large hemorrhages and rapid deterioration in neurologic status. Surgery may be delayed to minimize risk for vasospasm in the patient whose hemorrhage is small and whose neurologic status is stable.

c. Desired outcome: Preserve neurologic function by control of vasospasm.

4. Potential for fluid overload related to hypervolemic therapy
   a. Problem: Fluid overload increases oxygen demand of heart muscle and reduces cardiac output to ischemic brain tissue.
   b. Intervention
      i. Monitor CVP or PAD, as available, every 2 hours.
      ii. Auscultate heart and lung sounds every 2–4 hours for signs of fluid overload.
      iii. Monitor oxygen saturation and maintain optimal oxygenation by tailoring volume therapy to patient tolerance; ie, minimal crackles and no evidence of reduced cardiac output.
   c. Desired outcome: Maximize cerebral perfusion.

5. Potential for immobility related to activity restrictions or possible decreased level of consciousness.
   a. Problem: Decreased mobility can result in ineffective gas exchange, stasis of blood, musculoskeletal injury, infection, and skin breakdown.
   b. Intervention
      i. Incentive spirometry every 2 hours while awake. Monitor oxygenation and administer supplemental oxygen as required to maintain oxygen saturation greater than 90%.
      ii. Chest percussion and postural drainage may be necessary for patients with decreased level of consciousness. Physician approval for chest percussion may be required.
      iii. Perform range-of-motion exercises on all extremities every 4 hours. Maintain compression devices to lower extremities when ordered.
      iv. Support weak or paralyzed extremities in functional position during repositioning and at rest. Take special precautions to prevent any break in skin integrity in affected limbs.
      v. Monitor all intravenous access sites for evidence of infiltration or phlebitis.
      vi. Monitor temperature every 4 hours for elevations greater than 100.5°F.
      vii. Change securing devices and/or dressings for nasogastric, endotracheal, tracheotomy, and gastrostomy or jejunostomy tubes daily or according to set protocol.

    viii. Assist patients who are unable to reposition themselves independently with turns every 2 hours. Assist mobile patients with repositioning every 4 hours.

    ix. See national standards for treating skin breakdown in *Pressure Ulcer Guidelines* [1].

    x. Use an immobility scale to evaluate the need for pressure-relieving devices.

Guillain-Barré Syndrome

I. Definition: Acute rapidly progressive form of polyneuritis or inflammation of peripheral neurons. The process results in destruction of myelin, the protective sheath of the axon of the neuron (Fig. 11.2). The syndrome is often preceded by an upper respiratory tract infection, a viral infection, or a vaccination.

II. Etiology: Cell-mediated and humoral inflammatory response to virus. Infection leads to destruction of the myelin cells that insulate nerve fibers where conduction of impulses normally occur.

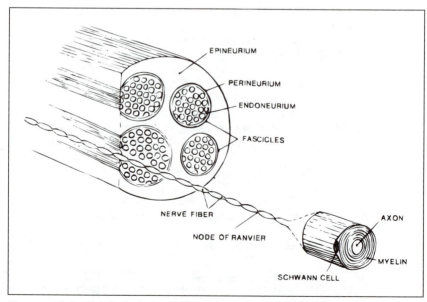

Figure 11.2 Histologic features of a peripheral nerve. (From *Medical Neurosciences: An Approach to Anatomy, Pathology, and Physiology by Systems and Levels* (3rd ed.). Westmoreland, B. F., et al. Boston: Little, Brown and Company, 1994. P. 331.)

III. Nursing process

A. Assessment

1. Signs and symptoms
   a. History: May be significant for a recent illness.
   b. Most patients have acute-onset weakness and paresthesia (numbness or sensory changes) in their legs related to ascending neuronal injury.
   c. Physical exam demonstrates the following:
      i. Usually awake and alert.
      ii. Motor weakness and diminished or absent reflexes due to neuronal injury.
      iii. May involve cranial nerves (ie, facial weakness; diplopia; difficulty talking, chewing, or swallowing).
      iv. Autonomic nervous system dysfunction may result in hypertension and bradycardia or tachycardia.
      v. Diminished deep tendon reflexes due to failure of the nerve to conduct impulse to muscle fiber.
      vi. Respiratory muscles may be involved, and breath sounds may be diminished or secretions retained.
      vii. Symptoms may worsen over the first 2 weeks following onset. May progress to complete paralysis. Resolution of symptoms may begin as early as 2–3 weeks after onset but may require 6–12 months or longer to realize final outcomes.

2. Diagnostic tests
   a. Lumbar puncture: Cerebral spinal fluid analysis may show an elevated protein count.
   b. Measure of respiratory parameters for vital capacity, negative inspiratory force, and tidal volume may be decreased.
   c. Electromyelogram evidences neuromuscular blockade.
   d. Nerve conduction studies show slowed conduction velocities.

B. Patient management

1. Impaired physical mobility related to paralysis
   a. Problem: Immobility predisposes to decreased venous return, pneumonia, decreased bowel motility, contractures, altered skin integrity.
   b. Interventions
      i. Explain all interventions to patient. Patients are usually alert though they may be unable to respond.
      ii. Anticipate use of plasmapheresis to remove antibodies involved in disease process. Plasma portion of blood is removed by centrifuge and replaced with albumin or donor plasma. Accurate weights are required to calculate exchanges. Access catheters are of large gauge, and sites must be monitored for bleeding. Normal coagulation may be altered for hours following the exchange.
      iii. Administer IV immunoglobulin as ordered.

---

immunoglobulin

Action May block action of antibodies involved in immune response.

Administration Guidelines Usually 1–2 mg/kg given in divided doses over 3–5 days. Infusion is started slowly and rate increased based on patient tolerance. Total dose is calculated by body weight.

Nursing Considerations Immunoglobulin is a large molecule and represents a volume load. Patients should be monitored for signs of fluid overload. Intravenous immunoglobulin is a pooled blood product and may cause allergic reactions. Monitor patient closely for symptoms of anaphylaxis. Premedications may be ordered for complaints of chills and headache.

---

   iv. Inspect lower extremities for signs of thrombophlebitis.
   v. Assess for signs of respiratory involvement.
   vi. Assess abdomen for bowel sounds, distention; track bowel function. Apply splints to affected limbs. Perform passive range of motion on affected limbs. Provide skin care to prevent breakdown.
   c. Desired outcome: Prevent complications related to immobility.
2. Retained secretions due to chest wall weakness.
   a. Problem: Ineffective airway clearance.
   b. Interventions
      i. Turn and position the patient at least once every 2 hours, and perform postural drainage and chest percussion to maintain a patent airway.
      ii. Assist patient with coughing and deep-breathing exercises, ie, incentive spirometry.
   c. Desired outcome: Clear breath sounds and expectoration of secretions.
3. Ineffective coping related to fear of dying.
   a. Problem: Patient is unable to effectively participate in therapies because of fears.
   b. Interventions
      i. Allow patient to express fears.
      ii. Educate patient as to the disease process and anticipated outcomes.
      iii. Identify and incorporate significant others in the plan of care.
      iv. Offer the support of the Guillain-Barré Association.
   c. Desired outcome: Patient and support persons will be integrated into the plan of care.

IV. Discharge planning

A. Consult social worker to evaluate the home environment.
B. Ensure that preparations have been made to accommodate functional status of the patient.
C. Transfer techniques, feeding methods, bowel and bladder elimination plans, and rest and exercise regimens should be reviewed with patient and family.
D. Contact a Guillain-Barré Support Group through the hospital or rehabilitation facility.

Increased Intracranial Pressure

I. Definition: Intracranial pressure is determined by the volume, compliance, and elastance of the contents of the intracranial vault. Normally contents include brain tissue, cerebrospinal fluid, and intravascular blood. Normal fluctuations in pressure occur as arterial blood pulsates, and the volume of venous drainage from the jugular veins varies because of changes in intrathoracic pressure during the respiratory cycle. Intracranial pressure also varies with normal activity. Elevated pressures are explained by the Monroe-Kellie hypothesis, which states that in a defined compartment such as the cranium, any increase in one component must result in a decrease in another component, or the pressure within the compartment will rise. "Compliance of the brain" refers to the brain's ability to tolerate increases in volume without increases in pressure. "Elastance" is the tightness of the intracranial cavity.

II. Etiology: Increases in intracranial pressure occur in response to increases in volume of one or more of the intracranial components (Fig. 11.3).

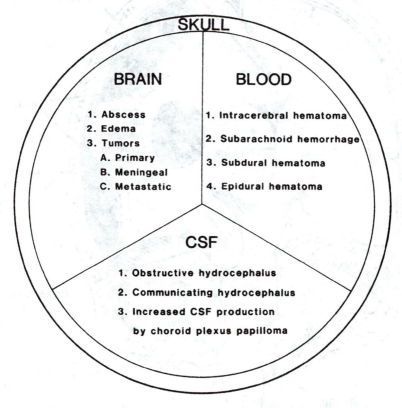

Figure 11.3 Increases in intracranial volume, resulting in increases in intracranial pressure. (From *Principles of Neurologic Diagnosis*. Montgomery, E. B., Wall, M., and Henderson, V. Boston: Little, Brown and Company, 1985. P. 157.)

III. Nursing process

A. Assessment

  1. Signs and symptoms

    a. Herniation syndromes (Fig. 11.4)

      i. Supratentorial

        ▪ Lateral herniation: Midline shift.

        ▪ Uncal herniation: Uncus of temporal lobe shifts toward/over the tentorial notch.

        ▪ Central: Downward herniation of the cerebral contents through the tentorial notch.

      ii. Infratentorial

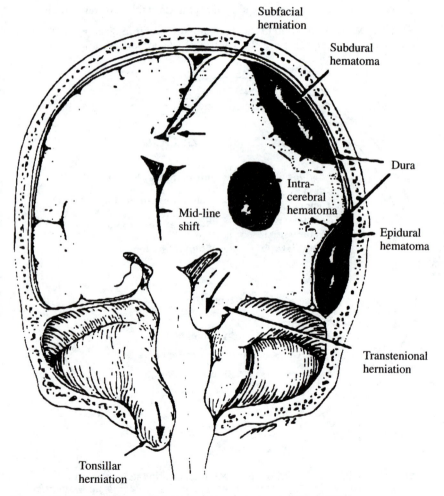

Figure 11.4 Herniation syndromes. (From Current concepts: Diagnosis and initial management of head injury. White, R. J., and Likavec, M. J. *N. Engl. J. Med.* 327:1508, 1992.)

- Upward: Tissue below the tentorium herniates upward through the tentorial notch.
- Tonsillar: Downward herniation of the cerebellar tonsil through the foramen magnum.
    iii. Extracranial: Herniation of tissue through a surgical or traumatic opening in the skull.
2. Associated signs and symptoms (Table 11.2)
    a. Measurement of intracranial pressure
        i. Epidural devices: In the epidural space.
        ii. Intracranial bolt: In the subarachnoid space; cannot drain cerebrospinal fluid (CSF).
        iii. Ventriculostomy: In the lateral ventricle; permits drainage of CSF to assist in control of intracranial pressure; risk for infection is higher.
    b. Cardiac monitoring
        i. ST-segment changes, U waves, Q waves, inverted or spiky T waves on ECG.
        ii. Supraventricular tachycardias from sympathetic dysfunction.
        iii. Systolic "surges" of blood pressure.
        iv. Cushing's triad (a very late sign): rising systolic blood pressure, widening pulse pressure, and bradycardia; indicative of pressure on the brain stem.
    c. Pulmonary
        i. Respiratory pattern changes: Apneic periods, Cheyne-Stokes respiration.
        ii. Neurogenic pulmonary edema.

Table 11.2 Signs of Increased Intracranial Pressure

	Early	Late
Level of consciousness	Subtle changes in orientation Changes in speech, slurring, difficulty finding correct words Increased restlessness or agitation Sudden quietness	Unarousable
Eye	Nystagmus Deviation of one eye Dysconjugate gaze Sluggish pupillary reaction Unilateral hippus Alternate constriction and dilation of pupil, "bouncing" reaction	Unilateral pupillary dilation Unusually small pupils "Blown pupil" Nonreactive
Motor	Unilateral muscle weakness Pronator drift Wrist flexion to noxious stimuli Dense weakness Resistance to passive movement—spasticity	Rigid posturing

   d. Gastrointestinal
      i. Increased risk for ulceration and bleeding.
      ii. High metabolic rate and increased nutritional requirements.
3. Diagnostic tests
   a. CT scan: Identifies hemorrhage, mass lesions (hematomas or edema), and the effect on intracranial structures.
   b. MRI: Differentiates soft-tissue changes.
   c. Skull x-ray: In traumatic injuries.
   d. Neurologic function testing: Early identification of herniation syndromes.
   e. ECG: Baseline.
   f. Volume pressure test: 1 mL sterile saline injected into ventricular catheter to evaluate compliance of the brain.
      i. Expected response: Less than 2-mm rise in intracranial pressure.
      ii. Abnormal response: Greater than 2-mm rise in intracranial pressure.
B. Patient management
   1. Risk for neurologic deterioration related to increased intracranial pressure.
      a. Problem: Loss of neurologic function may be permanent if pressure is unrelieved.
      b. Interventions
         i. Identify as early as possible any change in neurologic function.
            • Neurologic function exams every hour, or as indicated with the Glasgow Coma Scale (see Table 11.1).
            • Perform cranial nerve tests to evaluate motor function.
            ○ Cranial nerve III
              —Eyelid opening: Ask the patient to open eyes; observe for symmetry in the amount of visible eyelid when the eyes are open. In the patient who is unable to follow commands, observe response to noxious stimuli (eg, sternal rub).
              —Pupillary constriction in response to a bright light beamed directly into the eye. May be more easily observed if the room is darkened and eye is viewed from the side.
              —Eye movement: Up and out; up and in; down and out. Ask the patient to follow an object held 10 inches from the face and moved into the six cardinal positions of gaze. In the patient who is unable to follow commands, observe resting gaze and random movement of eyes when possible.
            ○ Cranial nerve IV: Down-and-in eye movement (see Cranial Nerve III).
            ○ Cranial nerve VI: Lateral eye movement (see Cranial Nerve III).
            ○ Cranial nerve VII: Facial symmetry. Observe the nasolabial fold (line from the nare adjacent to the mouth) and the corners of the mouth for symmetry during a smile or grimace. Weakness is demonstrated by flattening of the fold and droop of the corner of the mouth.
            ○ Cranial nerves IX and X: Swallowing. Be alert for any signs of difficulty in swallowing such as coughing, choking, or retention of food in mouth after a swallow attempt. If there

is suspected dysfunction the patient should receive nothing by mouth, and formal swallowing evaluations should be performed by qualified personnel.

- ○ Cranial nerve XII: Midline tongue. Ask the patient to stick out tongue. Weakness or paralysis is demonstrated by deviation to the affected side.
- ▪ Perform motor strength scoring.
- ○ 5: Normal strength.
- ○ 4: Offers resistance but can be overcome by examiner.
- ○ 3: Able to overcome gravity but offers no resistance to examiner.
- ○ 2: Cannot oppose gravity; moves only in horizontal plane.
- ○ 1: Flicker of muscle movement.
- ▪ Evaluate protective reflexes: These exams may adversely affect intracranial pressure.
- ○ Corneal: Drop saline into each eye.
- ○ Gag: Tongue depressor inserted to touch base of tongue or soft palate.
- ○ Cough: During endotracheal tube suctioning or by moving the endotracheal tube.

ii. Control intracranial pressure: Normal pressures range between 0 and 15 mm Hg and cerebral perfusion pressure (CPP) is greater than 60 mm Hg.

- ▪ P_{CO_2} between 25 and 30 mm Hg: Manipulate the diameter of cerebral vasculature to support cerebral perfusion. This range results in constriction of cerebral vessels and decreases in blood component of intracranial cavity.
- ▪ Monitor cerebral oxygen consumption via jugular bulb catheter to individualize cerebral oxygen requirements. Keep oxygen extraction ratio less than 40%.
- ▪ Control of mean arterial pressure (MAP): 50–170 mm Hg; anything outside this range disrupts the normal control of blood flow to the brain (autoregulation). CPP must be considered.
- ▪ Suppress cough and gag responses with 0.5 mg/kg; lidocaine IV or via endotracheal tube.
- ▪ Drain CSF via ventriculostomy catheter slowly to prevent rapid decompression of ventricle; abrupt appearance of grossly bloody fluid may indicate hemorrhage.
- ▪ Environmental controls
- ○ Head of bed elevation: Generally elevate 30–45 degrees. Current debate over elevation vs flat to facilitate cerebral perfusion. Measurement of cerebral oxygen requirement is the best reflection of intracerebral dynamics.
- ○ Neutral positioning and support to neck to facilitate venous drainage of blood through the jugular system.
- ○ Evaluate the effect of stimuli on maintaining intracranial pressure in a normal range of 0–15 mm Hg and absolutely below 20 mm Hg.

- ° It is critical that light, noise, and tactile stimuli be controlled based on the effect on measured intracranial pressure.
- ° Avoid prolonged stimulation of any kind.
- ° Nursing activities may need to be accomplished at brief intervals; avoid "clustering" together of several treatments and interventions.
- Calculate CPP as MAP − ICP. CPP must be maintained at 60 mm Hg or above.
- Glucose control: Elevations in serum glucose are associated with poor outcomes in brain-injured patients.
- Anticipate surgical intervention to remove hematoma, clot, tumor, abscess, or tissue that may be contributing to increased intracranial pressure.
- Administer pharmacologic agents to optimize cerebral perfusion.
- ° Administer diuretics.

---

diuretics
Action Used to minimize free water.
Administration Guidelines Furosemide 10–40 mg IV slowly.
  Mannitol 0.5–1.0 g/kg IV.
Nursing Considerations Avoid large or rapid changes in fluid balance; disrupted blood–brain barrier permits fluid shifts in cerebral tissue.

- ° Administer systemic pressors.

---

systemic pressors
Action Used to support BP as required for maintenance of cerebral perfusion pressure.
Administration Guidelines Dopamine 2–10 μg/kg per minute.
  Phenylephrine mix 100 mg per 250 mL; infuse at 100–200 mL/h until desired BP is obtained; then maintain at 40–60 mL/h as needed for BP support.
Nursing Considerations Increases in heart rate increase myocardial oxygen demand and should be minimized.

- ° Antipyretics are used to normalize temperature and thereby reduce oxygen demand. Acetaminophen 650–1000 mg every 4 hours.
- ° Administer sedatives.

sedatives

Action Used to decrease response to environmental stimuli and to prevent resistance to ventilator-delivered breaths.

Administration Guidelines Morphine 2–5 mg IV push every 2 hours. Benzodiazepines: Lorazepam 1–2 mg IV push; diazepam 2–5 mg IV push; midazolam 1–2.5 mg IV push every 2 hours.

Nursing Considerations Smaller doses will limit period of sedation and allow more accurate neurologic testing. When the brain is very tight, even minimal stimuli may result in intracranial pressure increases. The need for sedation should be monitored constantly.

- Therapeutic paralysis.

vecuronium, atracurium

Action Used to control isotonic muscle contraction as in posturing or Valsalva's maneuver.

Administration Guidelines Vecuronium 0.08–0.10 mg/kg bolus; repeat every 12–20 minutes, or 0.1 mg/mL continuous infusion. Atracurium 0.4–0.5 mg/kg bolus; repeat bolus of 0.8–0.1 mg/kg every 25–40 minutes or continuous infusion of 2–15 μg/kg per minute.

Nursing Considerations Multisystem support required: BP, air-way patency, corneal protection. Must be administered with a sedative.

- Administer pentobarbital.

pentobarbital

Action Used to reduce metabolic requirements of intracerebral tissue by inducing therapeutic coma.

Administration Guidelines 3–5 mg/kg loading dose; 1–3 mg/kg continuous infusion.

Nursing Considerations Slow to clear from adipose tissue. Multisystem support required: BP, airway patency, corneal protection.

- Administer steroids.

steroids

Action May be used to manage edema.

Administration Guidelines 10–12 mg every 6 hours, tapered over 1 week.

Nursing Considerations Must be tapered slowly because of the risk of adrenal insufficiency. Serum glucose monitoring is necessary. Risk of gastric ulceration is increased.

    c. Desired outcome: Maintain integrity of the cerebral hemispheres and associated structures, as evidenced by normal alertness, cognition, sensory interpretation, and movement.

2. Altered pulmonary function related to immobility and sedation.
    a. Problem: Adequate gas exchange is required to preserve function of cells in the ischemic areas of the brain.
    b. Interventions
       i. Monitor oxygen saturation; maintain greater than 90%.
      ii. Positive end-expiratory pressure (PEEP) may be required for adequate oxygenation: Its effect on intracranial pressure must be evaluated in each individual.
     iii. Suction patient based on assessment by auscultation rather than at a routine time interval.
     iv. Reposition as possible based on intracranial pressure. Weight shifting (ie, lifting patient and moving 2 or 3 inches so that weight is redistributed over soft tissue) is an acceptable alternative to a complete turn when patient's intracranial pressure does not tolerate side-lying position.

3. Altered GI function related to potential for ulceration, immobility, sedation
    a. Problem: Gastric/duodenal ulceration may threaten adequate oxygenation by decreasing hemoglobin through active bleeding or nutrition by preventing enteral feeding. Immobility and sedation cause decreased motility of bowel.
    b. Interventions
       i. Administer histamine H_2 blocker.

---

histamine H_2 blocker
Action Alters acid secretion in the stomach.
Administration Guidelines Ranitidine 50 mg IV three times daily. Cimetidine 300 mg IV every 6 hours.
Nursing Considerations Large doses may exacerbate asthma; separate antacid dosing by at least 1 hour.

---

      ii. Consult dietician to determine metabolic energy expenditure and nutritional needs.
     iii. Measure pH of gastric secretions and administer antacids for pH less than 5.
     iv. Give stool softeners and laxative daily to maintain normal elimination pattern.

IV. Discharge planning: Increased intracranial pressure is a serious and complex problem. Disability following this event is not uncommon and requires early intervention of a multidisciplinary team to plan efficiently for long-term possibilities. The team should include the following:

A. Neurosurgery
B. Neuropsychiatry
C. Physiotherapy

D. Nutrition support
E. Spiritual support
F. Nursing
G. Occupational therapy
H. Speech therapy
I. Social work
J. Neuropsychometrics

Myasthenia Gravis

I. Definition: Weakness of skeletal or voluntary muscles, often involving the muscles innervated by the cranial nerves. Muscle weakness patterns often involve the face and mouth, eyelids, eye movements, swallowing, neck, and muscles proximal to the trunk more than distal. It is characterized by a pattern of exacerbation and remission. Muscle weakness may cause respiratory failure.

II. Etiology: An autoimmune disorder in which antibodies block neuromuscular receptors for acetylcholine. Without acetylcholine, nerve transmission at the neuromuscular junction does not take place.

III. Nursing process

A. Assessment
  1. Signs and symptoms
    a. Common patient complaints
      i. Excessive weakness after usual activity.
      ii. Feels best in the morning or after a nap, then progressively weaker.
      iii. Ptosis (eyelid drooping) and diplopia (double vision).
      iv. May have difficulty chewing or swallowing ("the food just won't go down").
    b. Physical exam
      i. Level of consciousness, cognition, and coordination are unaffected.
      ii. Ptosis, unilateral or bilateral.
      iii. Masklike expression. Ask patient to show teeth; unilateral weakness will show in flattened lip line and nasolabial fold (Fig. 11.5).
      iv. Neck strength may be diminished. Ask patient to lift head from bed and hold it up; apply resistance with one finger.
      v. Assess each muscle group: Test only once to avoid tiring the patient.
      vi. Assess respiratory function with measured vital capacity and inspiratory force.
  2. Diagnostic tests
    a. Tensilon test: IV injection of edrophonium (Tensilon) dramatically improves muscle strength within 30–60 seconds and lasts for up to 30 minutes.

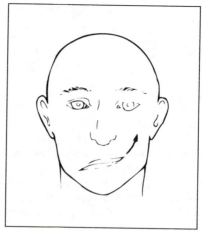

Figure 11.5 Facial expression defect associated with lesions of upper motor neurons. (Adapted from *Clinical Neuroanatomy for Medical Students* (3rd ed.). Snell, R. S. Boston: Little, Brown and Company, 1992. P. 454.)

---

edrophonium

Action Short-acting cholinesterase inhibitor.

Administration Guidelines 2 mg IV over 15–30 seconds; if no response, inject 8 mg.

Nursing Considerations May cause increased secretions, bradycardia, and bronchoconstriction. Keep 0.5 mg atropine available to counteract this response.

---

    b. Electromyelogram (EMG): May reveal decreases in muscle action potential with repeated stimulation.

    c. CT scan: To evaluate for the presence of thymoma (benign tumor of the thymus gland).

    d. Serum testing for acetylcholine receptor antibodies.

B. Patient management

    1. Ineffective airway clearance related to respiratory muscle weakness.

        a. Problem: Potential for respiratory failure.

        b. Interventions

            i. Monitor respiratory parameters every 4–8 hours; establish a trend for daily highs and lows. Anticipate intubation if vital capacity trend is downward or falls below 15 mL/kg, ie, less than 1 liter for a 70-kg person.

            ii. Monitor oxygen saturation to reflect effectiveness of gas exchange.

        c. Desired outcome: Anticipate episodes of weakness and allow for rest; anticipate need for intubation and perform in a controlled approach.

2. Increased risk for aspiration related to weak muscles of swallowing.
   a. Problem: Aspiration will further impair respiratory efforts.
   b. Interventions
      i. Maintain suction apparatus and Yankauer tube at bedside.
      ii. Consult speech pathologist to determine safety and effectiveness of swallow. Patient may require specific swallowing procedures for safe intake, ie, chin tuck then swallow or double swallow.
      iii. Pureed food and thickened liquids may be required. Medications may need to be delivered crushed in pudding.
      iv. Stay alert to patient complaints or difficulty swallowing; safe enteral intake may require a temporary feeding tube.
      v. Ensure head of bed is elevated during eating or feedings.
   c. Desired outcome: Maintain safe and adequate nutritional intake.
3. Activity intolerance related to muscle fatigue.
   a. Problem: Difficulty and discouragement with activities of daily living.
   b. Interventions
      i. Perform self-care measures at intervals, taking frequent breaks. Assist patient with designing a schedule to gain control over energy expenditure.
      ii. Coordinate the core of activity during medication peaks, when patient will be most successful in accomplishing tasks.
      iii. Incorporate rest periods into the plan for the day, especially during the hour preceding medication administration and the latter part of the day.
      iv. Allow patient to discuss concerns. Some activities that require repetitive use of the same muscle groups may be impossible to perform (ie, table tennis).
   c. Desired outcome: Patient will develop a schedule for activities of daily living that prevents excessive fatigue and discouragement.
4. Muscle weakness related to dysfunction at the acetylcholine receptor site.
   a. Problem: Risk for respiratory compromise.
   b. Interventions
      i. Administer medications and therapies as prescribed. Avoid medications that exacerbate myasthenia gravis (Table 11.3).

pyridostigmine
Action Inhibits action of cholinesterase, thereby prolonging the availability of acetylcholine at the myoneural junction.
Administration Guidelines 30–120 mg every 4 hours. Time span capsule is available for 8-hour action.
Nursing Considerations Should be administered promptly at four intervals. May be given with an anticholinergic drug to control increased secretion production.

Table 11.3 Medications To Be Administered with Myasthenia Gravis*

Antibiotics	Heart disease drugs	Rheumatic disease drugs
Clindamycin	Quinidine	Penicillamine
Colistin	Propranolol (Inderal)	Chloroquine
Kanamycin	Procainamide	**Anesthesia drugs**
Neomycin	Oxprenolol	Succinylcholine chloride
Streptomycin	Practolol	Curare and other relaxants
Tobramycin	Trimethaphan	Decamethonium
Tetracyclines	Lidocaine	Gallamine
Gentamycin	Verapamil	Ether
Polymyxin	Nifedipine	**Seizure drugs**
Bacitracin	Diltiazem	Dilantin
Bactrim/Septra	**Psychiatric drugs**	Trimethadione
Hormonal drugs	Chlorpromazine	**Ocular medications**
ACTH	Promazine	Timoptic
Corticosteroids	Phenelzine	
Thyroid hormone	Lithium	
Oral contraceptives		

Pain medications

Avoid those that cause respiratory depression or use low dosage; also check on contraindications for each muscle relaxant prescribed

Avoid (D5LR) lactated Ringer's intravenous solution if possible

Avoid hypokalemia

A drug alone may not cause any symptoms, but when it is taken with another drug causing neuromuscular transmission defect, the effect may become apparent.

---

*Note: These medications should be administered with extreme caution to a patient with myasthenia gravis. Ensure that physician is aware that patient is myasthenic.
Source: Donohoe, K. Nursing care of the patient with myasthenia gravis. *Neurol. Clin.* 12:369–385, 1994.

   ii. Anticipate the use of plasmapheresis to remove antibodies involved in disease process. Plasma portion of blood is removed by centrifuge and replaced with albumin or donor plasma. Accurate weights are required to calculate exchanges. Access catheters are large gauge, and sites must be monitored for bleeding. Normal coagulation may be altered for hours following the exchange.

  iii. Administer IV immunoglobulin as ordered.

---

immunoglobulin

Action May block action of antibodies involved in immune response.

Administration Guidelines 1–2 mg/kg in divided doses, administered over 3–5 days.

Nursing Considerations Immunoglobulin is a large molecule and represents a volume load. Patients should be monitored for signs of fluid overload. IV immunoglobulin is a pooled blood product and may cause allergic reactions. Monitor patient closely for symptoms of anaphylaxis. Premedications may be ordered for complaints of chills and headaches.

IV. Discharge planning

   A. Educate patient regarding disease pattern and management.

   B. Develop a daily plan to include as many usual activities as possible.

   C. Adapt daily schedule to include rest periods.

   D. Teach patient to recognize signs of crisis.

   E. Avoid strenuous exercise, extreme emotional upsets.

   F. Advise the patient to wear an eye patch for diplopia.

   G. Avoid very hot baths or showers, which may cause excessive weakness.

   H. Contact the Myasthenia Gravis Foundation at 1-800-541-5454.

Neurologic Infections: Meningitis and Encephalitis

   I. Definition: Meningitis is an inflammation of the membrane surrounding the brain, spinal cord, and nerves. Disease-causing organisms typically invade the central nervous system by way of the bloodstream, although direct contamination may occur in surgical procedures or traumatic injuries. Encephalitis is an infection in the cerebral hemispheres, brain stem, cerebellum.

   II. Etiology: Meningitis usually stems from a bacterial infection. Bacterial meningitis is an emergency and, without prompt medical treatment, can lead to death. Usual pathogens are *Haemophilus influenzae, Neisseria meningitides,* and *Streptococcus pneumoniae.* Viral meningitis has a limited course, and most patients recover fully. Encephalitis often is caused by a virus. The enteroviruses, herpes simplex type I, and arboviruses are the most common.

III. Nursing process

   A. Assessment

     1. Signs and symptoms

       a. Patient may have the following symptoms, which are primarily the result of irritation of the meninges:

         i. Severe headache.

         ii. Sore throat.

         iii. Stiff neck and back (nucchal rigidity).

         iv. Malaise.

         v. Altered level of consciousness.

         vi. Photophobia.

         vii. Chills.

         viii. Vomiting.

         ix. Seizures.

         x. Positive Kernig's sign (inability to extend lower leg when hip is flexed 90 degrees) and Brudzinski's sign (involuntary flexion of hips and legs when neck is passively flexed). These signs result from irritation of the spinal nerve roots.

       b. Physical findings

         i. May have decreased attention span or memory impairment

         ii. Unequal or sluggish pupils

         iii. Dizziness, facial weakness, and ptosis

         iv. Increased intracranial pressure

   2. Diagnostic tests
      a. Lumbar puncture: increased CSF pressure, increased protein and WBC count. Gram's stain and culture can identify the specific organism.
      b. A complete blood count may reveal an increased WBC count.
      c. For encephalitis, blood or CSF analysis can identify the virus and confirm the diagnosis.
B. Patient management
   1. Potential for increased intracranial pressure, hydrocephalus, cranial nerve dysfunction, seizure, and vasculitis related to infectious process.
      a. Problem: Altered physiologic function related to exudate formation from infectious process.
      b. Interventions
         i. Administer antibiotics *immediately*.
         ii. See "Increased Intracranial Pressure" (p. 300) for management.
         iii. See "Seizure Disorders" (p. 323) for management of seizures.
      c. Desired outcome: Prevent permanent neurologic injury.
   2. Altered comfort related to meningeal irritation.
      a. Problem: Pain causes anxiety and decreased coping and decision-making ability.
      b. Interventions
         i. Use a pain scale to evaluate discomfort and effect of interventions.
         ii. Minimize light in the environment.
         iii. Medicate with non-narcotic analgesics to relieve head and neck pain. Narcotics are avoided because they may alter level of consciousness and mask worsening symptoms.
      c. Desired outcome: Provide safe and optimal relief of discomfort.
   3. Potential for altered level of consciousness and/or seizures related to infectious process.
      a. Problem: Potential for injury.
      b. Interventions
         i. Increase observation of patients with decreased level of consciousness.
         ii. Maintain oxygen and suction equipment at bedside.
         iii. Keep bed in low position, side rails up.
      c. Desired outcome: Patient will remain free of injury during recovery period.

IV. Discharge planning

A. Persons who have come in close contact with the patient with meningococcal meningitis need antibiotic prophylaxis.
B. Rest and activity limited to tolerance may be required for some time following an uncomplicated brain or meningeal infection.
C. Severe cases require multiple supports and resources during a prolonged recovery phase, as in severe head injury.

Neurologic Injuries/Acute Head Injury

I. Definition: Head injury can be an insult to the scalp, face, skull, or intracranial tissue. Brain injury occurs when oxygen and glucose supplies to the brain tissue are interrupted. Between 60,000 and 75,000 head injuries require intensive-care treatment annually; two to three times that number require emergency treatment. The incidence of head injury is highest among persons 15–29 years old. Motor vehicle accidents, in conjunction with alcohol and/or drug use, are responsible for most head injuries. Still other injuries occur in association with urban and domestic violence and work-related falls.

II. Etiology

A. The mechanism of head and brain injuries can be categorized as direct or indirect.

    1. Direct forces: More likely to result in serious injury.

        a. Acceleration: A moving object strikes the head, eg, the swing of a bat. Contusion and hemorrhage may occur at the point of impact and in tissue opposite the impact.

        b. Deceleration: Moving head (riding in or on a motor vehicle) strikes an immovable object (tree, street, windshield).

        c. Rotation: Lateral blow causes brain tissue to rotate within the skull, resulting in shearing of neuronal axons and twisting of the brain stem.

    2. Indirect forces

        a. Blast: Pressure waves transmitted to brain tissue.

        b. Fall: Force transmitted through spinal column.

        c. Blunt trauma: Force at site of impact is transmitted through brain tissue.

        d. Penetrating trauma: Shock waves extend away from the wound into surrounding tissue.

B. Types of injuries

    1. External: Scalp or facial—abrasion, laceration, avulsion, or contusion.

    2. Contusion of brain

        a. Capillary hemorrhage and edema.

        b. Loss of consciousness and confusion.

        c. Injury at coup and contracoup locations.

    3. Concussion

        a. Brief loss of consciousness.

        b. Prompt recovery.

        c. Possible retrograde amnesia.

        d. Severity indicated by the length of time unconscious.

    4. Dural tear: Laceration on bony prominences over the frontal or temporal intracranial surfaces; may result in pneumocephalus or meningitis when external communication occurs.

    5. Fractures

        a. Linear, nondisplaced; represents 70% of all skull fractures.

        b. Depressed

            i. May be associated with dural tear.

            ii. May compress underlying brain tissue.

        c. Basilar

            i. Linear fractures may extend inward to anterior fossa.

            ii. Periorbital ecchymosis: Raccoon's eyes.

            iii. Subconjunctival hemorrhage.

        iv. Rhinorrhea.
        v. Epistaxis.
   d. Linear fracture extending along middle fossa.
      i. Ecchymosis behind the ear: Battle's sign.
      ii. Otorrhea.
      iii. Facial nerve palsies.
      iv. Hemotympanum.
   e. Linear fracture extending into posterior fossa.
      i. Possible hemorrhage, thrombosis, or traumatic aneurysm in internal carotid artery.
        ▪ Comminuted: More than one linear fracture radiating from a site of origin; may be depressed at the focus of the impact.
        ▪ Compound: Having direct communication with the outside or a cavity that opens to the outside.
        ▪ Penetrating: From a missile of any kind; open wound, contaminated, high incidence of infection.

6. Hematomas/Hemorrhages
   a. Epidural: Bleeding between the skull and the dura, often a result of a tear in the middle meningeal artery. Characterized by loss of consciousness at the time of injury; patient may regain consciousness for minutes or hours before developing neurologic deficits as a result of increasing pressure on the brain from the developing hematoma. Surgical removal of the hematoma and control of the source of bleeding are required.
   b. Subdural: Bleeding between the dura and the arachnoid layer of the brain. Caused by shearing forces to the small bridging veins or branches of arteries in the subdural space. May be acute or chronic. Acute hematomas may require immediate surgical intervention to reduce increasing intracranial pressure.
   c. Intracerebral hematoma: Bleeding from arteries into the brain tissue; again may require surgical intervention to reduce intracranial pressure. Represents significant trauma to the brain.
   d. Subarachnoid hemorrhage: Bleeding into the subarachnoid space from contused brain or large vessel trauma. Results in meningeal irritation and may cause hydrocephalus due to blood cells' clogging the reabsorption of CSF.

7. Diffuse axonal injury: Stretching, shearing of axon portion of the neuron. Characterized by immediate and prolonged loss of consciousness. May occur without any evidence of focal injury. Diffuse swelling and neurologic dysfunction follow. This injury may disrupt the reticular activating system, resulting in coma and vegetative state.

8. Brain stem injuries
   a. From rotational forces.
   b. Any combination of cranial nerve injuries.
   c. Cerebellar signs: Ataxia, lack of coordination.
   d. Risk for vertebral artery dissection.

III. Nursing process
A. Assessment
  1. Signs and symptoms
    a. Symptoms may be minimal.
      i. Slight headache.
      ii. Mild confusion.
      iii. Amnesia to recent events.
      iv. Dizziness.
      v. Superficial head or facial wounds.
    b. Agitation and severe confusion.
      i. Palpable irregularities in the skull.
      ii. Severe lacerations, contusions, or avulsions.
    c. Progressive decreases in level of consciousness: Focal neurologic signs, hemiparesis, ophthalmoplegia, pupil changes.
  2. Diagnostic tests
    a. CT scan: Identifies hemorrhage, mass lesions (hematomas or edema), and the effect on intracranial structures.
    b. MRI: Visualizes tissue density; cannot be used in gunshot wounds unless metal fragments ruled out by skull radiograph.
    c. Skull and cerebral spine x-ray to identify fracture/dislocation.
    d. Cranial nerve testing: Early identification of herniation syndromes (see Fig. 11.4).
    e. Blood and coagulation studies to identify hemoglobin needs; possible coagulopathy, renal function.
    f. Drug and alcohol screening.
    g. Baseline ECG.
    h. Evaluation of any other injuries.
B. Patient management
  1. Risk for neurologic deterioration related to increased intracranial pressure.
    a. Problem: Loss of neurologic function may be permanent if pressure is unrelieved.
    b. Interventions
      i. Identify as early as possible any change in neurologic function.
      ii. Neurologic function exams: Test every hour or as indicated.
        ▪ Test with Glasgow Coma Scale (see Table 11.1).
        ▪ Perform cranial nerve tests to evaluate motor function.
        ○ Cranial nerve III
          —Eyelid opening: ask the patient to open eyes; observe for symmetry in the amount of visible eyelid when the eyes are open. In the patient who is unable to follow commands, observe response to noxious stimuli (eg, sternal rub).
          —Pupillary constriction in response to a bright light beamed directly into the eye. May be more easily observed if the room is darkened and eye is viewed from the side.
          —Eye movement: Up and out; up and in; down and out. Ask the patient to follow an object held 10 inches from the face

and moved into the six cardinal positions of gaze. In the patient who is unable to follow commands, observe resting gaze and random movement of eyes when possible.

- ○ Cranial nerve IV: Down-and-in eye movement (see Cranial Nerve III).
- ○ Cranial nerve VI: Lateral eye movement (see Cranial Nerve III).
- ○ Cranial nerve VII: Facial symmetry. Observe the nasolabial fold (line from the nare adjacent to the mouth) and the corners of the mouth for symmetry during a smile or grimace. Weakness is demonstrated by flattening of the fold and droop of the corner of the mouth.
- ○ Cranial nerves IX and X: Swallowing. Be alert for any signs of difficulty in swallowing such as coughing, choking, or retention of food in mouth after a swallow attempt. If there is suspected dysfunction the patient should receive nothing by mouth, and formal swallowing evaluations should be performed by qualified personnel.
- ○ Cranial nerve XII: Midline tongue. Ask the patient to stick out tongue. Weakness or paralysis is demonstrated by deviation to the affected side.
- Perform motor strength scoring.
- ○ 5—normal strength.
- ○ 4—offers resistance but can be overcome by examiner.
- ○ 3—able to overcome gravity but offers no resistance to examiner.
- ○ 2—cannot oppose gravity; moves only in horizontal plane.
- ○ 1—flicker of muscle movement.
- Evaluate protective reflexes: Note: These exams may *adversely* affect intracranial pressure.
- ○ Corneal: Drop of saline into each eye.
- ○ Gag: Tongue depressor inserted to touch base of tongue or soft palate.
- ○ Cough: During endotracheal tube suctioning or by moving the endotracheal tube.
  - iii. Control intracranial pressure: Normal pressures range between 0 and 15 mm Hg. See "Increased Intracranial Pressure" (p. 300) under "Patient Management" for systems review.
2. Potential for CSF leak related to altered integrity of meninges.
  - a. Problem: Contamination of CSF can result in meningitis.
  - b. Interventions
    - i. Consider meningeal tears in basilar skull fractures.
    - ii. Monitor any fluid drainage from ears, nose, or open skull wounds for halo effect on gauze (a dark ring formation around a serous stain on the gauze, which would indicate that drainage is CSF.
    - iii. Monitor temperature every 4 hours for elevations greater than 100.5°F.
  - c. Desired outcome: early identification of CSF leak.

3. Potential for agitated behavior related to disorientation and perceptual deficits during the recovery process.

a. Problem: Safety risks.

b. Interventions

    i. Provide quiet, low-light environment.

    ii. Familiar people are often more successful in quieting a patient than health care personnel.

    iii. Provide warm, dry environment.

    iv. Maintain bed in low position. Mattresses on the floor may be required.

    v. Ensure close observation for attempts to remove invasive equipment, eg, tracheostomy tube.

    vi. Protect invasive equipment with difficult-to-remove (not restrictive to the point of annoyance) coverings, eg, abdominal binder for feeding tube.

    vii. Provide regular sleep and rest patterns.

    viii. Evaluate the need for any sedative or antipsychotic medications. When administered, evaluate the effect.

    ix. Head injury requires early intervention of a multidisciplinary team to plan efficiently for long-term possibilities. The team should include the following:

- Neurosurgery.
- Neuropsychiatry.
- Physiotherapy.
- Nutrition support.
- Spiritual support.
- Nursing.
- Occupational therapy.
- Speech therapy.
- Social work.
- Neuropsychometrics.

c. Desired outcome: Provide a safe and reassuring environment.

IV. Discharge planning

A. The goal is to plan placement in an environment that will support continued recovery of cognitive, motor, and sensory capacity. Recovery processes should support the involvement of family to the highest degree possible.

B. Even minor head injury can result in symptoms that persist for months and up to 1 year following the injury.

C. These persistent symptoms may require the patient to do the following:

1. Limit social interactions.

2. Limit work hours.

3. Take rest periods throughout the day.

4. Restrict environment to limited stimuli.

D. The symptoms include the following:

1. Headache.

2. Dizziness.

3. Numbness.

4. Tinnitus.
5. Sleep disturbances.
6. Depression.
7. Lack of coordination.
8. Cranial nerve deficits.
9. Difficulty with concentration.
10. Difficulty with household chores.
11. Sensory deficits related to taste and smell.
12. Memory problems.
13. Mild weakness.
14. Diplopia.
15. Hearing problems.
16. Blackout spells.
17. Fatigue.
E. A supportive and interactive environment that includes persons significant in the patient's life is required. Families need to be informed, to be accepted by the health care team, to feel hope, and to know that the people caring for their loved one are concerned [2].

Spinal Cord Injuries

I. **Definition:** Mechanical or biochemical disruption of neuronal tissue responsible for the communication of sensory and motor signals to and from the brain. The extent of injury depends on the initial insult and the early management of the injury. Mechanical disruption can occur from compression, shearing, twisting or kinking, contusion, hemorrhage, or laceration. Vertebral bodies may be dislocated to varying degrees and involve injury to major ligaments required for support of the bony spine.

A. Incomplete spinal cord injury
  1. Concussion: Profound shaking; all resultant deficits resolve within 48 hours.
  2. Anterior cord syndrome: Flexion/compression of the anterior segment of the spinal cord or interruption in the blood supply from the anterior spinal artery.
     a. Paralysis below the level of the injury.
     b. Loss of pain and temperature below the injury.
     c. Preservation of proprioception, touch, vibration and motion sense.
  3. Central cord syndrome: Corticospinal tract compression or edema.
     a. Motor weakness greater in upper extremities than lower.
     b. Varying sensory deficits in upper extremities.
  4. Posterior cord syndrome: Posterior (dorsal) columns injured in hyperextension.
     a. Loss of touch, position, and vibration sense.
     b. Preservation of motor skills but impairment related to sensory losses.
  5. Brown-Sequard: Transverse hemisection of the spinal cord, lateral compression of cord.
     a. Ipsilateral loss of motor, position, and vibratory sense.
     b. Contralateral loss of pain and temperature.
  6. Cauda equina: Compression of nerve roots at the "tail" of the cord.

      a. Pain or tingling sensation in lower extremity.
      b. Motor weakness along spinal segment affected.
      c. Diminished reflexes in lower extremity.
  B. Complete spinal cord injury: May result from any single or combination of compression, flexion-extension, rotational forces; loss of all sensory and motor function below the level of the injury.

II. Etiology

  A. Motor vehicle accidents (50%).
  B. Falls (16%).
  C. Sports-related impacts (16%).
  D. Gunshot, knife wounds (12%).
  E. Frequently alcohol- and drug-related.

III. Nursing process

  A. Assessment
    1. Signs and symptoms
      a. Loss of motor function due to corticospinal tract involvement.
      b. Loss of touch, temperature, pain, and position and vibratory senses due to spinothalamic tract and posterior column involvement.
      c. Loss of sympathetic innervation in injuries above the sixth thoracic vertebra (T6).
      d. Altered level of consciousness in associated head injury.
      e. Other associated injuries; chest, abdominal, musculoskeletal trauma.
    2. Diagnostic tests
      a. Neurologic findings immediately after injury.
      b. Therapy instituted at the scene and in emergency phase.
      c. Vital signs, sensorimotor function (Table 11.4, Fig. 11.6), and intake and output records.

Table 11.4 Motor Function Tests by Spinal Segments

Muscle	Function	Spinal Segment
Diaphragm/trapezius	Respiration/shoulder shrug	C4
Deltoid	Raise arms	C5
Biceps	Elbow flexion	C5,6
Wrist extensors	Raise wrist	C6
Triceps	Arm extension	C7
Flexor digitorum profundus	Finger flexion	C8
Hand intrinsics	Finger abduction	T1
Iliopsoas	Hip flexion	L2
Quadriceps	Knee flexion	L3
Tibialis anterior	Foot dorsiflexion	L4
Extensor hallucis longus	Great toe extension	L5
Gastrocnemius	Foot plantar flexion	S1

C, cervical; T, thoracic; L, lumbar; S, sacral.

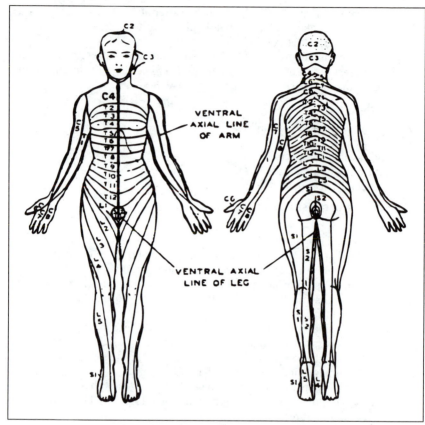

Figure 11.6 Sensory dermatomes. A map of the skin divided according to the areas of sensation received by spinal nerve roots. (From *Principles of Neurologic Diagnosis*. Montgomery, E. B., Wall, M., and Henderson, V. Boston: Little, Brown and Company, 1985. P. 233.)

  d. Complete cervical spine radiographs to include odontoid and seventh cervical vertebra (C7).
  e. CT scan for bony structure evaluation.
  f. MRI to evaluate narrowing or deformity of the vertebral canal, evidence of hemorrhage or tumor.
 B. Patient management
  1. Potential for life-threatening complications related to ineffective airway clearance and impaired gas exchange. Respiratory effectiveness may be compromised.
   a. Problem: Decrease in oxygen delivery to end organs and cells.
    i. Possible loss of consciousness and/or aspiration at the time of injury, related to head trauma.

    ii. Injuries at the level of T6 and above involve the muscles of respiration (ie, intercostal muscles), and therefore respiratory effort is compromised.

   iii. Injuries at T6 and above result in decreased sympathetic outflow below the level of injury. Therefore respiratory secretion production is abundant because of the absence of the drying effect of adrenalin.

   iv. Immobility imposed by supine positioning, required for initial spine stabilizing traction or bracing, further compromises respiratory effort.

    v. As a result of impaired sympathetic tone, gastric dilation occurs and restricts the movement of the diaphragm on inspiration.

   vi. Many of these patients require intubation and mechanical ventilation and eventual tracheostomy during the acute phase of injury.

  b. Interventions

    i. Airway protection with intubation performed with jaw thrust maneuver. No hyperextension of neck.

    ii. Chest physiotherapy with repositioning every 2 hours and as needed. To maintain spinal alignment, the head of bed cannot be lowered beyond 0 degrees (flat). Arm movement is limited to 90 degrees adduction. Patients may require chest physiotherapy to each side when repositioning, and then suctioning, to stabilize oxygenation.

   iii. Continuous measurement of oxygen saturation pulse oximetry; maintain greater than 90%.

   iv. Quad assist cough: An abdominal thrust performed by placing the heel of both hands, one on top of the other, halfway between the patient's xiphoid process and umbilicus and in the midline. A forceful push is delivered during the patient's exhalation to create a cough to facilitate airway clearance. Perform after chest physiotherapy, after ventilating patient, before suctioning, and as required to mobilize secretions.

  c. Desired outcome: Maintenance of adequate oxygenation as evidenced by maintenance of neurologic and end-organ function.

2. Prevent further neurologic impairment; related to mechanical or biochemical injury.

  a. Problem: Mechanical or biochemical injury may cause permanent disability.

  b. Interventions

    i. Sensorimotor exam: Includes all major muscle groups. Identify each muscle group (see Table 11.4). Performed every hour for 4 hours, then every 2 hours for 24 hours, and then every 4 hours, before and after all transfers and with any change in or loss of traction. Documented by spinal segments. Refer to a chart of muscle groups.

     ▪ Components

     ◦ Shoulder shrugs: trapezius.

     ◦ Arm lift: deltoids.

- Elbow flexion: biceps.
- Wrist flexion.
- Arm extension: triceps.
- Finger extension.
- Hip flexion: iliopsoas.
- Knee flexion: hamstrings.
- Knee extension: quadriceps.
- Foot extension.
- Foot flexion: gastrocnemius.
  - Graded 0–5: Full resistance to no movement.
- 5—normal strength.
- 4—can be overcome by examiner.
- 3—can overcome gravity but offers no resistance to examiner.
- 2—cannot oppose gravity; moves only in horizontal plane.
- 1—flicker of muscle movement.
  - Sensation of touch evaluated on each side of the body. Documented by spinal segments. Refer to a dermatome chart (see Fig. 11.6).

ii. Immobilization
  - Initial immobilization on a long spine board, with rigid cervical collar, and sandbags lateral to head.
  - External stabilization
  - Gardener Wells tongs: Check regularly for palpable pin on one side of tongs that indicates appropriate pressure exists to secure the tongs on skull.
  - Bifemoral traction: May be used to further stabilize the spine, especially if thoracic or lumbar fractures exist.
  - Maintain free-swinging weights.
  - Clean pin sites every 8 hours.
  - Must have position change at least every 2 hours, with spinal alignment maintained.
  - Surgical stabilization
  - Anterior approach: Monitor for impaired swallow or airway patency secondary to edema.
  - Posterior approach: Special consideration to incisional integrity.
  - Iliac crest bone graft: Often used as a donor site for stabilizing graft. May require attention for pain management.

iii. Fluid resuscitation: Conservative administration to avoid excessive edema at the site of injury. Goals:
  - Systolic blood pressure greater than 80 mm Hg.
  - Clear mentation in the absence of head injury.
  - Urine output greater than 30 mL/hr.

iv. Administer steroid therapy.

steroids
Action Stabilize cell membrane and inflammatory response.
Administration Guidelines Solumedrol 30 mg/kg over first hour;
then 5.4 mg/kg over next 23 hours.
Nursing Considerations Statistically better outcomes long term
in patients who have received therapy.

    c. Desired outcome: Maintenance of neurologic function as evidenced by
       normal neurologic exam.
  3. Altered cardiovascular function related to spinal shock.
    a. Problem: Overhydration may extend injury at the site; conversely,
       underperfusion may lead to extension of injury. Spinal shock may
       develop in injuries above the level of T6. The shock state occurs as a result
       of the absence of sympathetic tone below the level of injury. The response
       is vasodilation leading to decreased BP without change in volume, inabil-
       ity to regulate heat loss, and diminished ability to raise heart rate.
    b. Interventions
       i. Bradycardia: Responsive to atropine in usual doses if threatening
         cardiac output.

atropine
Action Blocks vagal tone to increase heart rate.
Administration Guidelines 0.5–1.0 mg IV push to maximum of
2 mg.
Nursing Considerations Slower administration and lower doses
may cause bradycardia.

       ii. Hypotension: Treated only if level of consciousness decreased or
         urine output less than 30 mL/h.
       iii. Poikilothermia: Monitor temperature every 2–4 hours; use heat
         or cold applications carefully; temperature decreases will lower
         heart rate.
       iv. Very high risk for deep vein thrombosis (DVT)
         ▪ Pneumatic compression boots.
         ▪ Heparin 5000 U SC twice daily.
    c. Desired outcome: Prevent cardiovascular compromise.

IV. Discharge planning

  A. Long-term rehabilitative programs must be identified early to obtain place-
     ment when the patient is medically stable.
  B. Psychosocial support persons should be identified and be kept informed.
     Community support groups may be useful to significant persons involved.
  C. Spinal cord injury can be an extensive handicap, requiring ongoing physical
     and psychological therapy for successful adaptations.
  D. Technological advances in acute therapy and rehabilitation have permitted
     many patients with spinal cord injury to drive, work, and function within
     their family units.

Seizure Disorders

I. Definition: Epileptic or seizure activity is caused by rapid and repeated abnormal electrical discharge from the neurons of the brain, resulting in impaired consciousness, abnormal movement, or sensation. Seizures are classified according to an internationally accepted method of classification that describes the way a seizure begins.

  A. International classification

    1. Partial (focal) seizures: Electrical activity begins in one region of the brain and a single hemisphere.

      a. Simple partial seizures: No impairment of consciousness.

      b. Complex partial seizures: Impaired consciousness.

      c. Evolving: Partial seizures progress to generalized seizures.

    2. Generalized seizures: Electrical activity has its onset in several parts of the brain simultaneously; involves deep regions and both hemispheres of the cerebrum.

      a. Absence (petit mal) seizures: Decreased awareness, may involve some mild motor activity (eg, eye fluttering).

      b. Atypical absence seizures: May have more activity than absence.

      c. Myoclonic seizures.

      d. Tonic seizures: Muscle contraction where there is excessive muscle tone.

      e. Tonic-clonic seizures: Alternating extensor rigidity and contraction.

      f. Atonic seizures (drop attacks).

Substantially increased metabolic demands during seizure activity can result in injury to the brain. Continuous or frequently recurring seizure activity is termed "status epilepticus." This pattern of seizure activity needs to be controlled as soon as possible to prevent the cascade of cellular events that may cause permanent brain injury.

II. Etiology: It is estimated that between 2 and 4 million Americans are affected by epilepsy. The extent of epilepsy is not well measured because of the lack of reported data on the disorder. Approximately 90% of cases begin in childhood, before the age of 20 years. A segment of the general population has a predisposition for epilepsy related to an inherited low threshold for seizures; in these patients the condition usually is controlled with medication. Acquired mechanisms for epilepsy are related to a specific process or insult to the brain; these patients may have more difficulty maintaining control of seizure activity.

  A. Pathologic processes that may result in seizure activity include the following:

    1. Tumor.

    2. Neurovascular abnormalities.

    3. Metabolic toxins: Electrolyte imbalances.

    4. Drugs.

    5. Inflammatory processes in the brain: Encephalitis, meningitis.

    6. Trauma: During birth or later.

III. Nursing process

A. Assessment
1. Signs and symptoms: To classify and treat effectively, it is useful to describe in terms of level of consciousness and motor activity changes what you see from beginning through the termination of the seizure event.
2. Diagnostic parameters: Diagnosis may be complicated due to the vast number of etiologic factors that may be involved.
    a. Blood chemistries: Electrolytes, blood urea nitrogen, blood glucose.
    b. Drug levels.
    c. Therapeutic levels of anticonvulsants.
    d. Levels of other drugs can alter the levels of anticonvulsant drugs.
        i. Alcohol.
        ii. Antibiotics, especially erythromycin.
        iii. Aspirin.
        iv. Calcium channel blockers.
        v. Birth control pills.
    e. CT scan to evaluate for mass or hemorrhage.
    f. Lumbar puncture: If infection is suspected.
    g. Electroencephalogram (EEG) to classify type of epilepsy.
    h. MRI.

B. Patient management
1. Potential for altered gas exchange.
    a. Problem: Altered gas exchange may cause permanent neurologic injury.
    b. Interventions
        i. Maintain oral airway and oxygen supply with delivery device at bedside.
        ii. Position patient on side during seizure activity to promote drainage of oral secretions.
        iii. *Do not put anything in the patient's mouth during a seizure.*
        iv. Monitor arterial blood gases or pulse oximetry for oxygenation data during seizure and postictal period.
        v. Initiate chest physiotherapy and postural drainage in the event of aspiration.
        vi. Have drugs for seizure control readily available. Often ventilation is impaired during the seizure but will improve when seizure activity abates.
    c. Desired outcome: Airway remains open, and oxygen saturation remains greater than 90%.
2. Potential for physical injury from uncontrolled seizure activity.
    a. Problem: Seizures may be violent and result in physical injury and increased metabolic demand for oxygen.
    b. Interventions
        i. Maintain bed in a low position, side rails up and padded.
        ii. Move objects away from patient during seizure activity.
        iii. Keep patient in an area where direct visualization is possible until recurrent seizure activity is controlled.

      iv. Family and staff can accompany patient when out of bed. Body restraints may be required for safety.

  3. Uncontrolled seizure activity

    a. Problem: Continuous seizure activity creates tremendous oxygen demand in brain tissue. Uncontrolled, this activity can lead to permanent brain injury.

    b. Interventions

      i. Administer drugs to control seizures.

---

lorazepam

Action Fast-acting anticonvulsant and muscle relaxer.

Administration Guidelines Up to 0.15 mg/kg intravenously. Dilute with equal portions of sterile water or saline. Do not give faster than 2 mg/min.

Nursing Considerations As with any major tranquilizer; contraindicated in narrow-angle glaucoma.

---

phenytoin

Action Inhibits spread of seizure activity. Stabilizes electrical threshold.

Administration Guidelines 300–400 mg daily in divided doses. Mix only in normal saline for intravenous administration; flush intravenous tubing with saline before and after infusion of drug. Rate of infusion should not exceed 50 mg/min to avoid hypotension and respiratory depression.

Nursing Considerations May cause drowsiness, GI upset, irritability, rash, anemia, nystagmus, fever, hirsutism, and gingival hyperplasia.

---

phenobarbital

Action Increase threshold for seizure activity.

Administration Guidelines 10–20 mg/kg intravenously. Give at a rate no faster than 50 mg/min.

Nursing Considerations Drowsiness, dizziness, fever, irritability, rash, ataxia, or anemia.

---

      ii. Measure drug levels of current antiepileptic drugs. If below or at low therapeutic range, anticipate a loading regimen based on the specific drug. If levels are high or high therapeutic, anticipate addition of an alternative antiepileptic drug. Evaluate administration regimens for any foods or drugs that may be interfering with absorption.

      iii. Seizure activity unresponsive to lorazepam and phenytoin may be treated with continuous IV infusion of phenobarbital or pentobarbital. This level of treatment is aggressive and requires endotracheal intubation, ECG monitoring, and anticipated hemodynamic support for hypotension. EEG monitoring is necessary to determine the effectiveness of therapy.

    c. Desired outcome: cessation and control of seizure activity.

IV. Discharge planning

  A. General health maintenance

    1. Educate patient regarding the importance of taking medications as prescribed.

    2. Educate patients in ways to avoid constipation, including high-fiber diet, high fluid intake, and routine bathroom use.

    3. Review with patient that menstruation may precipitate seizure activity.

    4. Encourage regular sleep patterns of 8 hours.

    5. Any activity in water should be monitored by another person.

    6. Excessive stress should be avoided.

  B. Physical activity

    1. Normal activity is encouraged. Some activities (eg, swimming) are best done in the company of another person who could come to the patient's aid in the event of a seizure.

    2. Driving depends on state law. Usually permissible if patient is seizure free for 1–3 years.

  C. Occupational concerns

    1. Potential injury to self or coworkers must be considered in making a job choice.

    2. Provide accurate information on the impact of the diagnosis on work environment. Access social work to assist with any financial concerns. Provide information regarding diet and exercise. Identify family supports and contacts with the Epilepsy Foundation of America at 1-800-332-1000.

References

1. *Pressure Ulcer in Adults: Prediction and Prevention.* U.S. Department of Health and Human Resources Public Agency for Healthcare Policy and Research. AHCPR Pub. No. 92-0047, May 1992.

2. Mathis, M. Personal needs of family members of critically ill patients with and without acute brain injury. *J. Neurosurg. Nurs.* 16:36–44, 1984.

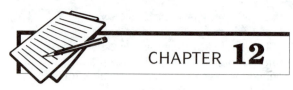

CHAPTER **12**

Renal Disorders

Merrily A. Kuhn

Acute Renal Failure

 I. Definition: A clinical syndrome associated with an abrupt decline in renal function. As glomerular filtration rate (GFR) decreases, the kidney is unable to excrete metabolic waste products. Diminished renal reserve results when there is 50% nephron loss, renal insufficiency when there is 75% nephron loss, and end-stage renal disease when there is 90% nephron loss. Acute renal failure is often rapidly progressive, although the process may be halted, treated, and reversible. However, end-stage renal failure may ensue.

Acute renal failure is often categorized as to its etiology: prerenal, intrarenal, or postrenal failure (Table 12.1).

 A. Prerenal failure or prerenal azotemia occurs acutely following a decrease in renal blood flow usually associated with a general decline in blood flow and/or perfusion throughout the body.

 B. Intrarenal failure or acute tubular necrosis is a complex disorder involving the renal cortex and medulla. Intrarenal failure is most often referred to as acute tubular necrosis. As the damage to the nephrons occurs, it is usually patchy in appearance. As damage occurs in the nephrons, cells are shed and begin to plug the tubules; thus, oliguria occurs. Gaps form along the tubular epithelium that allow some glomerular filtrate to reenter the circulation. Days to weeks later, the sloughed tissue begins to leave the tubes. The urine becomes cloudy with increasing larger amounts of debride. The kidney then enters a recovery period during which renal function may return to normal over a period of weeks to months.

 C. Postrenal failure is most often associated with obstruction of the urinary collecting system by blood, tumors, calculi, or by prostatic hypertrophy. Since urine is now impeded, there is a retrograde or "back-up" pressure that can predispose to nephron dysfunction. Postrenal failure can usually be reversed by removing the obstruction and flushing the kidney.

 II. Etiology: The etiology is dependent on the type of acute renal failure; therefore, each type is discussed.

 A. Prerenal failure is associated with any condition that generally or specifically reduces blood flow to the kidney. Hypotension, volume depletion, shock states, edematous disorders (such as congestive heart failure or even diuretic

Table 12.1 Acute Renal Failure

	Prerenal	Intrarenal	Postrenal
Etiology	Before the kidney—hypovolemia, hypotension, fluid and electrolyte imbalance, shock, trauma, CHF	Ischemic or nephrotoxic* processes, immunologic processes, long surgeries, endogenous protein secretion	Obstruction by stone or BPH, after the kidney
Blood urea nitrogen: creatinine ratio	14:1–20:1	20:1	10:1
Urine: Na$^+$ (normal 20 mEq or less)	Normal and usually less than 10 mEq/L	Increased; may be over 200 mEq/L	Normal
Specific gravity	Above 1.020	Fixed 1.010	Usually concentrated
Urine amount	Oliguric less than 300 mL/d	Small amount	Anuric less than 100 mL/d
Sediment	Rare	Blood, crystals	Sand Gravel
Urine/Serum osmolarity	Above serum	Equal to serum	Above serum
Proteinuria	Rare	Heavy (cortex) Small amount (medulla)	Minimal

CHF, congestive heart failure; BPH, benign prostatic hypertrophy; NSAIDs, nonsteroidal antiinflammatory drugs.
*Drugs associated with renal failure include aminoglycosides, cephalosporins, tetracyclines, thiazide diuretics, NSAIDs, contrast media, heavy metals, pesticides, amphotericin B.

therapy to relieve pulmonary congestion; cirrhosis of the liver or the nephrotic syndrome, which both may elevate portal venous pressure sequestering fluid in the mesenteric vascular system), bilateral renal artery disorders, prostaglandin inhibitors, and cyclosporine all may precipitate prerenal failure. Hydrostatic pressure is reduced, thus creating a decrease in renal blood flow (RBF) and GFR. Severe uncontrolled hypertension can also result in prerenal failure when patients are treated acutely with antihypertensive drugs. Even though blood pressure is not below a normal level, GFR is reduced, and the kidney fails. Symptoms may develop within hours to days of the initiating event. Failure to restore blood volume or blood pressure may lead to intrarenal failure or acute tubular necrosis.

B. Intrarenal failure: Two types of intrarenal failure may occur—cortical or medullary. Intrarenal cortical involvement is associated with infection, immunologic (such as postglomerulonephritis) or vascular disease and involves damage to the cortical nephrons (seven eighths of all nephrons are in the cortex and are the Na$^+$-losing nephrons). The inflammatory process and ultimately the release of antigen-antibody complexes result in damage to the basement membrane and the filtration process in the kidney. Medullar failure is usually associated with ischemic or nephrotoxic injury. Only one eighth of all nephrons are in the medulla. Medullary nephrons are Na$^+$-retaining nephrons.

C. Postrenal failure is associated with obstruction somewhere in the urinary system with stones, clots, or prostatic hypertrophy.

III. Nursing process

A. Assessment
1. Signs and symptoms: Several stages of acute renal failure occur.
   a. Onset: from beginning of problem to the presentation of symptoms; may only be minutes.
   b. Oliguric phase: Less than 400 mL/d of urine is produced secondarily to a decrease pressure or blood flow to the kidney. Generally lasts 1–3 weeks. The longer it lasts, the poorer the prognosis is. During the phase the damaged basement membrane is being shed, and the nephrons are being plugged by debris.
   c. Diuresis stage: Patients may eliminate 3–4 liters of fluid per day. At first it is almost like water, and, as the kidney recovers, the fluid becomes more concentrated and urinelike. The urine often becomes cloudy or even a muddy brown color, since the debris that had plugged the nephrons is flushed out of the kidney. The diuretic phase may last 1–3 weeks. The longer it lasts, the poorer the prognosis is.
   d. Recovery stage will last 3–12 months. Renal function continues to improve until recovery is complete.
      i. Prerenal failure
         - Severe vomiting, diarrhea, poor skin turgor, orthostatic hypotension, tachycardia: may all be found in the history and lead to the hypovolemia that precipitates prerenal failure.
         - Oliguria: Less than 400 mL/d of urine occurs as volume or pressure of blood moving through the kidney is reduced. Therefore, the amount of urine produced is reduced. Oliguria can occur in all three types of renal failure.
      ii. Intrarenal failure
         - Hypertension, tachycardia, distended neck vein, peripheral edema, pulmonary edema, tachypnea, dyspnea: All indicate fluid overload as the kidney begins to fail. Proteins are being lost in the urine, and, therefore, a hypoproteinemia occurs. A reduction in serum osmotic pressure allows fluid to leave the vascular system and enter the interstitium, leading to edema formation.
         - Changes in mental status, confusion, cerebral edema occur secondarily to fluid overload and electrolyte and acid–base imbalance.
      iii. Postrenal failure
         - Palpable, tender, distended bladder: related to the distended bladder
         - Anuria: Less than 100 mL/24 h is usually found in postrenal failure due to the obstruction that blocks urine flow.
2. Diagnostic parameters
   a. Serum tests (see Table 12.1 for specific test results)
      i. Creatinine above 1.5 mL/dL: The failing kidney is unable to excrete creatinine that is produced in the body with muscular activity.
      ii. BUN above 15 mg/dL: related to blood remaining in the kidney for

a longer period of time and thus has more time to absorb even the waste product urea. Blood urea nitrogen (BUN) may also be elevated secondary to the original injury and tissue damage.

iii. Azotemia: indicated increased serum urea levels and frequently increased creatinine levels as well.

iv. Na^+ less than 135 mg/L: associated with volume depletion that stimulates the release of vasopressin, which can override the osmotic control of vasopressin secretion and thus waste ingestion and retention exceed water loss.

v. Uric acid levels rise: Reabsorption follows Na^+ reabsorption and therefore increases in Na^+ elevated uric acid, lowered uric acid clearance, and elevated uric acid concentration.

vi. Uremia: indicates the consequences of renal failure resulting in retention of toxic waste, deficiency states, and electrolyte disorders.

vii. Hyperkalemia above 5 mEq/L: The kidney is the primary organ of excretion of K^+. If the kidney is not functioning properly, serum K^+ levels are elevated. As K^+ rises above 5.5 mEq/L, there may be profound effects on cardiac function such as tall, tented T waves; prolonged (PR) intervals; and shortened QT intervals. Hyperkalemia can also precipitate cardiac dysrhythmias.

b. Urine tests

i. Specific gravity: remains normal in postrenal failure or may increase in prerenal failure as less blood is flowing through the kidney and a concentrated urine is being produced. A urine specific gravity greater than 1.020 and a urine osmolality in excess of 500 mOsm/kg in the face of oliguria and a rising azotemia strongly indicate intrarenal function is intact. Specific gravity is fixed in intrarenal failure, since the kidney is not able to concentrate or dilute urine.

ii. Spot urine Na^+: generally about 20 mEq, since the kidney readily reabsorbs 95% of all the Na^+. In both pre- and postrenal failure, the kidney is still able to function, and therefore spot urine Na^+ remains near normal. In intrarenal failure, the kidney is unable to function, and large amounts of Na^+ are lost. A spot urine Na^+ may be over 200 mEq in intrarenal failure.

iii. Urine osmolality: above serum in both pre- and postrenal failure but less than 400 mOsm/L in intrarenal failure. Urine osmolality in intrarenal failure may eventually become isotonic with blood, since the kidney is unable to concentrate.

iv. Urine protein: The kidney usually does not secrete protein. In pre- and postrenal failure, renal function is still preserved; therefore, no proteinurea is found. In intrarenal failure, protein is lost in increasingly large amounts, since the tubules are damaged and protein is allowed to leak into the filtrate.

v. Urinalysis: usually normal in prerenal failure. In intrarenal failure, urinalysis is abnormal. The urine often contains white blood cell (WBC) and red blood cell (RBC) casts, protein, and may appear a dirty brown color. The urinalysis in postrenal failure may contain significant bacteria due to stagnation of urine, gravel, or stones again from stagnation of urine behind the obstruction and possibly blood from the stone moving or from the prostatic hypertrophy.

    c. Other

        i. Ultrasound will assist with the differentiation of acute renal failure.

B. Patient management

  1. Prerenal failure

    a. Fluid volume deficit related to extracellular dehydration (hypovolemia) and intracellular dehydration (hypernatremia).

      i. Problem: A patient experiencing prerenal failure is likely to be fluid volume depleted. Hypovolemia leads to hypotension and decreased perfusion to all organs and body tissues. Decreased intravascular volume triggers three compensatory mechanisms: the renin-angiotensin-aldosterone system, the thirst mechanism, and antidiuretic hormone (ADH) release.

     ii. Intervention

- Assess neurologic function, level of consciousness, behavioral changes.
- Assess hemodynamic function and monitor central venous pressure (CVP), pulmonary artery occlusion pressure (PAOP), and cardiac output (CO).
- Assess and monitor renal function, urinary output, results of lab work, BUN, creatinine, and urinary studies—urinalysis, specific gravity, osmolality, spot urine Na^+.
- Assess GI function and nutritional intake.
- Monitor serum protein.
- Monitor fluid balance.
- Administer intravenous (IV) fluids as ordered. Fluid challenges may be ordered to improve output. Goal of therapy is to restore volume without rapid shifts or alteration in electrolyte concentration. Isotonic saline or Ringer's lactate is usually the fluid of choice. Restore half of the estimated fluid loss in the first 12 hours and the other half in the next 24 hours.
- Monitor cardiac function while fluid is being restored.
- Administer vasopressors such as dobutamine/dopamine to increase blood pressure and improve blood flow to kidneys.

    iii. Desired outcomes

- Patient's condition will stabilize.
- Neurologic status: oriented to person, place, date; deep tendon reflexes brisk.
- Hemodynamic status will stabilize as follows: heart rate, arterial blood pressure within 10 mm Hg of baseline; CVP, PAOP, CO, and pulmonary artery pressure (PAP) return to normal.
- Body temperature normalizes.
- Body weight will stabilize within 5% of baseline.
- Serum levels return to normal: serum osmolality, Na^+, BUN, creatinine.
- Hourly urine output: >30 mL/h.

2. Intrarenal failure

   a. Excess fluid volume related to extracellular overhydration (hypervolemia), circulatory overload, and intracellular overhydration (hyponatremia).

      i. Problem: As intrarenal failure develops, a hypo-osmolar state (water excess or sodium depletion) develops. This intracellular volume excess leads to alteration in body function, particularly the brain.

     ii. Interventions

- Monitor neurologic function: for instance, level of consciousness, behavior, and restlessness.
- Monitor hemodynamic function, heart rate, presence of edema, peripheral pulses, CVP, PAOP, neck vein distention.
- Assess pulmonary function—auscultate for adventitious lung sounds, presence of productive cough.
- Assess heart sounds—the presence of third and fourth heart sounds indicate developing congestive heart failure (CHF)/coronary insufficiency.
- Assess renal function, urinary output, body weight (1 kg = 1 liter of fluid = 2.2 lb), lab values.
- Implement treatment for volume overload—fluid restriction, hypertonic saline solution to remove fluid from edematous tissue, administer diuretics as ordered.
- Administer loop diuretics.

---

furosemide (Lasix),
ethacrynic acid (Edecrin),
bumetanide (Bumex)

Action Increases excretion of extracellular fluid. These drugs increase renal blood flow and urine output but do not change GFR. These drugs may or may not prove helpful.

Administration Guidelines Instruct to take with meals to avoid GI upset. Administer early in day so sleep is not interrupted. Do not administer after 3:00 PM. Weigh and measure input and output daily. Instruct patient regarding foods high in potassium. Instruct patient regarding over-the-counter drug use, especially sodium-containing products. Administer IV products slowly over several minutes. Administer furosemide no faster than 4 mg/min. Administer furosemide deep intramuscularly (IM) at a maximum dose of 40 mg to minimize irritation. Do not use discolored solutions.

Special Considerations Monitor K^+ levels; administer K^+ as needed.

- Limit activity of patient to conserve energy.

     iii. Desired outcomes

- Patient's condition will stabilize
- Neurologic status: oriented to person, place, time; deep tendon reflexes brisk

- ○ Hemodynamic status will stabilize as follows: heart rate greater than 60 to less than 100 beats per minute, arterial BP within 10 mm Hg of baseline
- ○ Hemodynamics return to normal: CVP, PAOP, and CO.
- ○ Body temperature returns to normal.
- ○ Lab values return to normal: Na^+, K^+, BUN, creatinine, osmolality
- ○ Urine lab values return to normal: spot Na^+, osmolality, specific gravity
- ○ Body weight will stabilize with 5% of baseline.
- ○ Hourly urine output > 30 mL/h
- ○ Respiratory status: lung fields resonant and without crackles

3. All patients with acute renal failure

   a. Electrolyte imbalance related to hypernatremia and water deficit.

      i. Problem: Electrolyte disturbances occur most often related to a disturbance in water. Hypernatremia often occurs secondarily to water deficiency and can result in neurologic dysfunction.

      ii. Interventions

- Assess neurologic status: level of consciousness, deep tendon reflexes
- Assess cardiac function: Hemodynamic parameters such as CVP, PAOP, CO, and BP should all be returned to and maintained within normal limits.
- Administer loop diuretics as ordered.
- Administer IV fluids as ordered.
- Fluids such as isotonic or hypotonic solutions are administered slowly to prevent rapid changes in volume that could lead to cerebral edema.
- Offer oral fluids as tolerated.
- Monitor lab data: both serum and urine.
- Monitor renal function, input and output, daily weight, skin turgor.
- Monitor K^+ levels. Hyperkalemia often occurs as a result of decreased renal function. Measures may need to be taken to decrease K^+ quickly if cardiac dysrhythmias occur.
- Administer IV of glucose, bicarb, and insulin, which quickly moves K^+ into the cell.
- Administer exchange resin (such as Kayexalate), which exchanges K^+ for Na. Monitor both K^+ and Na^+ levels. Do not allow K^+ to move below 3.5 mEq/L or Na^+ to rise above 145 mEq/L.
- Dialysis or other renal therapy may be needed to restore K^+ and other electrolytes to normal. (See Appendix A for modalities and nursing care.)

     iii. Desired outcomes

- Patient's condition will stabilize.
- ○ Neurologic status: alert, oriented to person, place, date; absence of headache, muscle cramps, convulsions, coma

- ○ Hemodynamic status will stabilize as follows: heart rate greater than 60 to less than 100 beats per minute, arterial BP = within 10 mm Hg of baseline, CVP, PAP, and PAOP.
- ○ Body weight will stabilize within 5% of patient's baseline.
- ○ Serum studies will stabilize as follows: Osmolality, sodium, potassium, chloride, proteins, glucose, BUN, creatinine, hematocrit, and osmolality will return to normal.
- ○ Urine studies: Urine output greater than 30 mL/h, specific gravity, sodium return to normal.

b. Decreased CO related to dysrhythmias associated with hyperkalemia and decreased cardiac function such as heart failure.

    i. Problem: A decrease in cardiac output could be the cause or the result of acute renal failure. As cardiac output falls, all organ systems are at risk for hypoxia and decreased function.

    ii. Interventions

- Assess cardiac function and all hemodynamics; note neck vein distention, presence/absence of edema. Neck vein distention is noted in cardiac failure but is not present in hypooncotic edema.
- Assess GI function.
- Assess neurologic function, deep tendon reflexes, and muscle strength.
- Maintain adequate nutrition enterally or parenterally. Use renal formulas to reduce protein load on kidneys. Patients with acute renal failure may require 40–50 kcal/kg per day. Seventy percent dextrose and/or lipid solution may be used to provide calories while minimizing fluid volume.
- Monitor acid–base and lab results.
- Administer digoxin or diuretics as ordered.

---

digoxin

Action Increase the force of myocardial contraction; prolong refractory period of arterioventricular (AV) node, decrease conduction through sinoatrial (SA) and AV nodes; reduce heart rate; improve cardiac output; reduce preload.

Administration Guidelines Store in tightly closed containers and protect from excessive heat and light. Take apical pulse for 1 minute before administering (range should be 60–110 beats/min). Administer at the same time each day. (Noontime is best.) Administering with food delays but does not reduce absorption. Determine pulse deficit as ordered. Administer PO or IV (IM and SC irritating to tissues). Do not discontinue medication without checking with the physician. Full loading dose is not given if other digitalis product is given within 1 week; or digitoxin within 2 weeks. Administer IV bolus over at least 10–30 minutes to avoid increase in BP. IV solutions stable for 6 hours at room temperature.

- Administer vasopressors to raise blood pressure, positive inotropics to improve contractility, and/or dilators to reduce afterload.
  iii. Interventions
  - Patient's status will stabilize as follows:
    ○ Neuromuscular status: muscle strength intact; absence of muscle twitching or seizures; deep tendon reflexes brisk
    ○ Cardiovascular status: heart rate greater than 60 to less than 100 beats per minute, arterial BP = within 10 mm Hg of patient's baseline; CVP, PAOP, and CO return to normal
    ○ Electrocardiogram (ECG); regular sinus rhythm. All waveforms are normal.
    ○ Lab values return to normal: K^+, Na^+, blood gases.
    ○ Respiratory status: lung fields resonant with normal lung sounds
    ○ Renal function: urine output greater than 30 mL/h
  c. Potential for infection related to depressed immunologic system
  i. Problem: Patients with acute renal failure are at risk for infection due to protein depletion and depressed functioning of the immune system. It is important to protect the patient and prevent upper respiratory infections and urinary tract infections. One of the leading causes of death in patients with acute renal failure is sepsis.
  ii. Interventions
  - Assess for signs of infection.
  - Monitor body temperature, white blood count; obtain cultures as indicated: sputum, blood, urine, wound.
  - Monitor pulmonary function; encourage deep breathing and coughing.
  - Auscultate lungs for adventitious sounds of pulmonary congestion or increased secretions; encourage frequent position changes.
  - Monitor urinary function; monitor use of Foley catheter; perform perineal care and cleansing around catheter as per unit protocol; maintain the integrity of the closed drainage system; examine urine for cloudiness or unusual odor.
  iii. Desired outcomes
  - Patient's condition will stabilize as follows:
    ○ Afebrile
    ○ White blood count within physiologic range
    ○ Patient will verbalize a general feeling of well-being.
    ○ Absence of infection; negative cultures and absence of redness, swelling, and pain.

IV. Discharge planning

A. Identify patient's/family's usual coping mechanisms.
B. Encourage family's participation in care.
C. Teach patient about condition and why and how it is being treated.
D. Teach patient and family how to prevent complications of immobility. Encourage active exercises.
E. Teach about medication.

F. Teach about importance of follow-up visits.
G. Maintain adequate nutrition.
H. Institute measures to prevent skin breakdown.
I. Encourage verbalization about disease and outcomes.

Calcium Imbalance (Hypercalcemia/Hypocalcemia)

Calcium (Ca^{++}) is a primary intracellular cation that promotes normal neuromuscular irritability, strengthens capillary membranes, promotes normal muscle contractility (particularly in the heart and vascular system), and promotes transmission of nerve impulses. Ca^{++} is also essential for blood clotting and for building of bones and teeth (Table 12.2). Ca^{++} is also an important component in the activation of the complement system (part of the immune system that destroys bacteria and enhances the inflammatory response). The normal range of Ca^{++} is 8.5–10.5 mg/100 mL. An average 70-kg person has approximately 1200 g of Ca^{++} with more than 99% of it in the bone. Therefore, only 600 mg is distributed between

Table 12.2 Electrolytes

Electrolyte	Total Daily Dietary Requirements	Handled by Body	Functions
Calcium (Ca^{++})	0.8 g	Absorbed by ileum in the presence of activated vitamin D and PTH	Excites heart, inhibits ADH, necessary for nerve transmission, needed for muscle contraction, constituent of bone, necessary for blood clotting
Magnesium (Mg^{++})	300–460 mg/d with 25%–60% absorbed	Absorbed in jejunum and proximal ileum and excreted by kidneys	Maintains cardiac function and neuromuscular transmission, bone structure, clotting
Phosphorus (PO_4)	1000 mg	Most absorbed by small intestine passively. Small amount absorbed actively under the influence of 1,25-dihydroxycholecalciferol. Excreted by the kidney	RBC oxygen release, calcium excretion, component of bones and teeth
Potassium (K^+)	40 mEq	Absorbed by GI, filtered by kidney; 80% excreted in urine; 20% excreted feces	Maintains acid base balance, RBC transport, blood osmolarity
Sodium (Na^+)	2 g	Actively absorbed by GI tract and excreted by kidneys and skin	Maintains fluid volume, cell permeability, nerve irritability, blood osmolarity, cellular contraction

PTH, parathyroid hormone; ADH, antidiuretic hormone.

the intracellular and extracellular compartments. Regulation of Ca^{++} is through multiple feedback loops: gut absorption, bone resorption or release, and kidney function.

About 1000 mg is ingested daily. Absorption of Ca^{++} depends in part upon the presence of vitamin D and is controlled by the parathyroid hormone, calcitonin, and vitamin D steroids. Inactive vitamin D, made by skin, is activated into 1,25-dihydroxycholecalciferol by the kidney; 200 mg of Ca^{++} is absorbed primarily in the jejunum, and 800 mg of Ca^{++} is excreted in the stool. The Ca^{++} that is absorbed eventually is filtered by the kidneys, where 98% is reabsorbed. Ca^{++} requirements increase during early childhood, puberty, and after age 65.

There is an inverse relationship between calcium and phosphorus. When calcium is elevated, blood levels of phosphorus are lower. When blood levels of calcium are low, phosphorous levels are elevated.

Circulating Ca^{++} exists in three forms: 40% is protein-bound Ca^{++} (primarily to albumin); 15% is diffusible nonionized calcium (as phosphates, sulfates, or citrates, for example); and 45% is free ionized Ca^{++} that is physiologically active. The protein-bound Ca^{++} may decline rapidly in a critically ill patient who is starved. Hypoalbuminemia is also directly associated with decreased concentrations of ionized Ca^{++}. Acidosis decreases protein binding, whereas alkalosis increases protein binding. Elevation in free fatty acid levels (which also occur in critically ill patients) increases the binding of Ca^{++} to albumin, therefore making it difficult to estimate true serum Ca^{++}.

Hypercalcemia

I. Definition: Hypercalcemia occurs as the free ionized serum Ca^{++} level rises above 10.5 mg/100 mL.

II. Etiology: Increases in protein—either an actual rise in albumin such as in dehydration or abnormal binding proteins such as in multiple myeloma—may increase serum Ca^{++} levels. Acidemia decreases the amount of protein-bound Ca^{++}, thus increasing serum Ca^{++}. In other hospitalized patients, malignancy accounts for about 50% of cases of hypercalcemia. In the general population, hypercalcemia is often associated with hyperparathyroidism.

III. Nursing process

A. Assessment

   1. Signs and symptoms

      a. Flaccidity, neuromuscular weakness, tonicity, diminished deep tendon reflexes, depression, lethargy, confusion: Hypercalcemia slows nervous system conduction time.

      b. Renal calculi, flank pain: associated with Ca^{++} being precipitated into the urine, forming a stone, and the stone moving.

      c. Nausea, vomiting, thirst, anorexia: all related to a decrease in smooth muscle tone. The bowel may become hypoactive.

      d. Peptic ulcer disease, pancreatitis: Excessive vomiting and increased gastric acid secretion increase likelihood of ulcer formation.

e. Polyuria, nocturia, dehydration: related to increased osmotic load of Ca^{++} and loss of ability to concentrate urine. Dehydration may rapidly ensue.

f. Heart block, short QT and ST intervals, dysrhythmias: due to positive inotropic effect of Ca^{++} on heart. May also precipitate digitalis toxicity in patients also receiving digitalis products.

g. Hypertension: Ca^{++} demonstrates direct increase in peripheral vascular resistance.

h. Band keratopathy, increased Ca^{++} deposits in soft tissues: Increased levels of serum Ca^{++} may precipitate Ca^{++} out of the vascular system to cause crystallization.

2. Diagnostic parameters
   a. Serum tests
      i. Ca^{++} above 10.5 mg/100 mL: Symptoms may not occur until Ca^{++} exceeds 11 mg/100 mL. Ca^{++} above 15 mg/100 mL is an emergency situation.
      ii. Phosphate less than 2.5 mg/dL has a reciprocal relationship with Ca^{++}.

B. Patient management
   1. Electrolyte imbalance hypercalcemia related to impaired renal function (renal tubular acidosis), alkalemia, prolonged immobilization, hypophosphatemia, hyperparathyroidism, and others
      a. Problem: Ca^{++} is necessary for many bodily functions. It acts as a sedative on the body; therefore, most body systems become quiet or depressed.
      b. Interventions
         i. Monitor neurologic function: personality, level of consciousness, neuromuscular activity.
         ii. Monitor cardiovascular function changes in cardiac rate, ECG changes, BP, and changes in contractility.
         iii. Monitor respiratory rate and function.
         iv. Administer drugs to reduce serum Ca^{++} (gallium nitrate, etidronate disodium, pamidronate disodium, calcitonin–salmon, plicamycin).

---

gallium nitrate (Ganite)

Action Inhibits calcium resorption from bone possibly by reducing bone turnover.

Administration Guidelines Dilute, mix, and administer IV over a 24-hour period.

etidronate disodium (Didronel)

Action Blocks the growth of calcium crystals by binding to calcium phosphate. Decreases bone resorption and turnover.

Administration Guidelines Dilute in at least 250 mL of 0.9 NaCl. Infuse over at least 2 hours.

Special Considerations Pretreat with saline and loop diuretics to enhance Ca^{++} excretion.

pamidronate disodium (Aredia)

Action Inhibits bone resorption of Ca^{++}. Binds to bone surfaces and blocks mineral dissolution.

Administration Guidelines Administer by infusion pump over a 24-hour period.

Special Considerations Patients may have vigorous saline hydration to maintain urine output at 2000 mL/24 h. Monitor input and output hourly.

calcitonin–salmon (Cibacalcin)

Action Reduces bone resorption.

Administration Guidelines Rotate injection sites. Dilute with supplied diluent. Refrigerate reconstituted solution. Do skin test before first dose.

plicamycin (Mithracin)

Action Inhibits osteoclastic activity.

Administration Guidelines A single dose every 24 hours over 4–6 hours.

v. Monitor fluid volume: Dehydration may have precipitated hypercalcemia; overhydration may increase risk of CHF and pulmonary edema.

vi. Monitor acid/base and return to normal values.

vii. Monitor other serum levels: phosphate, sodium, and protein.

viii. Identify and treat underlying cause.

ix. Strain urine for stones.

x. Administer IV fluids (200–300 mL/h) with furosemide (Lasix 40–200 mg) as fluids increase GFR and increases Ca^{++} excretion. Furosemide also interferes with Ca^{++} reabsorption. This regimen will reduce Ca^{++} by 2–3 mg/100 mL in 24–48 hours.

xi. Avoid thiazide diuretics, since there is a decrease in excretion of Ca^{++}.

xii. Carefully monitor phosphate and proteins.

c. Desired outcomes
   i. Patient's condition will stabilize as follows:
      ▪ Neurologic status; alert, oriented to person, place, and time; verbalized comfort, without pain or headache.
      ▪ Cardiovascular status; heart rate within normal range, arterial BP within 10 mm Hg of patient's baseline, ECG; regular sinus rhythm, ST segment isoelectric, QT interval within normal range.
      ▪ Serum studies return to normal: calcium, phosphorus, sodium, potassium, magnesium, and proteins.
      ▪ Renal status: urine output > 30 mL/h.

IV. Discharge planning

A. Teach about course of condition and its future prevention.
B. Teach about diet that will reduce absorption of Ca^{++} from intestine. (Increase fruit and fiber to decrease Ca^{++}, avoid caffeine foods/drinks to decrease HCl production.)
C. Teach about stool softeners, increased exercise to increase bowel activity and prevent constipation.
D. Encourage normal exercises when medically appropriate.
E. Teach patients to avoid immobility.

Hypocalcemia

I. Definition: Hypocalcemia occurs when the serum Ca^{++} level is less than 8.5 mg/100 mL.

II. Etiology: Hypocalcemia is most often associated with a decrease in parathyroid hormone (PTH), or in the critical care patient it may be associated with a severe hypomagnesemia. PTH may decrease in patients after surgery on or removal of the thyroid gland. The usual onset is within 2 days of surgery. Alkalosis related to vomiting or hyperventilation will lower Ca^{++}. Chronic renal failure results in retained phosphate, which in turn causes hypocalcemia. In addition, due to a diseased kidney, the vitamin D prohormone, 1,25-dihydroxycholecalciferol, is reduced; thus, Ca^{++} cannot be absorbed from the gut.

Malignancies in the bone deplete Ca^{++} stores due to abnormal bone formation. Malabsorption in the GI tract can also result in hypocalcemia. Gastrectomy, small-bowel surgery or small-bowel disease, or a high-fat diet, will decrease absorption of Ca^{++}.

Acute pancreatitis can precipitate hypocalcemia because Ca^{++} is precipitated within the inflamed pancreas as well as being bound in fat autodigestion by trypsin. Most symptoms begin to appear when the Ca^{++} falls to less than 7.0 mg/100 mL.

III. Nursing process

A. Assessment/Findings
   1. Signs and symptoms
      a. Muscle spasm, paresthesia, tremors with mild falls in Ca^{++} and tetany, bronchospam and seizures with severe decreases in Ca^{++}: all due to increased excitability of muscle and nerve tissues.
      b. Chvostek's and Trousseau's signs: both early signs of hypocalcemia are related to increased excitability in muscles and nerve tissue.

   c. Prolonged QT: Due to prolongation the cardiac action potential of the QT lengthens above 0.45 seconds, torsades de pointe may develop.

   d. Decreased cardiac contractility: Due to a decreased level of Ca^{++} available inside the cardiac cell, there is a reduction in ability of the muscle fibers to contract forcibly.

   e. Vomiting, paralytic ileus, abdominal pain, tenderness, and distention: as bowel muscle function is decreased.

   f. Compromised respiratory function, limited thoracic cage movement: all related to less Ca^{++} available for muscle contraction.

2. Diagnostic parameters
   a. Serum tests
      i. Ca^{++}: less than 8.5 mg/100 mL.
      ii. Phosphate: greater than 4.5 mg/dL.
3. Urine tests
   a. None.
4. Other tests
   a. ECG: prolonged ST and QT intervals due to impaired myocardial contractility; may lead to dysrhythmias and cardiac arrest.

B. Patient management
1. Hypocalcemic electrolyte imbalance related to alkalemia associated with vomiting, alkali ingestion, or hyperventilation, chronic renal failure with hyperphosphatemia, vitamin D deficiency state, chronic malabsorption state, hypomagnesemia, acute pancreatitis, idiopathic hypoparathyroidism
   a. Problem: the symptoms of hypocalcemia are usually obvious and can result in major dysrhythmias, neuromuscular disorders, and even cardiac arrest.
   b. Interventions
      i. Monitor serum Ca^{++} levels.
      ii. Monitor cardiac rhythm, measure ST and QT intervals.
      iii. Administer Ca^{++} products such as calcium chloride, calcium gluceptate, or calcium gluconate.

---

calcium chloride (27% Ca^{++})

Action Maintains cell permeability and activates transmission of nerve impulses and contraction of cardiac, skeletal, and smooth muscle. Essential for bone formation and coagulation.

Administration Guidelines Administer calcium chloride not to exceed 0.7–1.5 mEq/min. Warm solution to body temperature before administering. Use small needles in large veins to minimize phlebitis.

Special Considerations Monitor for Chvostek's and Trousseau's signs.

calcium gluceptate (8.2% Ca^{++})

Administration Guidelines Not to exceed 2 mL (1.8 mEq/min).

calcium gluconate (9% Ca^{++})

Administration Guidelines Not to exceed 0.5 mL/min or 200 mg/min.

      iv. Monitor digitalis levels if patient is receiving digoxin. When Ca^{++} is replaced, digitalis may be potentiated.

      v. Monitor neurologic and mental status changes. (Chvostek's and Trousseau's signs may be positive.)

      vi. Maintain cool, quiet environment; limit stressors; sudden noises as all can decrease neuromuscular excitability.

      vii. Monitor respiratory activity, particularly for bronchospasm and laryngospasm.

      viii. Monitor tidal volume routinely.

      ix. Monitor phosphate and magnesium levels—correct as necessary. (Hypomagnesium may aggravate hypocalcemia.)

      x. Monitor for seizure activity.

      xi. Monitor acid–base balance and correct when necessary.

      xii. Handle patient carefully to reduce muscle spasm and pain.

      xiii. Monitor cardiac function and hemodynamic status, since myocardiac contractility may be reduced.

      xiv. Monitor serum protein. Hypoalbuminemia may predispose to hypocalcemia as calcium (45%–50%) is bound to albumin.

      xv. Monitor K^+. Hyperkalemia potentiates myocardiac irritability and the development of dysrhythmia.

      xvi. Monitor fluid balance and return to normal as needed.

  c. Desired outcomes

      i. Patient's condition will stabilize as follows:

- Neurologic status: alert, oriented to person, place, and time, absence of muscle spasms or cramping, tremors, seizure activity, or tetany
- Respiratory status: eupnea, unlabored respirations, full chest wall excursion, absence of adventitious breath sounds; crackles, wheezes, absence of laryngospasm, airway obstruction (bronchospasm)
- Cardiovascular status: heart rate greater than 60 to less than 100 beats per minute, arterial BP within 10 mm Hg of patient's baseline, ECG regular sinus rhythm
- Renal status: urine output greater than 30 mL/h (depends on previous status of renal function), lab values return to normal

IV. Discharge planning

A. Teach patient about how condition developed and how to prevent in future.

B. Maintain nutrition.

C. Teach about foods that are high in calcium, such as dairy products.

D. Increase intake of dietary calcium.

E. Increase activities and exercise level as soon as medically able.

F. Teach patients about medications, indication, action, side effects, administration guidelines, if they are to be continued at home.

Potassium Imbalance (Hypokalemia/Hyperkalemia)

Potassium (K^+) is primarily an intracellular cation. The average adult has 3400 mmol of K^+, with only 2% being found in the serum. Serum K^+ has a very narrow range of 3.5–5.5 mEq/L; therefore, even the slightest fluctuation in serum K^+ can affect bodily functions (see Table 12.2).

K^+ is closely regulated by two systems. Intracellular K^+ systems allow K^+ to move out of the cell during K^+ depletion states and into the cell after K^+ intake has occurred. Intracellular K^+ is regulated by acid–base balance, hormones, body fluid tonicity, exercise, and cell integrity (Table 12.3). External cellular K^+ balance is regulated by K^+ intake versus excretion. Normal K^+ intake ranges from 50 to 150 mmol. The kidney can still control K^+ balance even if the K^+ intake reaches 600–1000 mmol. However, the kidney does not have the ability to conserve K^+ when intake is reduced or loss is excessive (GI losses). The kidney controls K^+ primarily in the distal tubule. Magnesium (Mg^{++}) stores are necessary to maintain the physiologic transmembrane K^+ gradient. Therefore, if Mg^{++} decreases, the effects of hypokalemia, particularly on the heart are magnified.

Hypokalemia

I. Definition: Hypokalemia occurs when the K^+ level drops below 3.5 mEq/L.

II. Etiology: Hypokalemia is associated with increased GI losses such as diarrhea; increased renal losses associated with diuretics or renal tubular disorders; endocrine disorders such as diabetes and hyperaldosteronism; resistance to ADH; refeeding syndrome after prolonged starvation (glucose-stimulated hyperinsulinemia shifts K^+ into cells, rapidly decreasing extracellular K^+); drugs such as gentamicin, carbenicillin, ticarcillin, beta-blockers; other electrolyte disturbances such as Mg^{++} deficiency and hypercalcemia. Acute losses are present for less than 48 hours and usually arise from disorders of internal K^+ balance, and chronic losses are present for days to weeks and usually are related to abnormal external K^+ balance.

Table 12.3 Regulation of Internal Potassium Balance

	K^+ Moves Out of Cells	K^+ Moves Into Cells

Acid–base balance	Acidosis
	    Respiratory
	    Hyperchloremic metabolic
		Alkalosis
		    Respiratory
		    Metabolic

Hormones	Epinephrine Alpha-adrenergic agonist Aldosterone	Insulin Beta$_2$-adrenergic agonist
Body fluid tonicity	Hypertonicity	
Exercise	Yes	
Cell integrity	Cell lysis Acute tumor lysis Rhabdomyolysis	

III. Nursing process

A. Assessment
  1. Signs and symptoms
      a. Neurologic (apathy, depression, drowsiness): all related to inappropriate functioning of the Na^+–K^+ pump.
      b. Cardiovascular (hypotension, dysrhythmias, digitalis toxicity, peaked P waves, depressed ST segments, flattened T waves, and U waves): As K^+ decreases, hyperpolarization of the resting membrane potential occurs and leads to increased irritability and dysrhythmias.
      c. GI (nausea, vomiting, constipation, paralytic ileus, respiratory muscle weakness, may lead to respiratory arrest): All are associated with a decreased muscle tone. Muscle tone may be so reduced that respiratory arrest may ensue.
  2. Diagnostic parameters
      a. Serum tests
          i. K^+: less than 3.5 mEq/L
          ii. pH above 7.45: As K^+ shifts from the cells into the serum, H^+ is shifted into the cell. Since few K^+ ions are now available to exchange with sodium in the distal tube of the kidney, there is an increase in H^+ loss and, thus, alkalosis.
      b. Urine tests: none.
B. Patient management
  1. Electrolyte imbalance (hypokalemia) related to excessive GI losses, excessive renal losses, or drug therapy—such as gentamicin, steroids, diuretics
      a. Problem
          i. Hypokalemia decreases muscle tone, and increases cardiac irritability (throughout the body) and possibly dysrhythmias
      b. Interventions
          i. When serum levels are between 2.5 and 3.5 mEq/L, increase oral potassium intake with high K^+ foods or oral potassium supplements.
          ii. When serum levels are below 2.5 mEq/L, and when cardiac dysrhythmias are present, IV K^+ replacements may be necessary.
          iii. Administer potassium acetate or potassium chloride.

---

potassium acetate, potassium chloride
Action Maintain cellular acid–base balance, tonicity of cells particularly the heart. Transmission of nerve impulses necessary for cardiac muscle, renal function.
Administration Guidelines Do not administer undiluted. Do not add K^+ to hanging IV bottle. Administer a maximum of 10 mEq/h.

---

          iv. Monitor cardiac activity.
          v. Monitor neurologic function.
      c. Desired outcomes
          i. Serum K^+ levels return to normal.
          ii. Cardiac dysrhythmias are controlled.
          iii. Acid–base balance returns to normal.

IV. Discharge planning

A. Teach patient about condition and how it can be avoided in the future.

B. Teach patient about how to increase K^+ in the diet—banana, melons, instant coffee.

Hyperkalemia

I. Definition: Hyperkalemia occurs when the K^+ level rises above 5.5 mEq/L.

II. Etiology: Hyperkalemia is associated with acute renal failure during the oliguric stage and in chronic renal failure during the later stage when urinary output along with K^+ excretions are reduced; acute disruption of cellular integrity in traumas, massive hemolytic transfusion reactions, crushing injuries, burns and rhabdomyolysis, endocrine disorders such as Addison's disease; too much or too fast administration of K^+; medications that are high in K^+; secondary to acid–base abnormalities such as acidosis; or due to medications such as calcium channel blockers, nonsteroidal antiinflammatory drugs, angiotensin-converting–enzyme II inhibitors.

III. Nursing process

A. Assessment findings

1. Signs and symptoms

   a. Neuromuscular irritability, weakness, cramps—progressing to ascending flaccid paralysis of face and extremities—occur because there is suppression of activity of the Na^+–K^+ pump due to the elevation of K^+.

   b. Cardiac changes (tall extended T waves, wide QRS, reduced R amplitude, depressed ST segment, prolonged PR, heart block): due to hypopolarization; a decrease in negativity within the cell that leads to slowed response in the action potential leading to serious conduction delays and depressed responses.

2. Diagnostic parameters

   a. Serum tests

      i. K^+: above 5.5 mEq/L.

      ii. pH: less than 7.35 as a result of increased loss of H^+ ions in the urine.

   b. Urine tests

      i. None

B. Patient management

1. Electrolyte imbalance (hyperkalemia) related to acidemia, renal disease, endocrine disease.

   a. Problem: Hyperkalemia directly impacts the excitability of nervous and cardiac cells. Return K^+ levels to normal at the speed the imbalance occurred, since chronic hyperkalemia reduces K^+ at about 1 mEq/h.

   b. Interventions

      i. Correct underlying cause.

      ii. If K^+ is between 5.5 and 6.5 mEq/L with adequate renal function use exchange resins.

      iii. Administer sodium polystyrene sulfonate.

> ### sodium polystyrene sulfonate (Kayexalate)
> *Action* Exchanges sodium for potassium in the intestine.
> *Administration Guidelines* Watch for sodium overload. Use only fresh suspensions. Stir before use. Mix with water or syrup. Check for constipation. Do not expose to heat. Make certain patient expels medication within several hours, otherwise hyperkalemia will recur as the potassium is reabsorbed from GI system.

     iv. If K^+ is above 6.5 mEq/L and severe renal impairment is present, emergency measures may be needed.

     v. Administer 500 mL 10% glucose with 10 U regular insulin IV over 30 minutes. This quickly moves K^+ into the cell. It is a temporary treatment lasting for several hours.

     vi. Administer sodium bicarbonate 2–3 amp, in 500 mL glucose IV over 2–3 hours. Relieves the acidemia. As pH rises, K^+ is moved into the cell.

     vii. Administer 10% calcium gluconate, which relieves the cardiotoxic effects of K^+.

     viii. Administer diuretics such as furosemide (Lasix) or bumetanide (Bumex) to increase excretion of K^+.

     ix. Dialysis therapy may be necessary if kidney function is insufficient to eliminate K^+. Hemodialysis is more effective than peritoneal dialysis to remove K^+.

     x. Monitor cardiac function.

     xi. Monitor neurologic function.

     xii. Monitor renal function to ensure K^+ can be excreted.

  c. Desired outcomes

     i. K^+ returns to normal.

     ii. Acid–base balance returns to normal.

IV. Discharge planning

A. Teach patient about cause of condition and how to prevent in the future.

B. Teach patient about high-potassium foods and how to decrease in diet.

C. Teach patient that salt substitutes are made from K^+, so these products should not be used.

Magnesium Imbalance (Hypomagnesemia/Hypermagnesemia)

Magnesium (Mg^{++}) is the second most prevalent intracellular cation ranging between 1.5 and 2.5 mEq/L (see Table 12.2). One half of total body Mg^{++} is found in the bone with the other one half divided between the muscle and soft tissue. Therefore, serum levels are a poor reflection of body Mg^{++}. Mg^{++} is necessary for the control of many metabolic processes including oxidative phosphorylation; enzymatic activity; the production or maintenance of RNA, DNA, and ATP; and fat and protein metabolism. Mg^{++} and Ca^{++} counterbalance each other on vascular smooth muscle tone. Mg^{++} is regulated by parathyroid hormone

346 ▼ 12. Renal Disorders

(PTH). Mg^{++} is secreted and reabsorbed in the ascending limb of Henle. The kidney can excrete large quantities of Mg^{++}; therefore, a hypermagnesemia is unusual if the kidney is functional.

Hypomagnesemia

I. Definition: Hypomagnesemia occurs when the Mg^{++} level is less than 1.5 mEq/L.

II. Etiology: Hypomagnesemia may be associated with hypokalemia in about one third of all patients in the intensive care unit. Singe Mg^{++} maintains the adenosine triphosphatase (ATPase) system around the cell, when Mg^{++} levels fall, K^+ more readily escapes from the cell. Thus, this accounts for the increased sensitivity to digitalis. Cardiac dysrhythmias that occur are similar to those seen with hypokalemia.

Hypomagnesemia is also associated with excessive GI losses such as nasogastric suction, intestinal fistulas, and secondary to malnutrition, pancreatitis, and alcoholism. Hypomagnesemia can also be precipitated by hyperparathyroid disease, thyrotoxicosis, and toxemia of pregnancy. Drugs such as aminoglycosides, amphotericin B, cyclosporine, cisplatin, digoxin, and alcohol may also cause hypomagnesemia. Prolonged starvation or feeding Mg^{++} free formulas can also lead to hypomagnesemia. Diabetic ketoacidosis can lead to hypomagnesemia probably due to tissue catabolism.

III. Nursing process

A. Assessment
 1. Signs and symptoms
   a. Increased neuromuscular excitement, muscle weakness, tremors, muscle spasms, and possibly the eventual development of tetany and seizures; cardiovascular changes, flat or inverted T wave, ST-segment depression, and prolonged QT interval: all due to inhibition of the Na^+–K^+ ATPase pump that allows more K^+ to leave the cell and increases cell irritability.
 2. Diagnostic parameters
   a. Serum tests
     i. Mg^{++}: less than 1.5 mEq/L.
     ii. Potassium: less than 3.5 mEq/L.
   b. Urine tests
     i. None.
B. Patient management
 1. Electrolyte imbalance (hypomagnesemia) related to excessive GI losses, hyperparathyroidism, various drug, toxemia of pregnancy, or prolonged starvation.
   a. Problem: Hypomagnesemia leads to a decreased activity of the Na^+–K^+ ATPase pump, which allows more irritability of all cells in the body, particularly the heart and nervous system.
   b. Interventions
     i. Monitor and treat underlying pathology.
     ii. Assess for and establish seizure precautions.
     iii. Administer magnesium sulfate as ordered.

> **magnesium sulfate**
> *Action* Essential for activities of many enzymes and plays an important role in transmission of both neuro and muscular excitability. Decreases muscle contraction and produces vasodilation peripherally.
> *Administration Guidelines* Administer 10% solution undiluted at a rate of 1.5 mL/min. Mix 1–2 g in 100 mL D5W or NaCl and run as infusion of 3–20 mg for 5–48 hours.
> *Special Considerations* Observe for signs of Mg^{++} toxicity, flushing, hypotension, weakness, absence of deep tendon reflexes, drowsiness.

  iv. Monitor ECG for changes that indicate improving or worsening of hypomagnesemia.
  v. If patient is on digitalis, monitor digitalis levels carefully as hypomagnesemia will enhance digitalis effects and toxicity.
2. Desired outcomes
  a. Serum Mg^{++} levels return to normal.
  b. Cardiac dysrhythmias are controlled.

IV. Discharge planning

A. Teach patient about condition and how it can be avoided in the future.
B. Teach patient about how to increase Mg^{++} in the diet—nuts, soybeans, cocoa, seafood, whole grains, dried beans, peas and all green vegetables.

Hypermagnesemia

I. **Definition:** Hypermagnesemia occurs when Mg^{++} level rises above 2.5 mEq/L.

II. **Etiology:** Hypermagnesemia is an uncommon occurrence. It is usually secondary to massive delivery of Mg^{++} or with moderate Mg^{++} loading with renal dysfunction.

III. **Nursing process**

A. Assessment
  1. Signs and symptoms
    a. Neuromuscular blockade, decreased deep tendon reflexes, hypoventilation, hypotension, cardiac depression, heart blocks: all related to the effects of Ca^{++}, which is antagonized by Mg^{++}, thus, there is inhibition of acetylcholine release.
  2. Diagnostic parameters
    a. Serum tests
      i. Mg^{++}: above 4.8 mg/dL. When levels rise to 12–14 mg/dL, heart block and respiratory muscle paralysis are more likely to occur.
    b. Urine tests
      i. None.

B. Patient management
1. Electrolyte imbalance (hypermagnesemia) associated with renal disease or Mg^{++} overload.
a. Problem: Mg^{++} antagonizes Ca^{++} activity in the heart and nervous system and blocks the release of acetylcholine.
b. Interventions
i. Correct the underlying disorder.
ii. Monitor respiratory function.
iii. Monitor cardiovascular (CV) function.
iv. Administer medication to antagonize Mg^{++}, such as calcium gluconate.

---

calcium gluconate

Action Maintains neuromuscular excitability and is involved with neurochemical transmission.

Administration Guidelines PO: Oral form is best administered in the morning with a full glass of water or juice. Bitter, salty taste may be disguised by chilling or by adding ice chips; it may also be flavored with lemon or orange juice. IV: Carefully monitor to avoid infiltration. If infiltration occurs, infiltrate area with 1% procaine and hyaluronidase and apply warm, moist compresses. Monitor digitalized patient carefully when giving calcium, since calcium increases risk of digitalis toxicity. Do not put calcium in same IV bottle with bicarbonate, since a precipitate may form.

Special Considerations Monitor baseline QT interval periodically for changes.

---

c. Desired outcomes
i. Serum Mg^{++} levels return to normal.
ii. Cardiac dysrhythmias are controlled.

IV. Discharge planning
A. Teach patient about condition and how it can be avoided in the future.
B. Teach patient about foods high in magnesium so that they can be avoided.

Sodium Imbalance (Hypernatremia/Hyponatremia)

Na^+ is the primary extracellular cation accounting for 90% of the total cation content. The daily intake of Na^+ equals its loss from the body (see Table 12.2). Na^+ is primarily regulated by the kidney with 99% of the filtered Na^+ being reabsorbed within the nephron. Na^+ regulation within the kidney is regulated by the renin-angiotensin-aldosterone system, atrial natriuretic peptide, prostaglandins, vasopressin, sympathetic nervous system, dopamine, and glomerular filtration rate. Sodium regulation through the kidney occurs primarily in response to the regulation of extracellular fluid (ECF) volume. When ECF volume decreases, the thirst-ADH mechanism and the renin-angiotensin-aldosterone system are activated.

Na$^+$ is responsible for controlling ECF volume and generating sympathetic transmission in the nervous system, conducting electrical impulses to muscle fibers, and for regulating acid–base balance.

Hypernatremia

I. Definition: Hypernatremia occurs when the serum Na$^+$ level is above 148 mEq/L.

II. Etiology: Hypernatremia may be related to a rise in Na$^+$ and a fall in water—a hyperosmolar imbalance, or a rise in both Na$^+$ and water in extracellular volume excess.

A hyperosmolar imbalance is usually related to water loss such as with inadequate intake or to excessive loss of fluid through kidneys and skin. The rise in osmolality draws water from the intracellular space. Cellular dehydration activates ADH, which consequently conserves body water by reducing urine volume.

Hyperosmolar hypernatremia is also associated with diabetic ketoacidosis when there is high water loss because of the increased serum glucose. In addition, hyperosmolar hypernatremia occurs due to excessive GI losses such as diarrhea; excessive sweating; endocrine disorders such as diabetes insipidus, where there is excessive Na$^+$ reabsorption in excess of water; and when patients are given high protein tube feeding or total parenteral nutrition, which pulls excessive water from the intracellular space that is then eliminated by the kidney. Hyperosmolarity and hypernatremia can also be associated, although less commonly, with Na$^+$ excess without a proportional increase in water.

An extracellular volume excess may be associated with CHF or renal disease when the body is unable to eliminate extra water.

III. Nursing process

A. Assessment
  1. Signs and symptoms
    a. Extracellular volume excess
      i. Changes in mental status, restlessness, irritability, agitation, lethargy, coma, tremors: all associated with increased cellular irritability due to increased Na$^+$.
      ii. Increased T, increased metabolic rate: since there is increased activity of the Na$^+$–K$^+$ pump.
      iii. Extracellular volume excess, weight gain, hypertension, possible edema: all related to excessive water in the body.
    b. Hyperosmolar imbalance
      i. Poor skin turgor, weight loss, decreased blood pressure: related to loss of total body water and dehydration.
  2. Diagnostic parameters
    a. Lab tests
      i. Extracellular volume excess
        ▪ Na$^+$ above 148 mEq/L: increased urine, decreased urine specific gravity below 1.010, decreased serum osmolarity less than 280 mOsm/L: all related to excessive water in the body diluting the blood.

      ii. Hyperosmolar imbalance
- Na$^+$ above 148 mEq/L: decreased urine, increased urine specific gravity above 1.020, increased serum osmolarity above 395 mOsm/L, hematocrit increased, hemoglobin increased: all related to less ECF and the results of dehydration and the ability of the body to conserve fluid.
- Spot urine Na$^+$ greater than 20 mEq/L: related to increased excretion of excessive Na$^+$.

B. Patient management

  1. Hypernatremic electrolyte imbalance related to water deficit or a rise in Na$^+$.

    a. Problem: As serum Na$^+$ is elevated, there is increased activity of the Na$^+$–K$^+$ pump that increases the metabolic rate in the body. Other associated symptoms of hypernatremia depend on whether the water level in the body is increased or decreased.

    b. Interventions

      i. Assess neurologic activity: level of consciousness is affected by Na$^+$ and volume balance.

      ii. Monitor GI function—hypernatremia may slow activity; anorexia, nausea, vomiting, abdominal distention may occur.

      iii. Monitor vital signs and hemodynamic parameters.

      iv. Monitor hematocrit and hemoglobin for complications associated with hemoconcentration.

      v. Monitor renal function—urine: urinary output, specific gravity; serum: BUN, creatinine levels.

      vi. Monitor fluid level—skin turgor, total intake and output.

      vii. Administer fluids if patient experiences a hyperosmolar imbalance. Restore volume slowly.

      viii. Monitor respiratory function, particularly for pulmonary edema or adventitious lung sounds.

    c. Desired outcomes

      i. Patient's condition will stabilize; neurologic status: alert, oriented to person, place, date; absence of headache, muscle cramps, convulsions, coma.

      ii. Hemodynamic status will stabilize as follows: heart rate greater than 60 to less than 100 beats per minute; arterial BP within 10 mm Hg of baseline, CVP, PAP, PAOP, and CO all return to normal.

      iii. Body weight will stabilize.

      iv. Serum studies: osmolality, sodium, potassium, chloride, proteins, glucose, BUN, creatinine, hematocrit, and osmolality will stabilize at optimum levels.

      v. Urine studies: urine specific gravity, sodium, and osmolality all return to normal.

IV. Discharge planning

A. Teach patient about condition and how it can be prevented in the future.

B. Instruct patient to keep follow-up appointments.

Hyponatremia

I. Definition: Hyponatremia occurs when the serum Na^+ level is less than 134 mEq/L.

II. Etiology: Hyponatremia may be related to an actual lack of Na^+ (depletional, or an extracellular volume depletion) or to a water excess (dilutional, or a hypoosmolar imbalance). An extracellular volume depletion, associated with both a loss of Na^+ and water, may be related to hemorrhage, diarrhea, vomiting, kidney disease, third-degree burns, and excess use of diuretics. A hypoosmolar imbalance, associated with a gain in water that then dilutes Na^+, may occur in the syndrome of inappropriate antidiuretic hormone secretion in a patient on a very–low-Na^+ diet, or in a patient who received only dextrose as an IV solution.

III. Nursing process

A. Assessment findings

1. Both extracellular volume depletion and hypoosmolar imbalances
2. If Na^+ falls to 130–140 mEq/L, thirst, impaired taste, anorexia, dyspnea on exertion, fatigue, and a dulled sensorium occur.
3. If Na^+ falls to 120–130 mEq/L, severe GI symptoms, vomiting, and abdominal cramps occur.
4. If Na^+ falls below 115 mEq/L, confusion, lethargy, muscle twitching, and convulsions occur.
5. If Na^+ falls below 110 mEq/L, even if it occurs slowly, it may result in irreversible neurologic damage.

   a. Signs and symptoms

      i. Extracellular volume depletion
      - Poor skin turgor, dehydration, decreased blood pressure: all related to loss of both Na^+ and water.
      - No thirst: osmolarity does not change as both Na^+ and water are lost together; therefore, the thirst mechanism is not triggered.

      ii. Hyperosmolar imbalance
      - Edema, hypertension: related to the increase in body water.

   b. Diagnostic parameters

      i. Lab tests
      - Extracellular volume depletion: decreased urine, increased urine specific gravity, hematocrit increased, hemoglobin increased: all related to volume loss in the body and loss of extracellular fluid.
      - Increased urine, decreased urine specific gravity, hemodilution: all related to an increase in water.

   c. Electrolyte imbalance related to hyponatremia (depletional hyponatremia: sodium deficit; dilutional hyponatremia: water excess)

      i. Problem: As serum Na^+ is reduced, cellular activity slows.

      ii. Interventions
      - Monitor serum Na^+ and other electrolytes.
      - Restore Na^+ to normal levels by administering sodium chloride solution.

---

sodium chloride

Action Maintains fluid and electrolyte acid–base balance, and osmotic pressure.

Administration Guidelines Depends on type of product. Isotonic: 0.9%; 1–3 L/24 h. Use for hydration. Hypotonic: 0.45%; 2–4 L/24 h. Use for fluid replacement. Hypertonic: 3% higher; 200–400 mL/24 h. Use for Na^+ replacement. Administer slowly.

- Monitor hemodynamic status, support pressure with fluid if necessary.
- Monitor neurologic dysfunction.
- Monitor cardiovascular (CV) function with fluid excess monitor for development of CHF and pulmonary edema.
- Monitor fluid volume: If increased, reduce volume.
- Monitor renal function.
- Monitor weight.
- Administer diuretics such as furosemide (Lasix) if fluid overload exists.
- Monitor respiratory function: Assess for development of adventitious lung sounds.

iii. Desired outcomes
- Patient's condition will stabilize.
- Neurologic status: alert, oriented to person, place, and time; deep tendon reflexes brisk; seizure-free
- Body weight will stabilize.
- Serum and urine parameters will stabilize at optimum levels for patient.
- Hemodynamic status will stabilize within patient's baseline values.

IV. Discharge planning

A. Teach patient about condition and how to prevent in future.
B. Teach patient about how to increase sodium in diet if necessary.
C. Teach patient about fluid: either increasing fluids or decreasing fluids depending on the underlying condition.
D. Encourage patient to keep follow-up appointments.

Phosphorus Imbalance (Hypophosphatemia/Hyperphosphatemia)

Phosphorus is abundantly found in all tissues, primarily the bone. Phosphorus influences oxygen-carrying capacity of hemoglobin through 2,3-diphosphoglycerate (2,3-DPG) (see Table 12.2). When there is a reduction in 2,3-DPG, hemoglobin cannot unload oxygen. Phosphorus is important in maintaining cellular integrity and function, since it is part of ATP and ADP. Phosphorus is also an important component of phospholipids.

Total body phosphorus is about 1000 g; 85% is found in the bone. Normal serum level is 3.0–4.5 mg/dL, with the level highest in the morning. Phosphorus level is affected by carbohydrate (CHO) intake; as CHO intake increases, serum phosphorus decreases. Therefore, to obtain the most correct phosphorus level, a fasting state is required.

Phosphorus is primarily regulated by PTH and dietary phosphorus intake. A rise in serum PTH decreases tubular reabsorption of phosphorus and increases loss in the urine.

Hypophosphatemia

I. Definition: Hypophosphatemia occurs when the phosphate level falls to less than 3.0 mg/dL.

II. Etiology: Hypophosphatemia usually results from decreasing intestinal absorption, increasing renal excretion, or movement of extracellular phosphorus to the intracellular compartment. Critically ill patients who are starved frequently have a reduced intake of phosphorus, thus leading to a decreased intestinal absorption. In addition, people who consume a large amount of aluminum- or magnesium-containing antacids actually bind phosphorus in the intestine, and it becomes unabsorbable.

The kidney may excrete more phosphorus due to a deficit in tubular reabsorption (Fanconi's syndrome) but more commonly due to an extrinsic factor such as primary hyperparathyroidism. In addition, during the acute phase of acute tubular necrosis and postrenal transplantation, more phosphorus may be lost in the urine.

The cells may also increase the uptake of phosphorus. Most often this occurs in a critical care setting. Large glucose infusions stimulate insulin release or treatment of the diabetic with insulin promoting cellular phosphorus uptake.

Respiratory alkalosis can also precipitate hypophosphatemia. By increasing the pH, glycolysis activity increases, which in turn creates phosphorus-containing sugars, and phosphorus is lost. This process is enhanced when high-glucose IV solutions are administered concurrently with hyperventilation. Patients with rapidly repairing bone, cancers of the bone, or Burkitt's lymphoma may all experience hypophosphatemia as phosphorus is more rapidly utilized.

III. Nursing process

A. Assessment

1. Signs and symptoms
   a. All tissue ischemia and maybe even tissue necrosis, a shift of the oxyhemoglobin dissociation curve to the left, is due to a reduced oxygen transport from a reduction in the formation of 2,3-DPG.
   b. Muscle weakness rhabdomyolysis, muscle pain, respiratory failure, decreased myocardial function, smooth muscle weakness, paresthesias, increased nervousness: As phosphorus levels are reduced, cells are unable to produce sufficient ATP for cellular activity; therefore, all cellular function is decreased.
   c. Decreased leukocyte phagocytosis, increased likelihood of infection, thrombocytopenia, decreased platelet survival: due to decreased ATP activity in the WBC

d. Bone pain, pathologic fractures, and rheumatic complaints are all related to phosphorus loss from bones.
2. Diagnostic parameters
  a. Serum tests
    i. Phosphorus: less than 3 mg/dL
    ii. Calcium: above 10.5 mg/dL as hypophosphatemia directly stimulates 1,25-dihydroxycholecalciferol (1,25-DHCC) and increases Ca^{++} absorption in the kidney and from the bone.
    iii. pH: below 7.35, because a low phosphorus causes bicarbonate wasting in the kidney
B. Patient management
1. Electrolyte imbalance (hypophosphatemia) related to decreased intestinal absorption, increased renal excretion, or excessive movement of phosphorus from the extracellular to the intracellular compartment
  a. Problem: Since phosphorus is responsible for many activities in the body, tissue ischemia, muscle weakness, bone pain, and many other symptoms occur.
  b. Intervention
    i. Correct underlying problem. Monitor Po_2 and changes in tissue oxygenation.
    ii. Monitor acid–base balance.
    iii. Monitor symptoms of organ dysfunction: heart, lung, nervous system, mental changes, and in all smooth muscle.
    iv. Monitor platelets and bleeding.
    v. Limit venipunctures and other injury to tissue to prevent bleeding.
    vi. Prevent all sources of infection.
    vii. Protect skin from injury, no pushing, pulling, no pulling tape off the skin, careful transporting if necessary.
    viii. Administer foods high in phosphorus such as skim milk.
    ix. Administer oral products when phosphorus levels are moderately reduced (1.5–2.0 mg/dL).
    x. Administer potassium phosphate and/or sodium phosphate.

---

potassium phosphate, sodium phosphate
Action Phosphorus involved with energy transfer and carbohydrate metabolism. Necessary for proper development and functioning of RBC, WBC, and platelets. Necessary for production of 2,3-DPG production, which facilitates unloading of oxygen.
Administration Guidelines Administer only diluted. Use infusion pump. Do not give postoperatively until urine flow is reestablished. Give by IV infusion; never IV push or IM.

---

    xi. When severe symptoms exist, administer IV phosphorous products.

---

phosphorus (Nutra-phosphorus PO)
Action Helps regulate calcium metabolism; is a buffer to maintain acid–base balance; and is necessary to make healthy RBCs, WBCs, and platelets.
Administration Guidelines Administer with meals and bedtime. Mix with water for administration.

---

xii. Monitor cardiac ECG function. A low phosphorus lengthens the QT. If QT lengthens beyond 45 seconds, attempt to restore phosphorus level quickly.
  c. Desired outcome
    i. Phosphate levels return to normal.

IV. Discharge planning

A. Teach patient the cause of disturbance and how it can be prevented.
B. Teach patient the importance of increasing phosphorus intake.

Hyperphosphatemia

I. Definition: Hyperphosphatemia occurs when the serum phosphorus level rises above 5 mg/dL.

II. Etiology: Hyperphosphatemia is most often associated with increased intestinal absorption of phosphorus, impaired renal excretion, and movement of phosphorus from the intracellular to the extracellular compartment. Excessive phosphorus intake such as with phosphorus-containing laxatives may lead to increased absorption particularly in patients with ulcerative colitis.

Impaired renal excretion of phosphate is often a consequence of renal failure. When GFR is less than 30 mL/min, hyperphosphatemia can develop. Hypoparathyroidism can also impair renal excretion of phosphorus.

Whenever there is increased tissue catabolism (tumor lysis syndrome, rhabdomyolysis), more phosphorus moves from the cell to the extracellular fluid. Acute respiratory acidosis can also move phosphorus from the cell into the extracellular fluid.

III. Nursing process

A. Assessment
  1. Signs and symptoms. (The signs and symptoms of hyperphosphatemia are associated with the concurrent hypocalcemia.)
    a. Muscle irritability, positive Chvostek's sign and Trousseau's sign, bronchospasm, tetany, seizures: all related to a reduced amount of Ca^{++} available to muscle tissue
    b. Increased crystallization in major vessels and in kidney: due to elevated levels of phosphorus
  2. Diagnostic parameters
    a. Serum tests
      i. Phosphorus: above 4.5 mg/dL.
      ii. Calcium: below 8.0 mg/dL. Phosphorus and Ca^{++} are reciprocal to each other. As phosphorus increases, Ca^{++} decreases.

B. Patient management

1. Electrolyte imbalance (hyperphosphatemia) related to increased intestinal absorption, impaired renal excretion, and movement of phosphorus from inside to outside the cell

   a. Problem: Excessive phosphorus also leads to a concurrent hypocalcemia that ultimately results in increased muscular activity.

   b. Interventions

       i. Treat underlying pathology.

       ii. Monitor both serum phosphorus and Ca^{++} levels.

       iii. Monitor for increases in muscle tremor, twitching, tetany, and seizures.

       iv. Administer drugs to reduce phosphorus such as phosphate-binding antacids.

---

phosphate-binding antacids: aluminum hydroxide gel USP (Amphogel, Alu-Cap, Dialume), aluminum carbonate, basic (Basaljel), dihydroxyaluminum sodium carbonate NF (Rolaids)

Action Neutralize or reduce gastric acidity.

Administration Guidelines Aluminum hydroxide interferes with the absorption of phosphates from the intestine. When administering aluminum products continuously through a nasogastric tube, dilute them 1:2 to 1:4 with water.

---

   c. Desired outcome

       i. Phosphate levels return to normal.

IV. Discharge planning

A. Teach patient about electrolyte imbalances and how to prevent them in future.

B. Teach patient about proper use of antacids.

CHAPTER 13

Respiratory Disorders

Merrily A. Kuhn

Adult Respiratory Distress Syndrome

I. Definition: Adult respiratory distress syndrome (ARDS), first identified in the 1960s, most often complicates major surgery, trauma, or serious medical illness. It is estimated that there are 200,000 cases per year in the United States. Despite the increased amount of research and knowledge about ARDS, the mortality rate still remains at about 50% or higher.

In 1992, the American Thoracic Society and The European Society of Intensive Care Medicine defined acute lung injury as a "syndrome of inflammation and increased permeability that is associated with a constellation of clinical, radiologic, and physiologic abnormalities that cannot be explained by, but may coexist with, left atrial or pulmonary capillary hypertension." ARDS is the most severe end of acute lung injury. The criterion for acute lung injury is an arterial oxygen tension/fractional inspired oxygen ratio (PaO_2/FiO_2) less than 300 mm Hg and for ARDS is PaO_2/FiO_2 less than 200 mm Hg [1].

ARDS occurs when widespread bilateral pulmonary infiltrates, severe refractory hypoxemia, and a marked reduction in lung compliance (if a lung is compliant, it is not stiff) occur. ARDS has an acute onset that typically progresses to respiratory failure within 6 to 48 hours. It can occur in all age groups. The common end result of ARDS is disruption of pulmonary endothelial and epithelial barriers. Vascular permeability is increased, resulting in noncardiogenic pulmonary edema. Fluid, plasma proteins, and blood cells diffuse from the capillary bed into the pulmonary interstitium and alveoli. Surfactant is activated and its production by the type II alveolar cells is impaired as alveoli and respiratory bronchioles fill with fluid or collapse. Within 24 to 48 hours of the onset of ARDS, hyaline membranes form, and fibrosis progressively obliterates the alveoli, respiratory bronchioles, and interstitium. This process leads to alveolar collapse, decreased functional residual capacity, decreased lung compliance, decreased ventilation/perfusion ratio ($\dot{V}/\dot{Q}$) and intrapulmonary shunting. Today it is suggested that activation of the complement system, which in turn causes activation and accumulation of blood neutrophils in the lung, is essential to the development of ARDS. Neutrophils can damage endothelial cells and, thus, the basement membrane of the lung.

II. **Etiology:** ARDS, over the last 30 years, has been associated with many etiologies: septic syndrome, systemic inflammatory response syndrome, aspiration, diffuse bilateral pneumonia, bilateral lung contusion, near drowning, multiple fractures, extensive body burns, hypothermia and hyperthermia, pancreatitis, complications of pregnancy, disseminated intravascular coagulation, massive drug overdose, and massive blood transfusions. Sepsis is so commonly implicated in ARDS that this cause should be considered first in any patient with otherwise unexplained ARDS [2]. Gram-negative sepsis is usually implicated, but gram-positive sepsis and fungi also have been implicated. Severely injured or ill patients may have sepsis-induced ARDS from the gut in the absence of focal infection. Malnutrition and prolonged catabolism promote translocation of bacteria or endotoxin directly from the lumen of the intestine into the systemic circulation by impairing the barrier function of the gut mucosa and the phagocytic function of hepatic Kupffer's cells [2–4].

III. **Nursing process**

A. Assessment

1. Signs and symptoms

   a. Profound hypoxemia: Related to intrapulmonary shunting of atelectatic or fluid-filled alveoli. Recent information suggests that there is little correlation between the amount of fluid present and the severity of gas exchange. $\dot{V}/\dot{Q}$ abnormalities correlate best with hypoxemia. Hypoxemia often does not respond well to oxygen therapy but improves with positive end-expiratory pressure (PEEP) (Table 13.1). Hallmark finding is a PaO_2 less than 50–60 mm Hg with an FiO_2 of greater than 50%.

   b. Marked respiratory distress, dyspnea, tachypnea, use of accessory muscles, and increased work of breathing: Secondary to the severe hypoxemia, the lung attempts to move more oxygen. Fluid accumulates in the alveoli and alveolar spaces. The rapid, shallow pattern of breathing contributes to increased energy expenditure and the dyspnea.

   c. Increased cardiac output, warm skin, full-bounding pulse: Compensatory mechanisms, in an attempt to deliver the available but reduced amount of oxygen to the cells.

   d. Decreased pulmonary compliance: Less than 30 mL/cm H_2O—lung stiffens due to increased areas of consolidation/atelectasis. This decrease in compliance makes it more difficult to ventilate the patient. Increasingly higher levels of airway pressure are needed to move air, which increases the likelihood of lung and airway damage. Pulmonary compliance is normally less than 30 mL/cm H_2O. As the lung becomes more stiff, the compliance number decreases.

   e. Increased airway resistance: A hallmark finding is airway pressure above 50 mm Hg. The higher the airway pressure, the more difficult it is to ventilate the patient. Airway resistance increases the work of breathing and may delay weaning. If expiratory airway resistance is present, air trapping (auto PEEP/intrinsic PEEP/occult PEEP) may occur, which further increases airway resistance and increases the work of breathing.

Table 13.1 Diagnostic Findings in Phases of Adult Respiratory Distress Syndrome

	Exudative Phase (Injury)	Reparative Phase (Proliferation)	Fibrotic Phase (Repair and Recovery)
Pathologic findings	Increased permeability, pulmonary edema Many alveoli and alveolar ducts fill with exudates Neutrophils begin to migrate across damaged endothelium and release protease that damages the lung directly Platelet/fibrin thrombi develop	Increased permeability, pulmonary edema Many alveoli and alveolar ducts fill with exudates Alveoli begin to collapse and are obliterated; granulation tissue fills alveolar space preventing restoration of effective gas exchange Interstitial inflammation with granulocytes and mononuclear cells Pulmonary fibrosis begins in 8–10 days	Interstitial collagen accumulation and structural obliteration; significant pruning of the alveolar capillary network Up to 75% of patients are left with mild to moderate impairment—even those severely disabled with chronic obstructive pulmonary disease Pulmonary hypertension may continue
X-ray	Dense patching infiltrates with consolidation in both lungs (bilateral white out)	Ground-glass opacities, thick fibrosis, pulmonary barotrauma	Clearing of dense infiltrates
Time	6–48 h from initial insult	3–4 days	Continues for 6–12 months
Compliance	< 35 cm water	> 50 cm water	Returns to normal
Physiologic shunt	10–25%	20–40%	Returns to normal
pH	Alkalotic	Alkalotic Acidotic	Returns to normal
Arterial oxygen tension on room air	60 mm Hg	< 60 mm Hg	Returns to normal
Clinical findings	Tachypnea Dyspnea Fatigue	Tachypnea Dyspnea Fatigue Decreased sensorium Central cyanosis Adventitious lung sounds Hypotension Bradyarrhythmias	Symptoms gradually return to a normal state
Mortality rate	< 40%	50–70%	?

2. Diagnostic parameters: It is important to differentiate ARDS from other conditions such as acute left-sided congestive heart failure (CHF) or massive aspiration of blood. Measurement of the pulmonary artery occlusive pressure (PAOP) will assist with the differential diagnosis. ARDS has

a PAOP of under 18–20 mm Hg. Usually ARDS requires FiO_2 levels 60% or higher, and, even then, the PaO_2 is often below 60 mm Hg.

a. Serum tests

    i. Decreased PaO_2 < 80 mm Hg, increased arterial carbon dioxide tension ($PaCO_2$) > 50 mm Hg, pH alkalosis, arterial oxygen saturation (SaO_2) < 85% and falling: All related to failing lung function, exudates filling the alveoli, and accumulation of interstitial fluid, each of which decreases gas exchange.

    ii. Hematocrit (Hct)/Hemoglobin (Hgb): A reduced Hgb can adversely affect oxygen-carrying capacity.

b. Urine tests

    i. None.

c. Other tests

    i. Dead space/tidal volume ratio (normal 0.15–0.35): Often above 0.6, since the pulmonary units are poorly perfused due to progressive occlusion or obliteration of the pulmonary capillary bed.

    ii. Shunt ratio ($\dot{Q}_S/\dot{Q}_T$) is increased (> 5%): Due to alveolar and interstitial space being filled with exudate, which inhibits oxygen exchange. Shunt ratios above 50% are incompatible with life.

    iii. Chest x-ray findings (see Table 13.1): Lag behind physiologic findings by about 1 day.

    iv. Decreased functional residual capacity (volume of gas returning to lung at end-expiration): Due to increased fluid in air spaces and widespread atelectasis.

    v. Pulmonary artery occlusive pressure (PAOP): normally less than 18 mm Hg. Elevation to about 18 mm Hg indicates cardiogenic pulmonary edema rather than ARDS.

3. Patient management

a. Impaired gas exchange related to right-to-left shunting, $\dot{V}/\dot{Q}$ mismatch.

    i. Problem: Leads to severe hypoxemia, which can precipitate tissue ischemia and necrosis. The hypoxemia of ARDS is associated with a moderate-to-large shunt and responds poorly to increasingly larger concentrations of oxygen. PEEP or pressure support–inverse ratio ventilation (PS-IRV) may be necessary.

    ii. Interventions

       • Monitor neurologic status for changes in cognition and behavior.

       • Administer oxygen. A hallmark finding is a falling PaO_2 even with a coincident rising FiO_2. Patient is usually ventilated. FiO_2 is increased to maintain the PaO_2 above 60 mm Hg; that may necessitate FiO_2 of 100%.

       • Implement PEEP as indicated to open airways at end of expiration and reduce shunting. PEEP may increase PaO_2 without requiring a greater FiO_2. Overdistention and rupture of already damaged alveoli are major complications of increasing levels of PEEP. As maximal PEEP levels are reached, there is a reduction of venous return; thus, a reduction in oxygen occurs. Increasing fluids may improve cardiac output for a period of time. If

PEEP levels above 15 mm Hg are needed, and oxygen and cardiac output begin to fall, alternate ventilation techniques may be necessary.

- Implement PS-IRV. Pressure support uses a very sensitive demand valve, so, as the patient takes a breath, a set pressure is delivered, thus improving oxygen delivery. IRV reverses the inspiration phase to 2, 3, or 4 and the expiratory phase to 1, causing more gas to flow over a longer period. Patients experience a severe feeling of fullness. When the patient is being ventilated with PS-IRV, sedation and skeletal muscle relaxants are administered. Continue to monitor PAOP and fluids (see Appendix A).
- Discontinue pressure support when respiration status improves (see Appendix A).
- Administer skeletal muscle relaxants and sedative agents.

---

pancuronium bromide (Pavulon)

Action Nondepolarizing agent works by competitively inhibiting acetylcholine on the postsynaptic membrane. The drug does not change membrane potential and only affects skeletal muscles.

Administration Guidelines Initial: 0.04–0.10 mg/kg. Administer IV push over 60–90 seconds. Maintenance dose: 0.01 mg/kg as needed.

Nursing Considerations When a skeletal muscle relaxant is administered, it causes apnea and paralysis of all muscles, and, therefore, the patient needs to be intubated and ventilated. This drug is administered along with sedation, because it only paralyzes muscles and does not affect cognitive function. Patient should be unconscious before administration.

---

atracurium (Tracrium)

Action Nondepolarizing agent works by competitively inhibiting acetylcholine on the postsynaptic membrane. The drug does not change membrane potential and only affects skeletal muscles.

Administration Guidelines Initial: Undiluted 0.05–0.50 mg/kg. Administer IV push over 30–60 seconds. Maintenance dose: IV infusion 2–15 μg/kg/min (dilution 2 mL in 98 mL = 200 μg/mL; 5 mL in 95 mL = 500 μg/mL).

Nursing Considerations When a skeletal muscle relaxant is administered, it causes apnea and paralysis of all muscles, and, therefore, the patient needs to be intubated and ventilated. This drug is administered along with sedation, because it only paralyzes muscles and does not affect cognitive function. Patient should be unconscious before administration.

fentanyl citrate (Innovan)
Action Produces sleep, an unconscious state, and an amnesiac effect.
Administration Guidelines Undiluted or diluted in 5 mL of sterile
water or NaCl. Administer 0.1 mg over 1–2 minutes IV.
Maintenance dose: 2–20 µg/kg.
Nursing Considerations This drug renders the patient
unconscious so he or she is unaware of treatments being utilized.

alfentanil hydrochloride (Alfenta)
Action Produces sleep, an unconscious state, and an amnesiac effect.
Administration Guidelines Induction: 8–20 µg/kg. Maintenance
dose: 3–5 µg/kg increments or 0.5–1.0 µg/kg/min. (Mix 20 mL
alfentanil with 230 mL NaCl or 5% dextrose in water or lactated
Ringer's solution.)
Nursing Considerations This drug renders the patient
unconscious so he or she is unaware of treatments being utilized.

midazolam (Versed)
Action Produces sleep, an unconscious state, and an amnesiac effect.
Administration Guidelines Dilute 1 mg in 4 mL normal saline or
5 mg in 20 mL normal saline. Administer 0.15–0.35 mg/kg titrated
slowly over at least 30–60 seconds. Allow a full 2 minutes to be
effective.
Nursing Considerations This drug renders the patient
unconscious so he or she is unaware of treatments being utilized.

morphine (Duramorph, MS Contin, RMS, Roxanol, Oramorph)
Action Produces sleep, an unconscious state, and an amnesiac effect.
Administration Guidelines 2.5–15 mg IV q4h, or IV infusion 1–10
mg/h as needed. Dilute with at least 5 mL of normal saline.
Administer slowly, 15 mg of morphine over 3–5 minutes. Use
infusion pump. After 4 to 5 days discontinue dose slowly to prevent
withdrawal symptoms.
Nursing Considerations This drug renders the patient
unconscious so he or she is unaware of treatments being utilized.

- Monitor blood gases, mixed venous oxygen ($S\bar{v}o_2$), compliance,
  and peak inspiratory pressure to determine progress.
- Reposition patient often. Turning patient to new position temporarily improves ventilation status until pulmonary exudates
  fill new alveoli. The use of the prone position may also improve
  ventilation significantly [5,6].

- Prevent infection that can lead to multiorgan system failure.
- Administer antibiotics as ordered.
- Maintain fluid volume. Administer crystalloids and/or colloids as ordered. Maintain PAOP above 12 mm Hg.
- Maintain cardiac output; vasopressors may be necessary.
- Assess cardiovascular status. Hypoxia may lead to cardiac ischemia and dysrhythmias.
- Monitor breath sounds. During acute stage, many adventitious lung sounds are heard. As patient improves, lung sounds clear.
- Percuss over lungs for dullness. Dullness indicates areas of consolidation.
- Palpate over lungs for fremitus. Fremitus increases with fluid or consolidation.
- Monitor for the development of pneumonia. Superimposed pneumonias usually are caused by gram-negative bacteria. Often it is difficult to diagnose these infections in the presence of preexisting diffuse alveolar damage.
- Hypothermia: As the patient worsens despite therapies, controlled hypothermia may reduce total oxygen consumption and allow organs (such as the brain and kidney) to tolerate greater degrees of hypoxemia. This therapy still is controversial and needs further research [6–8].
- Administration of exogenous surfactant.

---

surfactant (Exosurf)

Action Replaces natural surfactant, a phospholipid substance, which normally keeps the alveoli from collapsing at the end of expiration. Surfactant improves $\dot{V}/\dot{Q}$ mismatches, reduces stiffness, and improves compliance [9–12].

Administration Guidelines Instill into the endotracheal tube in divided doses. Doses determined by weight; 10–50 mL may be administered.

Nursing Considerations Patients need to be suctioned and oxygenated during therapy.

- Reduce oxygen demands by pacing activities and scheduling rest periods, relieving anxiety and fever, and sedating the patient as necessary.
- Administer intravenous oxygen: A catheter with a large filter is placed in the vena cava. Oxygen is bubbled into the body through the filter. This therapy is still experimental but does seem to improve severe hypoxemia (see Appendix A) [13,14].

iii. Desired outcome
- Patient will be alert and oriented to person, place, time.
- Patient demonstrates appropriate behavior.
- Patient maintains effective cardiovascular function.
  - Blood pressure within 10 mm Hg of baseline.
  - Cardiac output: 5 L/min.

- ○ Without cyanosis, if preexisting pulmonary function normal.
- ○ Laboratory values: Hct/Hgb is returned to normal.
- ○ Maintain optimal arterial blood gases
- ○ Alveolar–arterial oxygen gradient $P(A\text{-}a)o_2$: <15 mm Hg on room air.

b. Ineffective airway clearance related to increased tracheobronchial secretions.

  i. Problem: Ineffective airway clearance leads to hypoxemia, increased airway resistance, and a decrease in dynamic compliance, each of which increases the work of breathing.

  ii. Interventions
  - ▪ Implement chest physical therapy to remove secretions.
  - ▪ Suction only as needed to remove secretions (do not discontinue PEEP or PS-IVR during suction—use special endotracheal adapters).
  - ▪ Monitor respiratory function by evaluating serial vital capacities and tidal volumes.
  - ▪ Monitor serial changes in airway resistance (peak inspiratory pressure).
  - ▪ Monitor serial changes in dynamic compliance.

$$\text{Dynamic compliance} = T_V = PIP - PEEP$$

  where T_V = tidal volume; PIP = peak inspiratory pressure; PEEP = positive end-expiratory pressure.

  iii. Desired outcome
  - ▪ Patient will be alert and oriented to person, place, time.
  - ▪ Patient will maintain effective alveolar ventilation.
  - ○ Breath sounds audible throughout anterior/posterior chest.
  - ○ Reduced to absent adventitious sounds.
  - ○ Arterial blood gas values stabilized.
  - ▪ Airway resistance and dynamic compliance return to normal.

c. Alteration in acid–base balance (respiratory alkalosis) related to tachypnea, hyperventilation.

  i. Problem: During the early phase of ARDS, respiratory alkalosis occurs. As alkalosis develops, there is a reduction in 2,3-diphosphoglycerate that decreases the ability to unload oxygen to the tissues; thus, tissue hypoxemia worsens.

  ii. Interventions
  - ▪ Monitor acid base or $S\bar{v}o_2$ frequently to evaluate current therapy.
  - ▪ Monitor calcium levels as pH rises—more Ca^{2+} is bound to protein, thus precipitating hypocalcemia. If Ca^{2+} falls to less than 8.5 mL/dL, neurologic symptoms may occur.
  - ▪ Monitor tidal volumes routinely.

  iii. Desired outcome: Patient's arterial blood gas values stabilize.

d. Change in nutrition status related to decreased oral intake and increased metabolic demand.

    i. Problem: A decreased nutritional intake leads to catabolism of visceral protein. The stressed individual does not adapt well to starvation: (1) glucose requirements increase as the body responds to stress; (2) a relative insulin resistance occurs, because the tissues are less responsive to insulin; and (3) the increased production of insulin, in turn, decreases liposis. The body, therefore, continues to catabolize protein for gluconeogenesis. Starvation negatively affects the immune system, wound healing, the respiratory system, and lean body mass in general.

    ii. Interventions
- Monitor nutrition status: serum prealbumin, transferrin, total lymphocyte count, and albumin; urine: 24 hours, urinary nitrogen excretion.
- Feed the patient as soon as hemodynamic stability is reached. Enteral feedings are best [15].

    iii. Desired outcome
- Positive nitrogen balance returns.
- All nutritional laboratory values return to normal.

IV. Discharge planning

A. Teach patient importance of follow-up visits and treatments.

B. Teach patient importance of preventing upper respiratory tract infection (URI).

C. Teach patient about any medications that will need to be continued at home—their action, side effects, interactions, and means of administration.

D. Teach patient about limitations and how he or she now can live a productive life.

Hypercapnic/Hypoxemic Acute Respiratory Failure

I. **Definition:** Acute respiratory failure (ARF) is a major cause of death in patients with chronic obstructive pulmonary disease (COPD), also known as chronic obstructive lung disease (COLD). COPD is a common disorder affecting an estimated 10 million persons in the United States. COPD includes chronic bronchitis and emphysema, which may occur independently or coexist. Both of these conditions disrupt air flow in either the airways or the lung parenchyma.

    In the patient with COPD, precipitating events that may lead to ARF include respiratory infection; myocardial infarction; use of sedatives; dehydration; electrolyte imbalance; inappropriate oxygen therapy; air pollution; and, less commonly, increased metabolic demand caused by nonrespiratory febrile illness [16].

    Acute respiratory failure occurs when respiratory function is so compromised that it can no longer maintain normal arterial blood gases. When the patient develops a pH less than 7.35, a decreasing Pao_2 less than 55 mm Hg, a rising $Paco_2$ greater than 50 mm Hg, and a decreasing Sao_2 less than 90%, all on room air, the patient is entering acute respiratory failure. The pH is helpful in assessing the degree of hyperventilation that is acute vs the degree that is chronic and compensated, because renal compensation by retention of bicarbonate takes time (usually several days). In acute respiratory acidosis without renal compensation, the pH drops by 0.08 for each 10-point rise in the $Paco_2$. In chronic respiratory acidosis with normal renal compensation, the pH drops by 0.03 for each 10-point rise in the $Paco_2$. This relationship between $Paco_2$ and pH is particularly helpful in assessing acute exacerbations in COPD patients, because they frequently present with acute, superimposed or chronic, respiratory acidosis [17]. With extreme elevation of $Paco_2$ (160 mm Hg), patient may remain alert. The reason for deep sleep is not the elevation of $Paco_2$ but physical exhaustion resulting from prolonged hyperventilation. The pH, as stated, is an accurate indicator of acute ventilation failure. Therefore, a worsening pH trend is most helpful in making the diagnosis of ARF.

A. Chronic bronchitis: Characterized by excessive, thick mucous secretion, hyperactive and hypertrophied goblet cells, hypoactive cilia, and chronic cough. When chronic bronchitis is complicated by an upper respiratory infection, this combination of symptoms predisposes the patient to acute respiratory failure. A diagnosis of chronic bronchitis is made after the patient experiences cough with productive sputum 3 months per year for 2 successive years.

As the disease progresses, small airways become inflamed and develop cellular infiltrates, which in turn reduce their diameter. Increasing airway resistance impairs airflow and increases the work of breathing.

B. Emphysema: Characterized by destruction of elastic tissue within the lungs. There are two types of emphysema: panacinar or centriacinar. Panacinar is characterized by enlargement and destruction of the alveoli. This variety often is seen with alpha$_1$ protease inhibitor deficiency. Alpha$_1$ protease protects the lung from elastase produced by alveolar macrophages and polymorphonuclear leukocytes, which break down elastin. When elastin is damaged, elastic recoil is reduced, reducing airflow and the epithelial surface area available for gas exchange.

Centriacinar is characterized by the loss of elastic recoil of the terminal bronchioles, making airflow more difficult. This variety is seen more often in smokers.

II. Etiology: ARF ensues when the lung is no longer able to compensate for the loss of elastic recoil. ARF usually is precipitated by an acute respiratory insult, such as a bacterial or viral infection, or other acute illness. Any disorder that impairs cough and clearance of secretions may contribute to the development of ARF.

A. Chronic bronchitis: Associated with chronic irritation of the bronchial walls, resulting from smoking, air pollution, and industrial irritants.

B. Emphysema: Associated with smoking and/or hereditary predisposition. Smoking is responsible in the majority of cases, but it also may complicate the deficiency of alpha$_1$-protease inhibitor.

III. Nursing process

A. Assessment

1. Signs and symptoms

   a. Dyspnea, poor lung sounds, possible adventitious lung sounds present (such as rhonchi or wheezes), minimal air exchange, confusion, drowsiness, coma: Related to a decrease in alveolar ventilation (a decrease in total minute ventilation) due to wasted or dead-space ventilation. Dyspnea also is associated with a decrease in gas diffusion, which is associated with damage to the alveolar bed or capillary wall.

   b. Profound hypoxemia, confusion, drowsiness: Related to intrapulmonary shunting of atelectatic or fluid-filled alveoli. Hallmark finding is a PaO_2 less than 50–60 mm Hg with an FiO_2 of greater than 50%.

   c. Marked respiratory distress, dyspnea, tachypnea, use of accessory muscles and increased work of breathing, forced abdominal contraction of muscles, shortness of breath: Secondary to severe hypoxemia, the lung attempts to move more oxygen. Fluid accumulates in the alveoli and alveolar spaces. The rapid, shallow pattern of breathing contributes to increased energy expenditure and dyspnea.

   d. Increased cardiac output, warm skin, full bounding pulse: Compensatory mechanisms. An attempt to deliver the available, reduced amount of oxygen to the cells.

   e. Increased airway resistance: A hallmark finding is airway pressure above 50 mm Hg. The higher the airway pressure, the more difficult it is to ventilate the patient. Airway resistance increases the work of breathing and, if the patient is ventilated, may delay weaning. If expiratory airway resistance is present, air trapping (auto PEEP/intrinsic PEEP/occult PEEP) may occur.

   f. Dead space/tidal volume ratio (normal 0.15–0.35): Often above 6.0, because the pulmonary units are poorly perfused due to progressive occlusion or obliteration of the pulmonary capillary bed.

   g. $\dot{Q}_S/\dot{Q}_T$ is increased ($> 5\%$): Due to alveolar and interstitial space being filled with exudate, which inhibits oxygen exchange. $\dot{Q}_S/\dot{Q}_T$ ratio measures the fraction of total cardiac output that is not oxygenated during passage through the lungs. A $\dot{Q}_S/\dot{Q}_T$ ratio of about 50% is incompatible with life.

   h. Increased pulmonary hypertension ($> 30/10$ mm Hg): Related to chronic hypoxia, hypercapnia, and respiratory acidosis. Pulmonary hypertension also may be associated with secondary polycythemia and destruction of the pulmonary vascular bed. Pulmonary hypertension increases the workload of the right ventricle and may precipitate right-sided heart failure.

   i. Cyanosis: A late sign of hypoxemia and an unreliable index of the state of arterial oxygenation. Cyanosis is correlated with the presence of 5-g or greater reduction in Hgb per 100 mL of blood. Anemic individuals with hypoxemia may never become cyanotic; polycythemic individuals may become obviously cyanotic with mild hypoxemia because they are already slightly blue-tinged from the increased amount of reduced Hgb in the blood.

2. Diagnostic parameters
   a. Serum tests
      i. Hypoxemia (Pao_2 < 60 mm Hg), hypercapnia ($Paco_2$ > 45 mm Hg), pH < 7.35: Related to an overall decrease in ratio of $\dot{V}/\dot{Q}$, increasing right-to-left shunt, and increasing the work of breathing. Impairment of gas exchange appears to be the major factor contributing to hypercapnia. Poorly oxygenated respiratory muscles are more fatigued and less functional. Ventilation usually improves as Pao_2 improves. Hypoxemia also causes anxiety and restlessness and may impair cognitive function, which decreases patient cooperation with treatments. Hypoxemia also decreases stroke volume index during rest or exercise. When $Paco_2$ is elevated on a chronic level, the central chemoreceptors frequently are less responsive to the respiratory stimulation of an elevated $Paco_2$. These patients are much more dependent on hypoxia-sensitive peripheral chemoreceptors to preserve respiratory drive. Hypoxemia also is a stimulus for constricting pulmonary arterioles and may lead to pulmonary hypertension.
      ii. Hct/Hgb: Often elevated as a compensatory mechanism. As severe hypoxemia occurs, RBC mass increases in an attempt to bring more oxygen to the tissue. This secondary polycythemia can actually increase the burden on the heart.
   b. Urine tests
      i. None.
   c. Other tests
      i. Total lung capacity (TLC): The maximal force of generating a breath is equal to the elastic recoil of the lung and is increased in emphysema as elastic recoil is lost. TLC remains relatively normal in bronchitis.
      ii. Functional residual capacity (FRC): Volume of gas remaining in the lung after a normal expiration. FRC is increased in emphysema because the outside recoil of the chest cage is substantially higher than inward recoil; therefore, the lung is not emptied properly. FRC remains fairly normal in bronchitis.
      iii. Residual volume: The volume of gas always remaining in the lung; significantly increased in both bronchitis and emphysema. In chronic bronchitis, air trapping occurs as small airways are narrowed or occluded. In emphysema, airways close early due to already maximal expiration.
      iv. Lung compliance increased due to the dilated alveoli/bronchioles.
      v. $\dot{V}/\dot{Q}$ mismatch: A normal compensatory mechanism to help minimize the $\dot{V}/\dot{Q}$ mismatch that occurs with hypoxia is vasoconstriction of the surrounding pulmonary vessels. When oxygen is administered, it may actually impair gas exchange by altering the distribution of blood flow. Oxygen may dilate the previously

constricted pulmonary vessels that surround poorly ventilated alveoli. A greater proportion of cardiac output is delivered to the poorly ventilated air sacs, and less blood is perfused to the already well-ventilated air, thus creating the mismatch.

vi. $P(A-a)O_2$ (normal 5–20 mm Hg): Estimates hypoxemia and intrapulmonary shunting. A value over 20 mm Hg indicates increased shunting.

vii. Peak inspiratory pressure (PIP) (normal >20 cm H_2O): Reflects the maximum inspiratory force or maximum inspiratory pressure that a patient can exert against a closed system from FRC. PIP is often above 50 cm H_2O. PIP pressure rises as more alveolar units become dead space, and $\dot{V}/\dot{Q}$ mismatch worsens. PIP above 50 cm H_2O necessitates intervention.

B. Patient management

1. Impaired gas exchange related to right-to-left shunting, $\dot{V}/\dot{Q}$ mismatch, impaired diffusion, alveolar hypoventilation.

   a. Problem: Leads to severe hypoxemia, which can precipitate tissue ischemia and necrosis. The hypoxemia of ARF is associated with a moderate-to-large shunt. Although oxygen therapy is necessary, it must be carefully controlled and administered to avoid suppressing the hypoxic drive to breathe.

   b. Interventions

      i. Monitor neurologic status for changes in cognition and behavior.

      ii. Administer low-liter–flow oxygen as appropriate. Use Venturi mask (24%) or nasal cannula prong (2–3 L/min). However, if PaO_2 is less than 40 mm Hg, 28% oxygen is appropriate. Nasal prongs are preferable because they are lightweight, well tolerated, and eliminate the "closed-in" feeling. It is irrelevant whether the patient is a mouth or a nose breather, because the nasopharynx effectively entrains oxygen flow from the nasal prongs. Do not overventilate. Maintain the $PaCO_2$ at about 55 mm Hg. Overventilation causes the kidney to excrete the excess base. Then when the patient is weaned, he or she quickly incurs an acute respiratory acidemia due to the acute rise in PCO_2. The patient often develops acute distress, and mechanical ventilation may need to be reinstituted [18].

      iii. As COPD worsens and as the patient develops ARF, it is necessary to discuss with the patient and family what treatments will be undertaken. Will the patient be intubated and ventilated, and will CPR be done? These decisions are often difficult. If aggressive therapy is chosen, intensive care unit (ICU) admission is appropriate. It is important not only to identify the patient's wishes but also to make sure that they are communicated to all caregivers.

      iv. Ventilate patient only if necessary because weaning often is very difficult. Mechanical ventilation is necessary only when the patient's response to adequate oxygen therapy and other interventions does not show improvement in PaO_2.

     v. Monitor blood gases or $S\bar{v}O_2$ (mixed venous oxygen) to determine progress.

     vi. Prevent complications related to rapid fall in $PaCO_2$.

     vii. Reposition patient often. Turning patient to new position improves ventilation status temporarily until pulmonary exudates fill these new alveoli. The use of the prone position also may improve ventilation significantly [5,6].

     viii. Prevent infection, which can lead to multiorgan system failure (MOSF).

     ix. Administer antibiotics as ordered.

     x. Maintain cardiac output; vasopressors may be necessary.

     xi. Assess cardiovascular status. Hypoxia may lead to cardiac ischemia and dysrhythmias.

     xii. Monitor breath sounds. During acute stage, many adventitious lung sounds are heard. As patient improves, lung sounds clear.

     xiii. Percuss over lungs for presence of dullness. Dullness indicates areas of consolidation.

     xiv. Palpate over lungs for fremitus. Fremitus increases with fluid or consolidation.

     xv. Monitor $P(A\text{-}a)O_2$. If above 20 mm Hg, there is need to improve ventilation to decrease shunting.

     xvi. Monitor $\dot{Q}_S/\dot{Q}_T$ ratio. If $\dot{Q}_S/\dot{Q}_T$ ratio rises less than 5%, the blood is not well oxygenated. Enhancing cardiac output and FiO_2 may improve the $\dot{Q}_S/\dot{Q}_T$ ratio.

     xvii. Monitor PIP. As pressure rises above 50 cm H_2O, the work of breathing increases. Institute treatment that will reduce PIP: bronchodilators and PS-IRV.

     xviii. Reduce oxygen demands by pacing activities and scheduling rest periods, relieving anxiety and fever, and sedating the patient as necessary.

c. Desired outcome

     i. Patient and family will be able to make appropriate decisions for acute and long-term care.

     ii. Patient will be alert and oriented to person, place, time.

     iii. Patient will demonstrate appropriate behavior.

     iv. Effective cardiovascular function maintained:
- Blood pressure within 10 mm Hg of baseline.
- Cardiac output: 5 L/min.
- Without cyanosis, if preexisting patient color was "pink."
- Laboratory values: Hct/Hgb returns to normal.
- Optimal arterial blood gases maintained. Very close to pre-ARF levels. PaO_2 55–60 mm Hg, and slightly acidotic.
- $P(A\text{-}a)O_2$: less than 15 mm Hg on room air.

     v. Effective respiratory function maintained.
- PaO_2 between 55 and 65 mm Hg and SaO_2 about 90% (hypoxic ventilatory drive is not reduced until about a PaO_2 of ≤ 60 mm Hg).

- pH slightly acidic, because respiratory acidosis greatly potentiates the hypoxic stimulus and the respiratory drive to breathe.

    vi. If patient was ventilated, change to Venturi mask or nasal cannula when possible.

2. Ineffective airway clearance related to increased, thick tracheobronchial secretions and ineffective cilia.

    a. Problem: Ineffective airway clearance leads to hypoxemia, increased airway resistance, and a decrease in dynamic compliance, each of which increases the work of breathing.

    b. Interventions

        i. Assess airway patency, chest and diaphragmatic excursion.

        ii. Assess use of accessory muscles and presence of intercostal retraction.

        iii. Auscultate breath sounds frequently.

        iv. Monitor color, consistency, and quantity of sputum.

        v. Obtain sputum for signs and symptoms when indicated.

        vi. Administer bronchodilators as ordered.

        vii. Assess fluid balance and state of hydration, including thickness of sputum. Administer fluids as indicated or ordered.

        viii. Implement chest physical therapy to remove secretions.

        ix. Suction only as needed to remove secretions.

        x. Monitor respiratory function by evaluating serial vital capacities and tidal volumes.

        xi. Monitor serial changes in airway resistance (PIP). As airway resistance increases, work of breathing increases.

        xii. Monitor serial changes in dynamic compliance.

$$\text{Dynamic compliance} = T_V = PIP - PEEP$$

where T_V = tidal volume; PIP = peak inspiratory pressure; PEEP = positive end-expiratory pressure.

    c. Desired outcome

        i. Patient will be alert and oriented to person, place, time.

        ii. Effective alveolar ventilation maintained.

- Patient demonstrates proper breathing techniques and effective secretion-clearing cough.
- Breath sound audible throughout anterior/posterior chest.
- Adventitious sounds reduced to absent.
- Arterial blood gas values stabilized.
- Risk of aspiration minimized.

        iii. Airway resistance and dynamic compliance return to normal.

3. Ineffective breathing pattern related to reduced maximum expiratory airflow

    a. Problem: Ineffective breathing pattern leads to increased work of breathing and increased oxygen consumption, which result in further hypercapnia and physical fatigue/exhaustion.

    b. Interventions

        i. Monitor respiratory function (rate, depth, pattern of breathing, pulmonary function tests). A rising respiratory rate above 30

breaths per minute (bpm) generally is accepted as a sign of ventilation-muscle decompensation and impending fatigue.
  ii. Teach pursed-lip breathing to emphasize pattern.
  iii. Change patient position often and use prone position; avoid flat position.
  iv. Decrease airway resistance to minimize the work of breathing.
  v. Improve respiratory muscle function.
  vi. Decrease anxiety.
  vii. Administer bronchodilators, antibiotics, and steroids as ordered.
  viii. Monitor for paradoxical inward movement of abdomen on inspiration, which may or may not indicate muscle fatigue.
c. Desired outcome
  i. Patient demonstrates effective minute ventilation: tidal volume, respiratory rate.
  ii. Vital capacity achieved.
  iii. Patient verbalizes ease of breathing.
  iv. Patient demonstrates pursed-lip and diaphragmatic breathing.
  v. Breath sounds audible throughout anterior/posterior chest.
  vi. Adventitious sounds reduced to absent.

4. Alteration in cerebral tissue perfusion due to changes in acid base balance
  a. Problem: Compromised hemodynamics and hypoxemia predispose to cerebral hypoxia with altered cerebral function.
  b. Interventions
    i. Assess ongoing neurologic function: mental status, level of consciousness; behavior appropriate?
    ii. Assess fluid and electrolyte status: body weight, intake and output (hourly urine output), serum electrolytes, blood urea nitrogen, creatinine.
    iii. Maintain a quiet, relaxed milieu: use a calm, reassuring approach; provide explanations of care.
  c. Desired outcome: Patient will demonstrate appropriate behavior and is oriented to person, place, and time.

5. Change in nutrition status related to decreased oral intake and increased metabolic demand.
  a. Problem: A decreased nutritional intake leads to catabolism of visceral protein. The stressed individual does not adapt well to starvation: (1) glucose requirements increase as the body responds to stress; (2) a relative insulin resistance occurs, because the tissues are less responsive to insulin; and (3) the increased production of insulin, in turn, decreases liposis. The body, therefore, continues to catabolize protein for gluconeogenesis. Starvation negatively affects the immune system, wound healing, the respiratory system, and lean body mass in general.
  b. Interventions
    i. Monitor nutrition status: Serum prealbumin, transferrin, total lymphocyte count, and albumin; urine: 24 hours, urinary nitrogen excretion.
    ii. Feed the patient as soon as hemodynamic stability is reached. Enteral feedings are best [15].

    c. Desired outcome
        i. Positive nitrogen balance is returned.
        ii. All nutritional laboratory values return to normal.
        iii. Body weight during acute episode maintained.

IV. Discharge planning

A. Teach patient importance of follow-up visits and treatments.
B. Teach patient importance of preventing URI.
C. Teach patient about any medications that will need to be continued at home—their actions, side effects, interactions, and means of administration.
D. Teach patient about limitations and how he or she can now live a productive life.
E. Encourage patient to develop own program for vigorous chest physiotherapy and bronchial hygiene.
F. Teach patient about how to use supplement oxygen effectively.
G. Work with dietitian to restore and maintain nutritional status.
H. Teach patient to monitor weight weekly.
I. Teach patient breathing techniques that may assist with proper ventilation (pursed-lip breathing, diaphragmatic breathing).
J. Encourage daily exercise.
K. Teach patient about disease process and how to prevent worsening of condition (avoidance of smoking or being in smoke-filled rooms for instance).
L. Encourage patient's significant others to express fear/concerns regarding patient's chronic disease and disruption in lifestyle.
M. Initiate referrals to social services or home health agencies if necessary.

Pneumonia

I. Definition: Pneumonia is a commonly occurring disease (2 million cases each year in the United States) and accounts for about 50,000 to 70,000 deaths per year in the United States; it also is responsible for extended mortality in the ICU. When ICU patients develop pneumonia as a complication of a preexisting condition, their mortality can reach 50%, and even 70% when pneumonia complicates ARDS.

    Predisposing factors include respiratory viral infections, alcoholism, age extremes, debility, immunosuppressive disorders and therapy, compromised consciousness, and dysphagia. The usual mechanisms include droplet infection, aspiration, hematogenous dissemination, or contiguous infections.

    When pneumonia develops, there is infection and inflammation of the lung parenchyma in the distant airways and acini. As the body produces its own attack on the infectious process, the area is flooded with inflammatory cells, polymorphonuclear leukocytes (PMNL), edema fluid, and fibrin to limit the spread. Recovery from pneumonia may be complete without sequelae, or it may progress to tissue necrosis, abscess formation, and scarring.

    Pneumonia may result from inhalation of viral, bacterial or mycoplasmal organisms, or from fungal or protozoan infections, chemical irritation, or nosocomial infection. Nosocomial pneumonias account for 10–20% of hospital-acquired infections and continue to be a major threat to any critically ill patient.

Pneumonia is generally classified into three types based on morphologic and roentgenologic characteristics.

A. **Alveolar, airspace, or lobar pneumonia:** Affects peripheral alveoli, resulting in puffy white infiltrates; often due to *Streptococcus* and *Klebsiella* pneumonias.

B. **Broncho-segmental, lobular pneumonia:** Staphylococci cause the inflammatory response in conducting airways and surrounding parenchyma, resulting in patchy areas of consolidation.

C. **Interstitial pneumonia:** Viruses or mycoplasmas cause inflammation in the interstitial space. These pneumonias may be acute or chronic (eg, chronic alveolitis).

II. **Etiology:** Various defense mechanisms (filtration of air, cough reflex, mucous secretion, pulmonary macrophages, and intact humoral immunity) maintain sterility of the lower respiratory tract. Due to a breakdown of the host defense mechanism, organisms enter and grow in the previously sterile environment. Factors that contribute to the impairment of host defenses include cigarette smoking, alcohol abuse, existing COPD, underlying malignancies, and concurrent URIs.

Most nosocomial infections in the patient in the ICU are due to gram-negative bacilli. However, many organisms may precipitate pneumonia. (Table 13.2 lists microorganisms, significant history of infection, and current drug regimen choices.) There is a high incidence of pneumonia in patients who are receiving histamine-2 (H_2) inhibitors or antacids. These drugs raise the normal sterile pH of the stomach from 1 to 4–5, which allows gram-negative microorganisms to flourish.

III. **Nursing process**

A. Assessment
   1. Signs and symptoms
      a. Adventitious lung sounds (crackles), abnormal bronchial breath sounds, increased fremitus, dullness to percussion, abnormal egophony: Related to infiltration of lung tissue by microorganisms, and the body's release of inflammatory cells (PMNLs), edema fluid, and fibrin. This group of symptoms is typical of lobar pneumonia. As pleural effusion develops, there is dullness to percussion, decreased breath sounds, and a pleural rub.
      b. Shaking chills, high fever: Compensatory mechanisms that occur as the body attempts to rid itself of the infection.
      c. Cough, increased sputum (productive or nonproductive depending on the type of pneumonia): Protective mechanisms that occur secondarily to increased mucus production to help cleanse the respiratory tract.
      d. Hyperventilation: Occurs as a compensatory mechanism to maintain adequate oxygenation.
      e. Pleurisy: Acute chest pain; indicates pleural complications.
   2. Diagnostic parameters (30–50% of patients have no identifiable pathogen, despite clinical impression of pneumonia)

Table 13.2 Pneumonias

Organisms	Comments	Treatments
Community acquired		
Streptococcus pneumoniae	Often preceded by URI; cough, rusty, blood-streaked sputum; shaking chills; often second infection; often seen in COPD or in nursing homes	Penicillin G or penicillin V or erythromycin Prophylaxis: pneumonia vaccine
Methicillin resistant *Staphylococcus aureus* (MRSA)	Purulent blood-streaked sputum, shaking chills, necrotizing pneumonia, thin-walled abscesses; creates cavities	Vancomycin
Gram-negative (most often hospital acquired; mortality is often 20–50%)		
S. aureus	Purulent, blood-streaked sputum, shaking chills; necrotizing pneumonia; thin-walled abscesses; creates cavities	Oxacillin, nafcillin, first-generation cephalosporins, clindamycin
Pseudomonas aeruginosa	Thick, yellow-green sputum; persistent cough, mucoabscesses; focal hemorrhages; most patients neutropenic and receiving broad-spectrum antibiotics	Ticarallin or piperacillin and aminoglycosides
Klebsiella pneumoniae	"Currant jelly" sputum; pleuritic chest pain; tissue necrosis; early abscess formation; common in alcoholics or in nursing homes	Aminoglycoside/cephalosporin combination
Escherichia coli	Often secondary to intraabdominal or genitourinary infections	Multiple antibiotics
Serratia marcescens	Associated with high mortality	Much resistance amikacin and third cephalosporins or imipenem plus cilastatin
Haemophilus influenzae	Often found in COPD	Second-generation cephalosporins or ampicillin with sulbactam; prophylaxis: *H. influenzae* vaccine
Protozoan		
Pneumocystis carinii	Found in immunosuppressed patient, often secondary to HIV	(Neutrexin), or trimethoprim-sulfamethoxazole, or pentamidine
Viral		
Viruses	Adenoviruses 7, 14, and 21 are associated with severe pneumonia and respiratory failure; mucopurulent sputum	Antivirals: Ribavirin (often course is not altered by administering drugs) Amantadine prophylactically

Table 13.2 *Continued*

Organisms	Comments	Treatments
Atypical		
Legionella pneumophila	Usually associated with large outbreaks from contaminated air conditioning systems or contaminated shower heads; prodromal symptoms—high fever, headache, myalgia, diarrhea	Erythromycin for 3 weeks to prevent relapse
Mycoplasma pneumoniae	Primarily affects children and young adults; often endemic; preceded by pneumonitis or bronchitis; fatigue and malaise often continue for several weeks; maculopapular rashes occur in 10–20% of patients	Tetracycline, erythromycin
Gram-positive		
Streptococci	Abrupt onset of fever, cough, chest pain; pleurisy common	Response to therapy is slow; penicillin G, cephalosporins, erythromycin, clindamycin

URI, upper respiratory tract infection; COPD, chronic obstructive pulmonary disease; HIV, human immunodeficiency virus.

    a. Serum tests
        i. Increased WBC count, increased PMNLs: White blood cells increase as a compensatory mechanism to combat infection. In addition there usually is increased release of stab/bands (immature neutrophils) that cause a shift to left, particularly in bacterial infection.
    b. Urine tests
        i. None significant.
    c. Other diagnostic tests (special culture techniques, serologic assays, or even lung biopsies are required to identify many pathogens [mycobacteria, mycoplasmas, anaerobic bacteria, chlamydia, viruses, fungi, and legionellae]).
        i. $\dot{V}/\dot{Q}$ mismatch: Occurs as the alveoli become filled with inflammatory exudate and gas exchange is impaired.
        ii. Chest x-ray: Pulmonary infiltrates tend to persist for days to weeks, whereas atelectasis usually resolves within 48 hours. Chest x-ray findings assist with the differentiation and location of pneumonia.
        iii. Sputum culture: May not be diagnostic, because sputum culture is positive only in 10–30% of patients. Sputum often is of poor quality and contaminated.
  B. Patient management
    1. Ineffective airway clearance related to tracheal/bronchial inflammation,

edema formation, increased sputum production, pleuritic pain, decreased energy, and fatigue.

a. Problem: Ineffective airway clearance eventually leads to worsening of the $\dot{V}/\dot{Q}$ mismatch, increased airway resistance, increased hypoxemia, hyperventilation, and worsening of the acid-base balance.

b. Interventions
  i. Assess rate and depth of respirations and chest movement.
  ii. Auscultate lung fields, noting areas of decreased/absent airflow and adventitious breath sounds (eg, crackles, wheezes).
  iii. Elevate head of bed; change position frequently.
  iv. Suction as indicated.
  v. Force fluids to at least 2500 mL/d (unless contraindicated).
  vi. Monitor effects of respiratory physiotherapy (eg, incentive spirometer, intermittent positive pressure breathing, blow bottles, percussion, postural drainage, particularly in surgical patients and patients with chronic disease).
  vii. Administer medication as indicated.
    - Mucolytics

---

acetylcysteine (Mucomyst)
Action Aerosol breaks disulfide bonds in respiratory mucus.
Administration Guidelines Taken orally; to prevent irritation of oral and pharyngeal tissues, have patient rinse mouth after treatment. When 25% of the drug remains in nebulizer, dilute with an equal amount of normal saline solution to minimize reconcentration. Have suction apparatus available for patients with ineffective cough. If wheezing occurs after treatment, inform the physician and suggest possible concurrent use of bronchodilator.
Nursing Considerations Unused portion should be capped tightly and discarded after 4 days (although purple discoloration does not affect potency). Encourage adequate hydration to decrease sputum viscosity.

  - Expectorants

---

guaifenesin, iodide preparations
Action Stimulates bronchial mucous glands to secrete less viscous mucus.
Administration Guidelines Withhold fluids for up to 30 minutes after administering to promote demulcent effects. Instruct patient not to chew capsules. Instruct in proper cough techniques. Contact physician if cough persists for a week or more.
Nursing Considerations Administer with fruit juice or milk to disguise bitter taste. Gastric irritation is decreased by giving drug with a whole glass of water after meals.

- Bronchodilators

---

epinephrine (Adrenalin, Sus-Phrine)

Action Relaxes smooth muscle via adrenergic stimulation.

Administration Guidelines Check dose and route carefully. Administer second dose as ordered 20–30 minutes after initial dose.

Nursing Considerations Avoid gluteal IM injection to prevent abscess. Discard any discolored solution. Discourage overuse of inhalers.

---

racemic epinephrine (Vaponefrin)

Action Local decongestant via adrenergic stimulation.

Administration Guidelines Deliver aerosol spray to back of throat.

---

ephedrine sulfate

Action Local decongestant via adrenergic stimulation.

Administration Guidelines Administer as ordered; if ordered every day, administer in morning to avoid insomnia. Teach patient to avoid increasing dose if tolerance develops and to inform physician. If bronchospasm is severe, consult physician (drug is effective only for milder forms of bronchospasm).

- Analgesics

---

acetaminophen (Anacin-3, Datril, Pandaol, Tempra, Tylenol)

Action Blocks pain impulses in the CNS that occur in response to inhibition of prostaglandin synthesis. Antipyretic action is caused by inhibition of hypothalamic neurons related to heart regulation.

Administration Guidelines Do not exceed the recommended dosage.

Nursing Considerations Severe or recurrent pain or high or continued fever may indicate serious illness. Poisoning or overdose may cause few early symptoms but requires immediate medical treatment.

---

meperidine (Pethidine, Demerol)
Action Inhibits ascending pain pathways in the CNS and alters pain perception.

Administration Guidelines Oral doses may be administered with food or milk to minimize GI irritation. Syrup should be diluted in half a glass of water. Oral dose is less than 50% as effective as parenteral. When changing to oral administration, dosage may need to be increased. IM is the preferred parenteral route for repeated doses. SC administration may cause local irritation. Dilute IV administration with at least 5 mL sterile water or 0.9% NaCl. Administer slowly, at a rate not exceeding 25 mg/min.

Nursing Considerations Rapid administration may lead to increased respiratory depression, hypotension, and circulatory collapse. Do not use IV administration without having antidote available.

---

     viii. Provide supplemental fluids, eg, IV, humidified oxygen and room humidification.

     ix. Monitor blood gases if necessary.

     x. Administer antibiotics (see Table 13.2).

  c. Desired outcome

     i. Patient demonstrates behaviors to achieve airway clearance.

     ii. Demonstrates patent airway with clearing breath sounds, absence of dyspnea, cyanosis.

     iii. Blood gases return to normal.

2. Impaired gas exchange related to alveolar-capillary membrane changes (inflammatory effects), altered oxygen-carrying capacity of blood (fever, shifting oxyhemoglobin curve), and altered delivery of oxygen (hypoventilation).

  a. Problem: Impaired gas exchange will decrease oxygenation to all tissues, leading to tissue hypoxia and other organ damage. Impaired gas exchange will worsen $\dot{V}/\dot{Q}$ mismatch and acid–base balance.

  b. Interventions

     i. Assess respiratory rate, depth, and ease; use of accessory muscles.

     ii. Observe color of skin, mucous membranes, and nailbeds, noting presence of peripheral (nailbeds) cyanosis or central (circumoral) cyanosis.

     iii. Assess mental status.

     iv. Monitor heart rate and rhythm.

     v. Monitor body temperature, as indicated. Assist with comfort measures to reduce fever and chills (eg, addition/removal of bedcovers, comfortable room temperature, tepid or cool water sponges).

     vi. Elevate head of bed and encourage frequent position changes, deep breathing, and effective cough.

     vii. Assess level of anxiety; encourage verbalization of concerns/feelings.

      viii. Observe for deterioration in condition, noting hypotension, copious amounts of pink/bloody sputum, pallor, cyanosis, change in level of consciousness, severe dyspnea, restlessness.

      ix. Administer oxygen therapy by appropriate means (eg, nasal prongs, mask, Venturi mask).

      x. Monitor arterial blood gases, ear/pulse oximetry readings.

      xi. If pneumonia does not clear with appropriate therapy, lung biopsy may be indicated.

      xii. Monitor $P(A-a)O_2$. If $P(A-a)O_2$ widens, it is a hallmark finding of an overwhelming pneumonia.

  c. Desired outcome

      i. Patient demonstrates improved ventilation and oxygenation of tissues: arterial blood gases within normal range, absence of symptoms of respiratory distress.

      ii. Participates in actions to maximize oxygenation.

3. Activity intolerance related to imbalance between oxygen supply and demand, general weakness, and exhaustion associated with interruption in usual sleep pattern due to discomfort, excessive coughing, and dyspnea.

  a. Problem: As activity levels are reduced, muscle strength and muscle tone deteriorate.

  b. Interventions

      i. Assess patient's response to activity. Note complaints of dyspnea, increased weakness/fatigue; note also changes in vital signs during and after activities.

      ii. Provide a quiet environment, and limit visitors as indicated. Encourage use of stress management and diversional activities as appropriate.

      iii. Assist the patient to assume comfortable position for rest and/or sleep.

      iv. Assist with self-care activities as necessary. Provide for progressive increase in activities during recovery phase.

  c. Desired outcome

      i. Patient reports or demonstrates a measurable increase in tolerance to activity, with absence of dyspnea, excessive fatigue.

      ii. Vital signs within patient's normal range.

4. Potential fluid volume deficit related to excessive fluid loss (fever, profuse diaphoresis, mouth breathing/hyperventilation, vomiting) and decreased oral intake.

  a. Problem: A fluid volume deficit leads to hypovolemia and an increased burden on the heart.

  b. Interventions

      i. Assess vital sign changes (eg, increased temperature/prolonged fever, tachycardia, orthostatic hypotension).

      ii. Assess skin turgor, moisture of mucous membranes (lips, tongue).

      iii. Note complaints of nausea/vomiting.

      iv. Monitor intake and output, noting color and character of urine. Calculate fluid balance. Weigh as indicated.

      v. Force fluids to at least 2500 mL/d or as individually appropriate.

      vi. Provide supplemental IV fluids as necessary.
    c. Desired outcome
      i. Patient demonstrates fluid balance evidenced by individually appropriate parameters (eg, moist mucous membranes, good skin turgor, prompt capillary refill), stable vital signs.

IV. Discharge planning

A. Teach patient about disease, its current treatments, and future prevention.
B. Encourage patient to avoid crowds, particularly if immunosuppression or chronic disease is present.
C. Teach about drugs that will be taken at home; teach importance of taking complete prescription of antibiotics.
D. Stress importance of continued follow-up care and visits.
E. Teach good coughing and pulmonary physical therapy techniques.
F. Emphasize importance of returning to daily exercise.
G. Teach patients susceptible to pneumonia the importance of vaccines for prevention.
H. Encourage nutritious diet high in protein for tissue repair.

Pneumothorax

I. Definition: A pneumothorax develops when air enters the intrapleural space, which is maintained by negative pressure. When enough air enters the space, the subatmospheric pressure is lost, and the lung collapses. The symptoms that ensue are dependent on the amount of air entering. A small amount of air may result in no or few symptoms, and it will usually absorb in a few days without treatment, but a large amount of air may lead to a complete pneumothorax and even cardiovascular collapse. Pneumothorax will complicate the recovery of any acutely ill patient. Full absorption of a large pneumothorax may take 2 to 4 weeks.

    The patient may experience several types of pneumothorax: (1) tension, (2) spontaneous, (3) hemothorax, (4) open, and (5) closed.

A. Tension pneumothorax: Occurs when the air in the intrapleural space is under positive pressure. A one-way movement of air into the intrapleural space occurs each time the patient inspires. Because of the "check valve" or "flap"-type injury, air cannot escape. Therefore, pressure rapidly increases until a mediastinal shift moves the heart, major vessels, and trachea onto the remaining good lung. This creates a medical emergency. If the patient is to survive, the pressure must be relieved quickly to prevent ensuing cardiopulmonary collapse. A tension pneumothorax occurs most often at the time of trauma.

B. Spontaneous pneumothorax: Occurs without antecedent trauma. Persons with emphysema, tuberculosis, asthma, or lung abscess may spontaneously rupture a bulla that is undetectable by clinical examination. The patient is usually male and 20–40 years of age. The pneumothorax occurs without associated exertion.

C. Hemothorax: Occurs when blood enters the intrapleural cavity. As the intrapleural cavity fills with blood, the lung is compromised and may be partially or totally collapsed. Hemothorax may occur secondary to trauma or as a postoperative complication to chest surgery.

Pleural blood often does not clot and may be easily withdrawn through a needle or water-sealed drainage.

D. Open pneumothorax: Occurs when a penetrating wound, such as bullet or knife wound, creates a communicating fistula between the outside air and the pleural space. Since air rushes in, the pneumothorax occurs quickly.

E. Closed pneumothorax: Occurs when the chest wall becomes airtight after penetration by a central line or thoracentesis needle. A closed pneumothorax can also occur in patients with ARDS who are being ventilated with high levels of PEEP or who have very high PIPs. Symptoms may present subtly.

II. Etiology: A pneumothorax may occur spontaneously in young healthy individuals, but more often it is associated with trauma or chronic lung disease (rupture of a pleural air pocket such as a bleb; or necrosis of the lung from COPD, tuberculosis, or neoplasm). Pneumothorax also may occur due to iatrogenic causes, such as secondary to mechanical ventilation with PEEP (barotrauma), unintentional puncture with subclavian line insertion, or during a thoracentesis or tracheostomy. Patients who develop a pneumothorax secondary to mechanical ventilation are at high risk for developing a tension pneumothorax.

III. Nursing process

A. Assessment
  1. Signs and symptoms
    a. Sudden sharp chest pain: Occurs in 80–90% of all patients because the collapsed lung causes pressure on the pleurital pleura, which is where pain fibers are located.
    b. Dyspnea: Occurs in 80–90% of all patients due to lung collapse.
    c. Nonproductive cough, abnormal chest wall movement: Occurs as lung collapses.
    d. Referred pain to the corresponding shoulder, across the chest, or over the abdomen. The pain may be acute and may mimic an "acute myocardial infarction" or "acute abdomen."
    e. Tactile fremitus/egophony: Decrease or are absent, since there is an absence of air in the lung.
    f. Unusual chest noise, diminished breath sounds, hyperresonant to percussion: Occurs because of the increase in trapped air in the pleural space. If the pneumothorax is small, these findings may not be present.
    g. Hamman's sign: A clicking or crunchy sound correlated to the heart beat. Most often heard with a left pneumothorax.
    h. Distended neck veins, distended liver: Occurs as central venous pressure (CVP) elevates and venous engorgement occurs.
    i. Displacement of cardiac dullness and apex beat, hypoxemia, and hypercapnia: Found in a tension pneumothorax, which indicates a mediastinal shift has already occurred. The shift will be away from the affected lung.

2. Diagnostic parameters
  a. Serum tests
    i. Arterial hypoxemia, acidic pH: As pulmonary dead space develops.
  b. Urine tests
    i. None.
  c. Other tests
    i. Vital capacity, tidal volumes, lung compliance: All reduced as lung function decreases. As the lung becomes stiffer, lung compliance decreases, thereby increasing the work of breathing.
    ii. Elevated peak airway pressure (PAP): Occurs as it becomes very difficult to inflate the collapsed lung. As PAP increases, the work of breathing also increases.
    iii. Elevated CVP: Blood becomes congested in the venous circuit, as it is not perfused well through the collapsed lung.
    iv. Chest x-ray: Usually characteristic, showing air without lung markings peripherally but limited by a sharp pleural margin with lung markings medially, indicating the position of the collapsed lung.

B. Patient management
  1. Ineffective breathing pattern related to air/fluid accumulation in the chest affects respiratory muscle mechanics and ability to inflate the lungs. Decreased lung expansion and increased work of breathing contribute to gas exchange abnormalities.
    a. Problem: As the lung collapses, normal ventilation/perfusion is compromised. Hypoxemia occurs quickly, which may lead to other organ failure. The course of treatment may be shortened by insertion of a chest tube to reexpand the lung and improve breathing pattern.
    b. Interventions
      i. Maintain position of comfort, usually with head of bed elevated to maximize lung expansion.
      ii. Assist with thoracentesis, which may be done on an emergency basis to relieve dyspnea. Fluid removal is limited to 1200–1500 mL to prevent cardiovascular collapse; although this is a rare occurrence.
        ▪ Encourage shallow, controlled breathing during needle insertion.
        ▪ Instruct patient not to cough or make any sudden movements.
        ▪ Apply firm pressure to site when needle is removed.
      iii. If the patient has a tension pneumothorax, air may be removed simply by inserting a 19-gauge or larger needle into the chest, followed by use of a three-way stopcock attached to a large syringe to withdraw air rapidly through the needle.
      iv. Prepare thoracic catheter and drainage system for insertion or reinsertion as indicated (see Appendix A for chest tube procedure).
      v. Once chest tube is inserted, do the following:
        ▪ Check suction control chamber for correct amount of suction (water level or regulator at correct setting, continuous bubbling in water-filled chamber, depending on type of chest drainage

unit). Add water as necessary or dial in correct negative pressure level on regulator.

- Check fluid level in water seal chamber or bottle and maintain at prescribed level.
- Drape tubing in a straight line from bed to drainage container. Coil extra tubing on bed. Check to make sure tubing has no dependent loops and is not kinked. Drain accumulated fluid as necessary.
- Assess underwater seal chamber for air leak; leak is indicated by bubbling in water seal chamber.
- Monitor water seal chamber for "tidaling" (fluctuations) of fluid level. Fluid should fluctuate 2 to 6 cm during ventilation.
- Monitor placement of chest tubes. Anterior chest tube drains fluid such as blood. Posterior chest tube drains air.
- Milk tubing gently from patient to bottle, if ordered.

   vi. Assess lung function every 1 or 2 hours.
   vii. Encourage deep breathing, coughing, and position changes.
   viii. Monitor and/or graph serial arterial blood gases.
   ix. Administer oxygen as indicated.
   x. Administer prophylactic antibiotics.

c. Desired outcome: Adequate ventilation/gas exchange as evidenced by respiratory parameters within patient's normal range and reestablishment of usual breathing pattern.

2. Multifactor potential for injury: The patient with a hemothorax or pneumothorax is at risk for complications associated with insertion and maintenance of a chest drainage system. Maintenance of intrapleural negativity is essential in order to prevent complications of hemothorax or pneumothorax. Various situations may occur that impair optimum elimination of fluid/air, or they may cause atmospheric air to enter the pleural space. Occasionally emphysema (also a predisposing factor) may result from invasion of microorganisms after chest tube insertion. Injury and surgical trauma or arterial rupture may result in hypovolemia or shock.

a. Problem: As pain increases, respiratory rate and cardiac output increase as compensatory mechanisms to increased anxiety.

b. Interventions

   i. Review reason for chest tube placement and location of thoracic catheter.
   ii. Anchor thoracic catheter to chest wall and provide for extra length of tubing before turning or moving patient.
   iii. Secure tubing connection sites with bands or tape.
   iv. Pad banding sites with gauze or tape.
   v. Secure drainage unit in stand or cart, or attach to side rails of bed. Place in low-traffic area.
   vi. Provide safe transportation if patient needs to be sent to procedures outside the unit. Disconnect from suction source and transport patient, or maintain on continuous suction and have procedure performed at bedside.

vii. Check water seal chamber to verify fluid is at correct level and to assess for leaks.

viii. Observe insertion site, noting skin condition, presence and/or odor of drainage from thoracic catheter. Change sterile occlusive dressing as indicated.

ix. Obtain drainage samples for analysis by allowing fluid to collect in dependent loop of tubing and inserting small-gauge needle that is attached to a syringe.

x. Observe for unusual change or increase in bloody drainage. Monitor vital signs.

xi. When patients have a hemothorax, fibrinolytic enzymes (streptokinase-streptodornase) may be instilled through an intercostal drainage tube to lyse fibrinous adhesions.

c. Desired outcome: Complications are prevented or minimized.

3. Impaired gas exchange related to right-to-left shunting, $\dot{V}/\dot{Q}$ mismatch.

a. Problem: Leads to severe hypoxemia, which can precipitate tissue ischemia and necrosis.

b. Interventions

i. Monitor neurologic status for changes in cognition and behavior.

ii. Administer oxygen. Patient is usually ventilated. FiO_2 is increased to maintain the PaO_2 above 60 mm Hg.

iii. Monitor blood gases or $S\bar{v}O_2$ to determine progress.

iv. Reposition patient often. Turning patient to new position improves ventilation status temporarily until pulmonary exudates fill these new alveoli. The use of the prone position also may improve ventilation significantly [5,6].

v. Prevent infection, which can lead to multiorgan system failure.

vi. Administer antibiotics as ordered.

vii. Maintain fluid volume. Administer crystalloids/colloids as ordered. Maintain PAOP above 12 mm Hg.

viii. Maintain cardiac output; vasopressors may be necessary.

ix. Assess cardiovascular status. Hypoxia may lead to cardiac ischemia and dysrhythmias.

x. Monitor breath sounds. As condition improves, lung sounds clear.

xi. Reduce oxygen demands by pacing activities and scheduling rest periods, relieving anxiety and fever, and sedating the patient as necessary.

c. Desired outcome

i. Patient will be alert and oriented to person, place, time.

ii. Patient demonstrates appropriate behavior.

iii. Effective cardiovascular function maintained.

- Blood pressure within 10 mm Hg of baseline.
- Cardiac output: 5 L/min.
- Without cyanosis, if preexisting pulmonary function normal.
- Laboratory values: Hct/Hgb returned to normal.
- Maintain optimal arterial blood gases.
- $P(A-a)O_2$ less than 15 mm Hg on room air.

4. Alteration in comfort, acute pain due to placement of tube within pleural/ potential space is irritating to nerve endings and original chest injury.

   a. Problem: As the patient breathes, the chest tube moves within the pleural space, which can result in pain.

   b. Interventions

      i. Monitor and evaluate changes in or development of sudden chest pain.

      ii. Assist with position changes, providing extra length of tubing. Place padding around insertion site when patient is turned on side.

      iii. Encourage patient to support thoracic catheter insertion with pillows when coughing.

      iv. Medicate patient before planned activities as indicated.

      v. Administer narcotics or sedatives to promote relaxation and relief of pain.

   c. Desired outcome: Patient verbalizes and/or demonstrates decreased pain.

IV. Discharge planning

A. Teach patient the importance of follow-up visits.

B. Teach patient the importance of preventing URI.

C. Teach patient about any limitations and how he or she can still live a productive life.

D. Teach patient about condition and if there is anything he or she can do to prevent recurrence.

Pulmonary Embolism

I. Definition: A pulmonary embolism arises from blood or other masses (tumor cells or fragments, fat emboli) that dislodge themselves in the venous circulation, move up and down the vena cava, and pass through the right heart into the lung vascular system. It is estimated that 90 to 95% of all pulmonary emboli originate in the deep veins of the lower extremities.

Pulmonary emboli is the most common cause of sudden, unexpected death in the hospitalized patient. The older the patient and the more acutely ill, the greater the risk. Pulmonary embolism is seen frequently as a complication in the ICU. In patients who are at high risk, it is important to institute early prophylactic measures, such as low-dose heparin, early ambulation, sequential compression stockings, low molecular weight dextran, and adequate hydration.

Pulmonary embolism affects approximately 500,000 people yearly in the United States. Mortality ranges from 10 to 30%; the earlier the diagnosis, the lower the mortality rate. Of clinical significance is the fact that up to two-thirds of cases of acute pulmonary emboli are misdiagnosed. The patient often is treated for other conditions, and therefore the true problem is not addressed. Pulmonary embolism is a diagnosis often made on autopsy. Missed diagnoses certainly influence patient outcome.

Large emboli that lodge in the major pulmonary arteries may cause immediate death secondary to vasovagal shock, right ventricular failure, or pulmonary failure. Cyanosis and cardiovascular collapse are ominous consequences of massive pulmonary emboli. Single, small emboli may resolve spontaneously.

About 20% of patients who develop a pulmonary embolism also develop a pulmonary infarction. The lung has a dual blood supply so this percentage is small. Pulmonary infarction is most likely in older patients, patients who have sepsis or an inflammatory process in the lung, patients with preexisting COPD and pulmonary vasculitis, or in patients with reduced blood supply to the lungs, such as patients with CHF and shock states. Within 12 hours of immobilization, hemorrhage occurs. Hemorrhagic consolidation and atelectasis occur within 24 hours, and necrosis and swelling later. In some cases, necrotic tissue may liquefy and form a cavity, which can be found on chest x-ray. Repair of tissue begins in 2 weeks, and necrotic tissue is replaced gradually with scar tissue.

II. Etiology: More than 100 years ago, Virchow suggested a triad of problems that leads to venous clot formation and pulmonary embolism: (1) stasis of blood flow, (2) vessel wall injury, and (3) hypercoagulability of blood. Stasis of blood flow frequently occurs in critically ill patients due to immobility and reduced cardiac function, which precipitate thrombus formation. Vessel wall injury may be precipitated by frequent venipuncture, or other injury to the blood vessel secondary to trauma or surgery. Hypercoagulability of the blood may be associated with activation of the clotting cascade secondary to disease, trauma, surgery, or hypovolemia.

Persons who may have a higher incidence of deep-vein thrombosis and thus a high likelihood of developing pulmonary embolism include patients with cardiovascular disease, particularly peripheral vascular disease, or who have atrial fibrillation; persons who are immobile for long periods of time (during automobile or airplane travel or prolonged bed rest); or persons having pelvic surgery or taking birth control pills. Occasionally, an embolism arises within the lung in the pulmonary arterial system (as in pulmonary vasculitis) and is associated with infarctions, foreign bodies, and immunologic responses.

Pulmonary embolism may also be produced by fat as a result of multiple fractures of the lower extremities; amniotic fluid secondary to difficult or complicated labor; air entering the venous system; tumor from fragmented pieces of malignant tissue; foreign material such as pieces of bullet, sutures, or tips of indwelling catheters that might have broken off; septic emboli from infarcted tissue; and parasitic emboli.

III. Nursing process

  A. Assessment findings

    1. Signs and symptoms

      a. Bronchospasm, hypocapnia, dyspnea: Occurs as the lung attempts to compensate for a $\dot{V}/\dot{Q}$ mismatch. Due to the bronchospasm, there is increased airway resistance, which increases the work of breathing and results in dyspnea.

      b. Dyspnea, pleuritic chest pain, diminished breath sounds, crackles, pleural friction rub: All related to acute pulmonary emboli and its resultant effect on lung function.

  c. Fixed splitting of second heart sound (S_2), right ventricular heave, right-sided fourth heart sound (S_4), jugular venous distention, atrial dysrhythmias, hypotension: All reflect right heart insufficiency and/or failure and a delay in closure of the pulmonic valve.

  d. Murmur over lung field: Reflective of turbulent blood flow through a pulmonary blood vessel that is partially occluded by an obstruction.

  e. Hemoptysis, fever, pleuritic chest pain: May occur in the presence of pulmonary infarction and is frequently caused by pure blood. (This finding may help with the differential diagnosis of pneumonia. When hemoptysis occurs with pneumonia, the blood is mixed with sputum.)

  f. Syncopal episodes: Associated with severe reductions in cardiopulmonary function, reduction in cardiac output, and thus a reduction in cerebral blood flow.

  g. Pleural effusion: Occurs when pulmonary embolism extends to the pleura. This is accompanied by a pleural friction rub. A low-grade fever is usually present.

  h. Mild to severe chest pain: Usually associated with pulmonary infarction involving the pleura.

  i. Friction rub: Occurs when the pulmonary embolism extends to the pleura.

2. Diagnostic parameters

  a. Serum tests

    i. $P_{O_2} < 60$ mm Hg, respiratory alkalosis pH > 7.45, $P_{CO_2} < 35$ mm Hg: Related to $\dot{V}/\dot{Q}$ mismatch and altered surfactant levels that can lead to alveolar collapse. Changes in P_{CO_2} and pH are associated with compensatory mechanisms.

  b. Urine tests

    i. None.

  c. Other tests

    i. Electrocardiographic (ECG) changes: S in lead I, Q and T in lead III, and possibly a right bundle branch block (RBBB) pattern in V_1. The first three changes are referred to as the McGinn White syndrome and all are associated with pulmonary embolism. RBBB pattern occurs when there is a sudden rise in pulmonary vascular resistance (PVR) that puts an acute burden on the right ventricle. ECG also helps to differentiate myocardial infarction.

    ii. Increasing pulmonary vascular resistance > 250 mm Hg: Chemical mediators released from the pulmonary embolism cause vasoconstriction in the pulmonary vasculature. This increase in PVR puts a burden on the right side of the heart that may actually precipitate right-sided failure. An elevated PVR also reduces the volume of blood moving through the lung vascular system, thus reducing total cardiac output and P_{O_2}.

    iii. Normal ventilation scan/abnormal perfusion scan: A typical finding in pulmonary emboli. Air exchange continues to occur normally, but perfusion is decreased in the area of the pulmonary emboli.

    iv. Chest x-ray: May be normal but may demonstrate hemidiaphragmatic elevation, showing areas of reduced ventilation associated with tachypnea and increased airway resistance due to bronchospasm. Hamptom hump, a peripheral wedge-shaped parenchymal lung defect with accompanying pleural effusion, may be evidence of pulmonary embolism.

    v. Lung scan: May or may not be beneficial in diagnosing pulmonary embolism.

    vi. Pulmonary angiogram: A definitive test for pulmonary emboli; rarely performed in the acute time period.

    vii. Dead space is elevated: Ventilation continues, but, due to a lack of perfusion, the blood is not oxygenated.

   viii. Duplex Doppler ultrasound: To lower venous system, may be able to identify the source of the deep vein thrombosis.

    ix. Echocardiography of the right ventricle: May identify the source of a mural thrombus, or the result of right ventricle hypertension such as increased right-sided pressures, or the presence of tricuspid regurgitation.

B. Patient management

  1. Impaired gas exchange related to altered pulmonary blood flow, $\dot{V}/\dot{Q}$ mismatching, right-to-left shunting.

    a. Problem: Impaired gas exchange is associated with $\dot{V}/\dot{Q}$ mismatch occurring with the pulmonary embolism. Hypoxemia leads to reduction in organ function throughout the body.

    b. Interventions

      i. Monitor signs and symptoms of hypoxia, air hunger, changes in vital signs, and cognitive function.

      ii. Monitor blood gases or $S\bar{v}O_2$ to determine baseline level and then to follow therapy. $S\bar{v}O_2$ of less than 60% indicates therapy is necessary.

     iii. Administer oxygen as ordered and treat $\dot{V}/\dot{Q}$ mismatch. Increasing the FiO_2 may be helpful. If the patient is ventilated, increasing the tidal volume and adding PEEP may improve the $\dot{V}/\dot{Q}$ mismatch.

     iv. Intubate and ventilate if indicated.

      v. Assess breath sounds frequently to determine the presence of normal/abnormal breath sounds, adventitious sounds, or the presence of friction rubs.

     vi. Assess level of fatigue as this is often associated with worsening hypoxemia.

    vii. Monitor for signs and symptoms of extension or recurrence of pulmonary embolism, such as sudden or exacerbated chest pain, more respiratory difficulties or tachycardia, or worsening of acid–base results.

      viii. Assist patient to comfortable resting position. Change position often as this may temporaly improve acid–base results as gas distribution in lung is altered.

      ix. Administer analgesics to reduce pain and anxiety. Control of pain and anxiety may improve oxygenation by improving ventilation and reducing oxygen consumption.

   c. Desired outcome

      i. Patient will maintain optimal arterial blood gas parameters: pH, Pa_{O_2}, Pa_{CO_2}, bicarbonate.

      ii. Cognitive ability is normal.

2. Decreased cardiac output related to pulmonary arterial hypertension, right-sided congestive heart failure (cor pulmonale), decrease in left ventricular end-diastolic pressure, and systemic arterial hypotension/hypovolemic shock.

   a. Problem: Pulmonary embolism may result in the development of pulmonary hypertension, which in turn compromises blood flow through the lung. The right side of the heart may not be able to maintain adequate pressure, and it begins to fail. Blood flow to the left side of the heart is compromised, and cardiac output fails.

   b. Interventions

      i. Assess for signs and symptoms of right-sided failure: Neck vein distention, right-sided third heart sound (S_3), elevated CVP, edema of the lower extremities. Failure of right ventricle may precipitate left-sided failure.

      ii. Monitor pulmonary arterial pressure: > 25–30 mm Hg indicates pulmonary hypertension.

      iii. Administer medications to support and maintain output of right side of heart.

---

dobutamine (Dobutrex)

Action Increases force of cardiac contraction and improves cardiac output; increases coronary blood flow and stroke-work index; improves ejection fraction; decreases pulmonary artery output pressure.

Administration Guidelines IV: 2.5–10.0 μg/kg body weight per minute initially. Adjust rate to effect desired response. Up to 40 μg/kg/min has been used in some instances; however, this increases potential for toxicity.

Nursing Considerations Monitor closely for infiltration. If infiltration occurs, 5–10 mg of phentolamine (Regitine) should be administered to infusion site.

dopamine (Intropin)

Action Increases blood pressure and heart rate and has a positive inotropic effect on the heart; also increases mesenteric blood flow and improves renal perfusion. Improves pulmonary artery output pressure.

Administration Guidelines IV: 2–5 μg/kg body weight per minute initially in patients likely to respond to minimum treatment; 5–10 μg/kg/min initially may be required to correct hypotension in the seriously ill patient. Gradually increase by 5–10 μg/kg/min at 10- to 30-minute increments until optimum response occurs. Average dose is 20 μg/kg/min; dose over 50 μg/kg/min has been required in some instances but is not recommended.

Nursing Considerations Monitor closely for infiltration. If it occurs, 5–10 mg of phentolamine (Regitine) should be administered to infusion site.

morphine (Duramorph, MS Contin, RMS, Roxanol, Oramorph)

Action Reduces preload returning to the heart. Reduces anxiety; controls pain.

Administration Guidelines Direct IV: 2.5–15.0 mg. Repeat every 2 to 4 hours as necessary. May be titrated to achieve pain relief with lowest dose (eg, pain relief in myocardial infarction: 1–3 mg every 5 min until desired response; 10 mg is adequate for most needs. Dose must be individualized based on response and tolerance. To enhance the analgesic effect, explain therapeutic value of medication prior to administration. Regularly administered doses may be more effective than administration as needed. Analgesia is more effective if given before pain becomes severe.

Nursing Considerations Instruct patient on how and when to ask for pain medication when needed. Medication may cause drowsiness. Advise patient to call for assistance when ambulating or smoking. Advise patient to make position changes slowly to minimize orthostatic hypotension.

    iv. Monitor for normal/abnormal breath sounds.
    v. Monitor urinary output as it is a good indication of cardiac output.
    vi. Administer vasodilators if left-sided failure.

392 ▼ 13. Respiratory Disorders

> ### nitrates
> *Action* Relax smooth muscle, thereby producing generalized dilation. Relieve spasm of normal and diseased arteries. Reduce venous tone, thereby reducing preload and decreasing myocardial oxygen demand.
>
> *Administration Guidelines* Mix in 5% dextrose in water (D5W) or normal saline solution (NS) only. Use proper tubing as recommended by the manufacturer. Titrate dosage to desired hemodynamic function. Titrate infusion upward every 3 to 5 min following blood pressure and pulse measurement.
>
> *Nursing Considerations* Closely monitor heart rate, blood pressure, and obstructive pressure. Patients with low obstructive pressure are likely to be sensitive to the hypotensive effects of nitrates.

    c. Desired outcome: Patient will maintain stable hemodynamics: Heart rate, CVP, PAP, PAOP, cardiac output, systemic arterial blood pressure within 10 mm Hg of baseline.

3. Alteration in tissue perfusion related to thromboembolic disorder, deep venous thrombosis, and pulmonary embolism.

    a. Problem: Decreased tissue perfusion leads to tissue hypoxemia and decreased organ function throughout the body.

    b. Interventions

        i. Assess for signs and symptoms of venous thrombosis (tenderness, inflammation, pain, warmth, edema).

        ii. Measure circumference of extremities daily.

        iii. Apply sequential compression stockings to extremities to prevent further thrombus formation; apply before any surgical procedure.

        iv. Encourage active exercise of extremities hourly.

        v. Teach patient to avoid positions that compromise blood flow in extremities (eg, crossing legs).

        vi. Encourage deep breathing and coughing.

        vii. Assist with therapies to prevent further clot formation (heparin/coumadin), dissolve clots (thrombolytics), remove clots (embolectomy). When patients are not candidates for any of these therapies, implantation of a vena cava filter that strains blood as it moves up the vena cava can prevent significantly sized blood emboli from reaching the pulmonary vasculature.

        viii. Administer heparin and enoxaparin sodium as ordered.

> ### heparin
> *Action* Binds to circulating antithrombin III and allows antithrombin III to become 1000 times more effective in inhibiting thrombin. (As the clotting cascade is activated, thrombin is produced, which produces more clotting.) Heparin also blocks factor X early in the cascade, which prevents the completion of the cascade and the clot.

Administration Guidelines Administer about 25 μg/kg/h for pulmonary embolism. Monitor partial thromboplastin time (PTT) to adjust subsequent doses. Maintain PTT at about 1½ times the control level. Monitor for bleeding. If bleeding occurs, stopping the heparin usually controls the bleeding. If more rapid clotting is necessary, administer protamine sulfate (1 mg of protamine neutralizes 90–110 μg of heparin); inject slowly IV not to exceed 50 mg in a 10-min period. Monitor PTT carefully. Monitor for thrombocytopenia and even thrombosis, which may occur 5 to 10 days after the start of therapy. (This reaction may be an immune reaction to heparin.)

Nursing Considerations Heparin IV; starts in 5 minutes, peaks in 2 hours, and is gone in 6 hours. Therefore, clotting studies normalize rapidly when heparin is discontinued.

---

enoxaparin sodium (Lovenox)

Action Interferes with the clotting cascade to retard clot formation. Interferes with stages I, II, and III.

Administration Guidelines Administer SC only; not intended for IM administration. Administer deep SC with patient lying down. Introduce whole length of needle into skin fold. Hold skin fold throughout injection. Do not mix with other drugs. Alternate injections into left and right anterolateral and posterolateral abdominal wall.

---

    ix. Administer warfarin when acute condition has stabilized.

---

warfarin (Coumadin)

Action Inhibits the action of vitamin K–dependent clotting factors II, VII, IX, thus prolonging the prothrombin time (PT). The action takes 2 to 3 days to begin.

Administration Guidelines Administer 10–15 mg PO for 3 days, then 2–10 mg daily based on PT. Warfarin usually will be administered for 6 weeks to 6 months.

Nursing Considerations Monitor PT and maintain at 1.25 to 1.50 times the control level. This lowered PT level decreases the risk of complications. Teach patient about reducing vitamin K (the antagonist)-rich foods in the diet: fat of meat, green leafy vegetables.

---

    x. Monitor closely for petechiae, ecchymosis, hematuria, and hematemesis.

    xi. Administer thrombolytics as ordered (Table 13.3).

    xii. Monitor for active bleeding with all thrombolytic drugs. (See Chap. 5 for more detail about thrombolytics.)

  c. Desired outcome: Patient will remain without recurrent pulmonary embolism and will demonstrate absence of pain, stable vital signs (for specific patient), and stable arterial blood gases.

4. Anxiety related to sudden, acute respiratory insufficiency with disruption of lifestyle; pain, hemoptysis; knowledge deficit regarding illness and its prognosis; intensive care setting.

   a. Problem: Anxiety increases oxygen requirements throughout the body. If pulmonary dysfunction exists, anxiety may lead to increased hypoxemia.

   b. Interventions

      i. Assess for signs and symptoms of anxiety (tachycardia, anorexia, nausea, diarrhea, finger tapping).

      ii. Initiate intervention to reduce anxiety.
         - Relieve pain.
         - Listen to patient.
         - Maintain comfort.
         - Allow liberal family visits.
         - Reassure family members.

      iii. Assess readiness of patient and family to learn about condition and treatments.

      iv. Involve patient and family in decision making regarding care whenever possible.

   c. Desired outcome

      i. Patient verbalizes feeling less anxious.

      ii. Patient demonstrates a relaxed demeanor.

      iii. Patient performs relaxation techniques with assistance.

      iv. Patient verbalizes familiarity with ICU routines and protocols.

IV. Discharge planning

A. Determine how patient usually copes in an acute situation.

B. Explain to patient how to identify and prevent further episodes of deep-vein thrombosis.

C. Provide support to patient and family in an attempt to reduce anxiety and improve coping skills.

D. Teach patient about the importance of taking warfarin and the need for frequent laboratory work (ie, PT) to assess for therapeutic dose. Teach about diet (reduce vitamin K foods, green leafy vegetables, and fat of meat).

E. Teach measures to minimize bleeding risks (wearing shoes, gentle flossing and brushing of teeth, safety razors, etc) during anticoagulant therapy.

F. Encourage exercise when physician approval is given.

G. Teach patient about importance of continued medical follow-up.

H. Teach patient to maintain hydration; hypovolemia may increase likelihood of further thrombi formation.

I. Teach patient and family what symptoms need to be reported to physician.

J. Teach patient about condition and what can be done to prevent future recurrence.

Table 13.3 Thrombolytics

Drug	Action	Source	Side Effects	Administration Guidelines for Pulmonary Embolism
Tissue plasminogen activator	Cleaves plasminogen with clot; requires systemic fibrinolysis; more rapid (?)	Recombinant DNA technology	Bleeding (nonantigenic)	IV infusion of 100 mg over 2 h
Streptokinase	Combines with circulating plasminogen to form activator complex; cleaves plasminogen to produce plasmin	Cultures of streptococci	Bleeding; antigenic; cannot be used again for at least several months; systemic fibrinolysis	IV bolus of 250 IU over 30 min followed by maintenance dosage of 100,000 IU for 12–24 h
Urokinase	Cleaves circulating plasminogen directly; more rapid (?)	Human urine or recombinant DNA technology	Bleeding (nonantigenic)	4400 IU/kg IV over 20 min followed by maintenance dosage of 4400 IU/kg/h for 12–24 h

References

1. Bernard, G., Artigas, A., Brigham, K. L., et al. The American-European Consensus Conference on ARDS: Definitions, mechanisms, relevant outcomes, and clinical trial coordination. *Am. J. Respir. Crit. Care Med.* 149:818–824, 1994.

2. Hansen-Flaschen, J. Adult Respiratory Distress Syndrome. In R. Carlson, M. Geheb (eds.), *Medical Intensive Care.* Philadelphia: Saunders, 1993. Chap. 73.

3. Runcie, C., Ramsay, G. Intraabdominal infection; pulmonary failure. *World J. Surg.* 14:196–203, 1990.

4. Deitch, E. A., Ma, W. J., Ma, L., et al. Protein malnutrition predisposes to inflammatory-induced gut-origin septic states. *Ann. Surg.* 211:560–570, 1990.

5. Jacobson, A. Prone to oxygenate. *Am. J. Nurs.* 93:20, 1993.

6. East, T. D. The magic bullets in the war on ARDS: Aggressive therapy for oxygenation failure. *Resp. Care* 38:690–704, 1993.

7. Baker, T., Zellinger, M. Trends in caring for the patient with respiratory disease: A kaleidoscope of changes. *Am. J. Nurs.* (Suppl):11–17, 1993.

8. Kuhn, M. Multiple trauma with respiratory distress. *Crit. Care Nurs.* 14:68–72, 1994.

9. Seager, W., Gunther, A., Walmath, H., et al. Alveolar surfactant and adult respiratory distress syndrome: Pathogenetic role and therapeutic prospects. *Clin. Investig.* 71:177–190, 1993.

10. Jacobson, W., Park, G. R., Saich, T., et al. Surfactant and adult respiratory distress syndrome. *Br. J. Anaesth.* 70:522–526, 1993.

11. Steinberg, K. P. Surfactant therapy in the adult respiratory distress syndrome. *Resp. Care* 38:365–372, 1993.

12. Sinski, A., Corbo, J. Surfactant replacement in adults and children with ARDS—An effective therapy? *Crit. Care Nurs.* 14:54–59, 1994.

13. Vaca, K. J., Reedy, J. E., Lohmann, D. P., et al. Nursing care of the patient with an intravascular oxygenator. *American Journal of Critical Care* 2:478–488, 1993.

14. Durbin, C. G., Jr. Intravenous oxygenation and CO_2 removal device: IVOX. *Resp. Care* 37:147–153, 1992.

15. Kuhn, M. *Pharmacotherapeutics: A Nursing Process Approach* (3rd ed.). Philadelphia: F. A. Davis, 1994. Pp. 254–288.

16. Shapiro, B. A., Kacmarek, R. M., Crane, R. D., et al. *Clinical Application of Respiratory Care* (4th ed.). St. Louis: Mosby–Year Book, 1981. P. 418.

17. Curtis, J., Hudson, M. Acute Respiratory Failure in Chronic Obstructive Pulmonary Disease. In C. Carlson, M. Geharb (eds.), *Medical Intensive Care.* Philadelphia: Saunders, 1993. P. 794.

18. Grossbach, I. The COPD patient in acute respiratory failure. *Crit. Care Nurs.* 14:32–40, 1994.

CHAPTER 14

Patients Undergoing Transplantation

Brenda Shelton

I. Definition

A. Organ transplantation is the process of transferring a functioning organ from one person to another in order to replace a nonfunctional, diseased organ. Organ transplantation has become the treatment of choice for end-stage organ disease. The donated organ is called a graft. Organ transplant patients most likely to require intensive care intervention include those receiving heart, lung, heart–lung, liver, pancreas, islet cells, kidney–pancreas, and bone marrow transplants. Discussions pertinent to each are included in this chapter.

B. There are three types of grafts.
  1. Isograft: A graft transplanted into an identical histocompatible recipient (eg, twin sibling).
  2. Allograft: A graft transplanted into a recipient of the same species but not necessarily of identical histocompatibility.
  3. Autograft: A graft transplanted from one area of the recipient's body to another (eg, skin transplant).

C. There are four types of organ transplants.
  1. Cadaveric: The donor is genetically different than the recipient, and the donor has been pronounced brain dead but is medically supported to maintain organ perfusion.
  2. Syngeneic: The organ donor is a living, blood-related individual with an identical genetic match.
  3. Autologous: The graft is "self"-donated.
  4. Allogeneic: The organ is donated from a genetically different living donor.

D. Criteria for matching donor and recipient: There are protocols or institutionalized variations in the applications of these transplantation criteria; in some centers, transplantation is contraindicated in a patient who may be considered eligible for transplantation elsewhere.
  1. Human leukocyte antigen (HLA) match: More emphasized in bone marrow transplant (BMT).
  2. ABO compatibility: All major organ transplants except BMT, islet cells.
  3. Mixed lymphocyte count: Done with living related donors and whenever else possible. Positive mixed lymphocyte reaction predicts increased incidence of rejection.

4. Equivalent donor/recipient organ size.
5. No active infections in donor or recipient (particularly human immuno-deficiency virus infection or hepatitis).
6. Donor criteria (ideal, but not applied uniformly in all transplant centers)
   a. No history of intravenous (IV) drug use.
   b. Core temperature greater than 32°F.
   c. Laboratory tests within normal limits.
   d. No history of metastasizing cancer, except basal cell carcinoma or an isolated brain tumor.
   e. For cardiac transplant, donor must have normal 12-lead electrocardiogram, echocardiogram, creatine phosphokinase, and creatine phosphokinase MB isoenzyme.
   f. For liver transplantation, normal transaminases are required.

II. Organ transplant immunology

A. HLA matching
   1. All persons have their own genetic universal product code called the HLA, which distinguishes their body cells from foreign cells.
   2. HLAs are proteins on the outside of cells that distinguish an individual's cells from other cells.
   3. This universal product code is used to match the donor and recipient as closely as possible to prevent rejection by the recipient.
   4. HLAs are divided into class I or major antigens (A, B, C) and class II or minor antigens (D, DP, DQ, DR).
      a. Normal immune response is to respond to foreign HLA.
      b. Class II antigens stimulate helper T cells.
      c. Helper T cells stimulate B cells to produce antibodies against class I antigens on foreign tissue.
B. HLA typing
   1. Used to match donor/recipient for reduced likelihood of rejection.
   2. Tissue typing for class I antigens.
   3. Mixed lymphocyte culture (MLC) is used to detect class II antigens with living donors. It takes days to obtain these results, but whenever time permits or if multiple donors are available, the potential donor who has the lowest MLC response is the preferred donor. Theoretically, a highly positive reaction indicates an increased risk of poor graft survival; however, the predictive value of the MLC in solid organ transplant such as kidney transplantation is unknown [1].

III. Nursing process: assessment

A. Signs and symptoms of engraftment include return of normal organ function.
B. Signs and symptoms of rejection
   1. Definition: An immune response against transplanted tissue; often both humoral and cellular mediated
   2. Hyperacute rejection
      a. Occurs within minutes.
      b. Characterized by the recipient's antibodies adhering to the vascular endothelium of the graft, triggering complement, and clotting.

    c. Signs and symptoms: Rapid, widespread vascular thrombosis causes severe graft necrosis and organ failure.

    d. No curative treatment except retransplantation.

3. Acute rejection

    a. Occurs hours to days following transplantation.

    b. Antigens on the recipient's macrophages process the antigens on the transplanted organ. The B and T lymphocytes become sensitized to these antigens and trigger humoral and cellular responses causing injury to the graft. Cytotoxic T cells cause lysis and direct injury to the graft; lymphokines produce activated T cells that enhance graft rejection.

    c. Signs and symptoms: Pain, tenderness over graft site, decreasing graft function, fever, malaise.

    d. Treatment with immunosuppressive medications.

4. Chronic rejection

    a. Occurs months to years after transplantation.

    b. Involves the minor histocompatibility antigens.

    c. Results in proliferation of endothelial and mononuclear cells with narrowing of the vascular arterial bed in the graft and other organs.

    d. Signs and symptoms: Gradual loss of graft function.

    e. Rejection signs and symptoms unique to the organ transplanted.

C. Initial posttransplant assessments are uniform whether solid organ surgical procedure or BMT.

1. Immediate postoperative care (except BMT, islet cells).

    a. Immediate monitoring for signs of hyperacute rejection by thrombosis or organ.

    b. Routine cardiopulmonary critical care monitoring based on length of anesthesia, fluids lost, complexity of organ resection, or prior medical history. Many of these monitoring parameters are not needed with routine kidney transplantation.

       i. Cardiac monitoring.

       ii. Oxygen saturation monitoring and arterial blood gas analysis.

       iii. Vascular volume assessments: Blood pressure, central venous pressure, weight, intake and output.

       iv. Blood chemistry monitoring.

       v. Hematology monitoring.

    c. Presence of pain.

    d. Monitoring of incision and drain sites for excess or abnormal drainage, signaling altered vascular integrity or rejection symptoms.

    e. Breath sounds, lung expansion, ability to cough, and deep breathing signaling atelectasis or early pneumonia.

    f. Temperature monitoring to detect potential infection. Other symptoms of infection are not usually appreciable due to immunosuppressive therapy.

IV. Nursing process: planning

A. Potential alteration in tissue perfusion

1. Problem: In the posttransplant period, failure to engraft leads to ischemia and dysfunction of the engrafted organ. Symptoms of failure to engraft

are particular to each type of transplant (see Tables 14.1 through 14.5); however, some nursing care is universal for all transplant patients experiencing potential rejection. Altered tissue perfusion in the posttransplant period also may be caused by reduced perfusion of the graft, so careful evaluation of graft circulation is essential.

2. Etiology: Hyperacute, acute, or chronic transplant rejection phenomena are the usual cause; however, inadequate vascular volume or postoperative shock may also produce ischemic graft symptoms.

3. Interventions
   a. Monitor engrafted organ's function carefully, especially during the first 2 weeks when severe rejection phenomenon is most common.
   b. Administer antirejection medications (immunosuppressives) as ordered. Regimens and doses vary greatly among organs, types of transplant, and transplant centers (see Tables 14.1 through 14.5).
   c. Administer IV fluids, blood components, or vasopressors as ordered to maintain vascular volume and adequate perfusion of the engrafted organ. Specific goal mean arterial pressure (MAP) differs with various types of transplants. The literature reports goal MAPs from 60 to 75 mm Hg.

4. Desired outcome: Normal graft function demonstrated by normalization of organ function, and normal mental status.

B. Potential for infection
   1. Problem: Patients who have undergone organ transplantation must be given immunosuppressive medications to prevent graft rejection, but the most serious adverse effect of these drugs is potential for infection. Additional risks for infection are associated with the surgical procedure, administration of anesthetic agents, and invasive therapy (eg, Foley catheters, central venous catheters) required to ensure recovery.
   2. Etiology: Patients undergoing organ transplantation are prone to infection due to immunosuppressive medications used to prevent rejection, exposure to nosocomial infections in the intensive care unit (ICU), and many breaks in the barrier defense (ie, during operative procedure; with IV lines, catheters, and drains). The administration of broad-spectrum antibiotics kills undesirable microbes but also destroys normal flora and encourages the growth of resistant microorganisms.
   3. Interventions
      a. Protect from environmental infection risks (eg, sterile technique; avoid assignments with patients having resistant infections; clean multipatient equipment prior to use).
      b. Maintain meticulous hygiene of the patient (including dental care, frequent cleansing, sheet changes).
      c. Consider carefully the need for invasive lines, realizing infection risks.
      d. Avoid unnecessary invasive procedures such as intramuscular injections or nasogastric tubes. Attempt to maintain barrier defense whenever possible.
      e. Measure body temperature at least once every 2 to 4 hours. Hyperthermia may be the only symptom of infection in the immunosuppressed patient.

f. Implement institutional "immunosuppressive precautions," such as daily dressing changes, use antimicrobial soap, or other unique measures.

g. Obtain body fluid cultures as ordered with febrile episodes or as a surveillance measure.

h. Administer antibiotics as ordered, and monitor medication levels, reporting new fevers or abnormal serum antibiotic levels.

4. Desired outcome

a. Patient is afebrile.

b. No cultures positive for microbes.

c. Normal leukocyte count and differential.

d. No wound drainage.

C. Alteration in comfort, postoperative pain

1. Problem: Most solid organ transplants (kidney, kidney–pancreas, pancreas, liver, heart, lung, heart–lung) require a major surgical procedure involving resection and anastomosis of the engrafted organ. Most patients require a large chest or abdominal incision that produces considerable postoperative discomfort.

2. Etiology: Pain is caused by extensive tissue damage required during the surgical procedure and is enhanced with immobility during a prolonged surgical procedure. Intensive care routines (eg, weights, dressing changes), pulmonary hygiene measures, and indwelling lines exacerbate this discomfort.

3. Interventions

a. Assess patient's perception of comfort at least every shift using a quantitative scale that reflects when the discomfort is worse or relieved by interventions (eg, visual analog scales).

b. Administer pain and sedating medications to relax the patient and to decrease oxygen consumption, which may contribute to cellular hypoxia.

c. Premedicate the patient with analgesics prior to coughing and deep breathing or early ambulation.

d. Monitor for common adverse effects of analgesics (especially opiates): hypoventilation, excessive sleepiness, hallucinations, confusion, constipation, urinary retention, nausea, headache, lower diastolic blood pressure, or itching.

e. Augment pharmacologic agents with other comfort measures such as positioning, pillows, or relaxation exercises.

4. Desired outcome

a. Patient denies discomfort.

b. Patient verbalizes relief of discomfort with ordered analgesics.

c. Absence of analgesic adverse effects.

d. Patient is able to perform mobility and breathing exercises as required.

D. Potential alteration in gas exchange

1. Problem: Patients undergoing transplantation often require assistance with ventilation and oxygenation.

2. Etiology: Prolonged anesthesia, which is common with some transplant surgeries, reduced independent ventilation and decreases vital capacity, which can impair gas exchange. Many patients also have complex postoperative courses with large chest or abdominal incisions and limited physical activity, which contribute to this problem and therefore compromise gas exchange. Last, immunosuppressive therapy administered to patients to prevent graft rejection predisposes patients to the risk of infectious lung processes when hypoventilation and atelectasis occur.

3. Interventions
   a. Place patient in high Fowler's or reverse Trendelenburg's position to provide maximal ventilation and oxygenation.
   b. Encourage coughing and deep breathing postoperatively.
   c. Early ambulation posttransplant.
   d. Assess respiratory rate, quality, and breath sounds frequently in the early posttransplant period.
   e. Monitor fluid status and cardiovascular tolerance to fluids to assess for hypervolemia or heart failure, which contributes to altered oxygenation.
   f. Assess arterial blood gases, oxygen saturation, and capnography as needed for indications of respiratory decompensation.
   g. Assess and manage pain to promote maximal respiratory effort and minimal medication-induced respiratory suppression.
   h. Assess sputum, breath sounds, sputum cultures as ordered.
   i. Monitor sputum, breath sounds, and temperature for evidence of pulmonary infections.
   j. Change respiratory care equipment daily to prevent infection.
   k. Turn patient every 2 to 4 hours to ensure adequate ventilation and circulation throughout both lungs.

4. Desired outcome
   a. Arterial oxygen saturation (SaO_2) greater than 90%.
   b. Arterial oxygen tension (PaO_2) is greater than 60 mm Hg by arterial blood gas analysis.
   c. Patient is afebrile.
   d. Patient has minimal clear sputum.
   e. Patient's chest x-ray is clear, without infiltrates.

E. Altered skin integrity
   1. Problem: Patients undergoing transplantation have prolonged illnesses and recovery periods that alter mobility and nutrition, both of which influence skin integrity. Altered resistance to infection from immunosuppressant medication also contributes to the risk of altered skin integrity and its subsequent infectious complications.
   2. Etiology: The etiologies of altered skin integrity cover a broad range of problems related to critical illness and the transplant process itself. Surgical wounds are often large, involve several major muscle groups (except routine kidney transplant), and are accompanied by multiple drains that may cause skin excoriation; more subtle causes include coexisting immune suppression. Multiple IV lines and catheters are necessary for immediate postoperative care and monitoring, but they contribute to the problem of altered skin integrity. The prolonged recuperative period for most patients may predispose them to immobility or altered nutrition, which inhibits wound healing and increases risk of intraoperative or incisional infection.

3. Interventions
   a. Assess skin every shift for breaks in integrity, evidence of pressure, or poor wound healing. Attempt to observe catheter sites every shift.
   b. Administer skin lotions to maintain skin integrity.
   c. Change sterile dressings daily. Be certain that wound drains do not leak on the skin.
   d. Use paper tape, hypoallergenic tape, DuoDerm (ConvaTec, Bristol-Meyers-Squibb, Princeton, NJ), or other skin preparation products if necessary to prevent skin breakdown.
   e. Perform passive or active range of motion to enhance circulation and joint mobility.
   f. Perform assessment and cultures of every catheter site, wound, break in skin integrity, and orifice with temperature spike.
   g. Attempt to keep all skin surfaces clean and dry. Moist, dark areas are likely to enhance microbial growth. Fungal skin infections are common in the immunocompromised host.
   h. Use topical antimicrobial agents as ordered for skin infections. Recognize that skin excoriations may be infectious in nature, and, if ordered, use antifungal powder in skin folds.
   i. If the patient is immobilized for an extended period of time, obtain splints for extremities to prevent contractures.
4. Desired outcome
   a. Wound heals without complications (infection, dehiscence, evisceration).
   b. No pressure breakdown areas occur.
   c. No evidence of infection at suture site or invasive IV lines and catheters.
F. Altered nutrition, less than requirements
   1. Problem: The prolonged hospitalization and recovery process in transplantation frequently interferes with adequate nutrition.
   2. Etiology: During transplantation, a long surgical procedure, prolonged recovery period, disruptions in barrier integrity, and immunosuppression contribute to a clinical situation in which the patient is unable to meet his or her metabolic demands. Even with initial parenteral supplementation, followed by enteral supplementation, caloric and nutrient needs often are not fully met during the posttransplant period. Complications in this time period accentuate this problem.
   3. Interventions
      a. Maintain intake and output records at least every shift.
      b. Weigh daily.
      c. Obtain nutrition consultation on all transplant patients.
      d. As diet progresses, monitor calorie counts and nutrition intake.
      e. Encourage vitamin supplementation as the patient's condition improves.
   4. Desired outcome
      a. Patient shows a less than 10% weight loss in the immediate posttransplant period.
      b. Maintain a caloric intake matching the assessed needs.

G. Altered health maintenance

1. Problem: The process of transplantation requires multiple changes in family structure and the patient's ability to provide self-care, which may interfere with normal health maintenance.

2. Etiology: Prolonged hospitalizations and recovery periods, multiple surgical wounds, and immunosuppressive therapy all serve to alter family relationships and the patient's ability to fulfill normal roles and functions. Physical needs may be extensive and may require skilled assessment and care even after discharge from the hospital.

3. Interventions

   a. Reassess need for organ support, such as medications or dialysis, after successful engraftment.

   b. Assess family and patient's perceptions of role changes and the patient's care needs after discharge.

   c. Plan for skilled or unskilled nursing care, equipment, and supply needs after discharge.

   d. Assess family dynamics and identify potential problems in patient and family adjustment after discharge.

   e. Assess family's ability and willingness to learn how to care for patient's physical needs and to fulfill patient's previous responsibilities. Make referrals as appropriate.

   f. Refer to posttransplant support groups as available and appropriate to patient needs.

   g. Teach patient and family that immunosuppression is for life and explain implications.

   i. Infection prevention is a priority for these patients (see Chap. 9 for more information on the immunosuppressed patient).

   ii. Dose-limiting adverse effects of each agent should be emphasized.

   iii. Immunosuppressive therapy increases risk of developing secondary malignancies (especially lymphoproliferative types).

   h. Assess financial resources and need for referral to social worker or financial counselors. This may include assessment of limitations of insurance after the transplant procedure.

   i. Assess and refer to mental health professional those patients or families who demonstrate a high risk for ineffective coping.

4. Desired outcome

   a. Patient and family express evidence of adjustment and planning for postdischarge needs.

   b. Patient and family demonstrate effective coping mechanisms.

   c. Patient and family have established financial plan for funding the transplant and posttransplant care.

V. Nursing process: interventions

A. Managing patients receiving immunosuppressive therapy

1. Goal of therapy is to suppress rejection phenomenon.

2. Most immunosuppressive therapy is continued for life after transplantation.

3. Immunosuppressive agents are used to suppress the immune response.

4. Doses of these agents are widely variable and dependent on several factors
   a. Whether the agent is being used as prophylaxis against rejection or as treatment of rejection symptoms.
   b. Which type of transplant (eg, heart transplant uses higher doses of immunosuppressive agents).
   c. Timing after transplant influences the dose: Higher doses are used in the immediate posttransplant period, and doses are reduced at a later time.
   d. Degree of HLA match may influence the drug doses in some circumstances (eg, in non–HLA-matched BMT, the immunosuppressive doses are higher than when a match is present; transplantations between identical twins may require minimal immunosuppressive therapy [see Table 14.6]).

VI. Nursing process: overview

A. Heart transplantation (Table 14.1).
B. Lung transplantation (Table 14.2).
C. Liver transplantation (Table 14.3).
D. Kidney-pancreas transplantation (Table 14.4).
E. Bone marrow transplantation (Table 14.5).
F. Immunosuppressive agents (Table 14.6).

Table 14.1 Heart Transplantation

Feature	Specifics
Indication	End-stage heart disease from an irreversible weakened or damaged cardiac muscle (eg, cardiomyopathy, myocarditis, valve disease, coronary artery disease, congenital heart disease)

Eligibility	1. Age < 65 years (not always a clear age cutoff)
	 2. Expected survival < 1 year
	 3. Compliant, well-motivated individual
	 4. Heart failure: NYHA classifications
	    a. Class III—marked physical limitations due to cardiac symptoms with less than ordinary activity
	    b. Class IV—symptoms of chronic heart failure at rest
	 5. Inoperable coronary artery disease with intractable anginal symptoms
	 6. Malignant ventricular arrhythmias unresponsive to medical or surgical treatment

Contraindications	1. Pulmonary infarction within the past 8 wk 2. Severe pulmonary hypertension with fixed pulmonary vascular resistance > 6–10 U 3. Significant functional impairment of other vital organs that is not reversible (eg, coagulation abnormality, chronic bronchitis, prerenal azotemia, or hepatic abnormalities) 4. Alcohol/drug abuse, mental illness, or inability to stop smoking

Process	1. Orthoptic
	    a. Most common
	    b. Donor's heart is anastomosed to remnant left and right atrial cuffs following removal of the diseased heart

Table 14.1 *Continued*

Feature	Specifics

Process (*cont.*)	2. Denervation—normal heart function controlled by the autonomic nervous system
	   a. Denervation of heart causes absence of parasympathetic stimulation; therefore, patient has faster resting heart rate. In the event that a patient develops bradycardia, give isoproterenol or epinephrine, *not* atropine, which acts on parasympathetic nerves
	   b. Denervated hearts are slower to respond to exercise, requiring longer warm-up and cool-down periods
	   c. Orthostatic changes are common secondary to venous pooling, causing a sudden loss of preload and the heart's inability to produce a compensatory tachycardia
	   d. Denervated hearts do not respond to Valsalva maneuvers such as carotid massage
	   e. Orthotopic transplant patients often have two P waves, but conduction from the recipient's atria stops at the suture line

Early complications Acute rejection *Treatment:* immunosuppressive therapy	*Signs/symptoms* 1. Fever 2. Dysrhythmias 3. Crackles auscultated in lungs 4. Elevated jugular venous pulsations 5. Increased pulmonary vascular resistance 6. Elevated right atrial or pulmonary artery pressures; increased systemic vascular resistance, low cardiac output 7. Gallop, murmur, or muffled heart sounds 8. Peripheral edema 9. Decreased urine output 10. Hypotension 11. Syncope 12. Decreased exercise intolerance 13. Malaise 14. Shortness of breath 15. Dyspnea
Decreased cardiac output secondary to transient myo-cardial dysfunction and heart dener-vation *Treatment:* supportive therapy to enhance myocardial function	*Signs/symptoms* 1. Dysrhythmias 2. Signs and symptoms of inadequate cardiac output—hypotension, oliguria, weak thready pulses, cool extrem-ities, cyanosis, dyspnea 3. Signs and symptoms of heart failure—dyspnea, crackles, fluid retention, weight gain, increased right atrial pressure, increased pulmonary artery pressures, decreased cardiac output, increased jugular venous pulsations, tender hepatomegaly, gallops and murmurs on cardiac auscultation
Surgical complications *Treatment:* symptomatic support	*Signs/symptoms* 1. Cardiac tamponade 2. Coagulopathies 3. Intraoperative or postoperative myocardial infarction 4. Low cardiac output shock

Table 14.1 *Continued*

Feature	Specifics
Early complications (*cont.*)	
Infection of graft *Treatment:* antimicrobial therapy	See Potential for infection, p. 400 See Chap. 9 for additional information on immunosuppression
Late complications	
Chronic rejection *Treatment:* immunosuppressive agents	*Signs/symptoms* 1. Persistent hypotension or hypertension 2. Dependent, peripheral edema 3. Chronic weight gain 4. Increasing intolerance to exercise 5. Increasing problems with shortness of breath and/or dyspnea
Graft atherosclerosis	*Signs/symptoms* Development of an accelerated form of coronary artery disease, speculated to be the result of chronic rejection
Lymphoproliferative diseases due to immunosuppressive therapy	*Signs/symptoms* 1. Lymphadenopathy 2. Extreme leukocytosis, including WBC blasts 3. Multisystem organ dysfunction

Discharge/home health	1. Immunosuppression is required for life
	2. Daily monitoring of blood pressure, heart rate, temperature, and weight to follow trends
	  a. Hypertension may signal rejection or adverse reaction to cyclosporine
	  b. Weight changes can alter cyclosporine levels and weight gain, and peripheral edema may signal rejection
	3. Presently the only diagnostic tool for determining rejection is the endomyocardial biopsy
	  a. Done on an outpatient basis or overnight stay to monitor for dysrhythmias
	  b. May be done monthly, then tapered to less often
	4. Frequent monitoring of blood work is performed to ensure adequate cyclosporine levels and WBC count

NYHA, New York Heart Association.

Table 14.2 Lung Transplantation

Feature	Specifics
Indication	End-stage pulmonary disease
Eligibility	1. Life expectancy 12–18 months 2. All other organs functionally normal or have reversible damage 3. Age < 55–60 years 4. Organ matching criteria—ABO compatibility, comparable lung size, some institutions match for cytomegalovirus antibody status 5. Adequate financial and social resources

Table 14.2 *Continued*

Feature	Specifics
Contraindications	1. Atherosclerotic heart disease 2. Irreversible renal or hepatic failure 3. Recent history (past 6 months) of current drug or alcohol abuse 4. Insulin dependent diabetes with end-organ damage 5. Cigarette smoking within past 6 months 6. Active human immunodeficiency virus infection or hepatitis B or hepatitis C infection 7. History of metastasizing malignancy 8. Prior thoracic surgery (some centers) 9. Severe pleural adhesions or fibrosis that would hinder lung resection

Process	1. Single lung transplants—chronic obstructive lung disease, restrictive lung disease, pulmonary hypertension (some centers)
	  a. Double-lumen endotracheal tube is utilized for unilateral independent lung ventilation
	  b. Posterolateral thoracotomy incision is performed, and fifth rib is removed
	2. Double-lung transplants—chronic obstructive lung disease, septic lung disease, or generalized bronchiectasis (including cystic fibrosis), pulmonary hypertension (some centers)
	  a. Has evolved to be similar to single-lung transplants using contralateral lung ventilation
	  b. Anterior transverse thoracosternotomy incision is performed
	3. Heart–lung transplant—in conditions where heart failure is not expected to resolve with transplantation of lungs only
	  a. Intussusception of donor bronchi into recipient, bronchi with overlap of one to two cartilaginous rings. This reduces ischemia of the anastamosis.

Early complications
  Acute rejection
  Treatment:
  immunosuppressive
  therapy
	Signs/symptoms
	1. Low-grade fever ($> 99.4°F$)
	2. General malaise
	3. Tachycardia
	4. Shortness of breath, dyspnea on exertion
	5. Cough
	6. SaO_2, diminished from baseline, particularly with exercise ($> 3\%$)
	7. Decreased PaO_2 or increased $PaCO_2$
	8. 10% decrease in FVC and FEV_1
	9. Perihilar infiltrate on chest x-ray
	10. Slight increase in WBC count

Surgical complications
  Treatment: based on
  presenting
  complication
	Signs/symptoms
	1. Bleeding at anastomosis site
	2. Pulmonary hypertension
	3. Atelectasis
	4. Pneumonia

Table 14.2 *Continued*

Feature	Specifics
Early complications (*cont.*) Infection of the graft *Treatment:* antimicrobial therapy	Often the organ is transferred from the donor. Cytomegalovirus infection is common in this transplant, if cytomegalovirus status has not been used as transplant eligibility criteria; infection and rejection symptoms are difficult to distinguish in lung transplant
	Signs/symptoms 1. Breath sounds on auscultation reveal coarse sounds: gurgles, crackles, and wheezes. 2. Decreased PaO_2, respiratory acidosis 3. Persistent pulmonary edema 4. Fever 5. Decreased FVC and FEV_1 6. Increased pulmonary artery pressures 7. Alterations in sputum quantity, color, or odor
Bleeding *Treatment:* positive pressure ventilation, blood component therapy	*Signs/symptoms* 1. Hemoptysis 2. Crackles on auscultation 3. Patchy pulmonary infiltrates on x-ray 4. Hypoxemia
Late complications Chronic rejection *Treatment:* immunosuppression	Symptoms same as for acute rejection, but develop more slowly; bronchiolitis obliterans may occur as a late complication associated with chronic rejection—Characterized by a fibrotic inflammatory process causing progressive reduction in pulmonary compliance and vital capacity
Lymphoproliferative disease *Treatment:* antineoplastic therapy	*Signs/symptoms* 1. Lymphadenopathy 2. Extreme leukocytosis, including WBC blasts 3. Multisystem organ dysfunction
Discharge/home health	1. Large wound may require complex home care; surgical clips are removed about 4 weeks postop 2. Signs and symptoms of rejection should be reported to coordinator as early as possible a. Activity should be gradually increased b. Ambulation of approximately 1 mile/d while maintaining an oxygen saturation above 90% is the goal for second to third postoperative week c. Patient must use a handheld spirometer to measure FVC and FEV_1; results are recorded daily; if pulmonary function decreases > 10%, the physician or coordinator should be notified d. Lung function is monitored periodically (about every 3 months) through pulmonary function laboratory spirometer tests e. Periodic bronchial biopsies via bronchoscopy to assess for rejection 3. Patients are referred to a pulmonary rehabilitation program that requires gradual increase in aerobic exercise about three times a week for about 3 months after transplant; likely to include walking, bicycling, upper body ergometer, and physical therapy for strengthening 4. Follow-up laboratory testing includes once to three times weekly chemistry panel, complete blood count

PaO_2, arterial oxygen tension; $PacO_2$, arterial carbon dioxide tension; SaO_2, arterial oxygen saturation; FVC, forced vital capacity; FEV_1, forced expiratory volume in 1 second.

Table 14.3 Liver Transplantation

Feature	Specifics
Indication	End-stage liver disease, such as Budd-Chiari syndrome, primary biliary cirrhosis, sclerosing cholangitis, alcohol-related cirrhosis, chronic active hepatitis, or isolated hepatoma
Eligibility	1. End-stage liver disease (alcohol-related, metabolic disturbances, hepatitis) 2. < 1 year expected survival 3. Age 1–70 years 4. Hepatoma without metastases 5. Evidence of alcohol rehabilitation 6. Bilirubin concentrations > 10 mg/dL, serum albumin < 2.5 mg/dL, and prothrombin time > 5 sec beyond control 7. Recurrent variceal bleeding despite sclerotherapy 8. Ascites refractory to medical therapy
Contraindications	1. Active infections such as human immunodeficiency virus 2. Severe cardiopulmonary dysfunction 3. Advanced chronic renal insufficiency due to hepatic disease 4. Any active extrahepatic malignancies

Process	1. Orthotopic liver transplantation—diseased liver is removed and replaced with the donor liver
	2. Heterotopic liver transplantation—diseased liver remains in place, and the donated liver is grafted in place (performed less often)
	3. Two types of biliary anastomoses
	  a. Choledochodedunostomy—preferred method of donor common duct anastomosis to recipient common duct
	  b. Roux-en-Y choledochojejunostomy—used when the common bile duct is diseased, involved donor common bile duct being anastomosed to the recipient's jejunum
	4. Cadaver livers are partially resected for small-framed recipients and children
	5. Living related donor "cut-down livers" are used for children or others as a last effort at transplantation

Early complications Acute rejection *Treatment:* immunosuppressive agents	*Signs/symptoms* 1. Hypotension after the first 24 hours postoperatively; diastolic and mean arterial pressures will be low 2. Fever or prolonged postoperative hypothermia 3. Decreased bile drainage or very light or dark muddy-colored bile drainage 4. Serum albumin < 2 mg/dL more than 72 hours postoperatively 5. Clay-colored stools following T-tube internalization 6. Increased serum bilirubin and hepatic transaminases 7. Right upper quadrant tenderness or pain

Table 14.3 *Continued*

Feature	Specifics
Early complications (*cont.*)	8. Dark tea-colored urine secondary to increased urinary bilirubin 9. Sudden, severe hyperglycemia or hypoglycemia more than 72 hours postoperatively 10. Fatigue 11. Uncorrectable coagulopathies (despite continuous replacement therapy, vitamin K supplementation) with or without overt bleeding
Surgical complications *Treatment:* correct underlying cause	*Signs/symptoms* 1. Hypothermia beyond normal postoperative period may actually signal rejection; may be related to transfusion therapy in operating room 2. Pulmonary insufficiency or difficulty in discontinuation of mechanical ventilation—problem worsened if liver tenderness, ascites, or other signs of acute rejection are present
Clotting abnormalities *Treatment:* support of coagulation until normal clotting returns	*Signs/symptoms* 1. Overt bleeding 2. Occult blood in stool, urine, emesis/nasogastric drainage 3. Petechiae 4. Easy bruising 5. Gum bleeding (oozing) 6. Inability to achieve hemostasis after injury or break in barrier (eg, venipuncture) 7. Bleeding around existing lines or old puncture sites 8. Flank/back mottling and tightness signal bleeding from anastomosis
Electrolyte and acid–base abnormalities *Treatment:* parenteral support for electrolyte disturbances	*Signs/symptoms* 1. Initial hyperglycemia should resolve within 72 hours 2. Early postoperative period shows hypokalemia, but normalizes in 24–72 hours 3. Alkalosis—both respiratory and metabolic
Renal insufficiency from increased hepatorenal pressure *Treatment:* maintain renal perfusion and minimize renal insults	*Signs/symptoms* 1. Oliguria 2. Concentrated urine with elevated urinary bilirubin 3. Increased blood urea nitrogen and creatinine 4. Altered clearance of medications—antibiotics, sedatives, narcotics, neuromuscular blocking agents
Hypotension from vasodilation related to abnormal liver function *Treatment:* provide IV fluids and vasopressor agents to support perfusion pressure	*Signs/symptoms* 1. Low diastolic BP 2. Low mean BP 3. Full, bounding pulses
Infection of the graft *Treatment:* antimicrobial therapy	*Signs/symptoms* 1. Fever 2. Worsening coagulopathies 3. Uncontrollable hypoglycemia or hyperglycemia

Table 14.3 *Continued*

Feature	Specifics
Late complications Chronic rejection *Treatment:* immunosuppressive agents	*Signs/symptoms* 1. Persistent jaundice 2. Somnolence, confusion, coma, seizures, asterixis, or other symptoms of hepatic encephalopathy 3. Elevated serum ammonia levels 4. Fluid retention (especially ascites) 5. Persistent pleural effusions 6. Hepatorenal syndrome is the progressive renal failure that occurs simultaneously with worsening hepatic function 7. Persistent respiratory and metabolic alkalosis 8. GVHD manifests as nausea, vomiting, diarrhea
GVHD *Treatment:* immunosuppressive agents	Donor immunocompetent T lymphocytes accompany the donor liver and recognize the recipient's tissue as foreign. These cells attempt to destroy the self-tissue. Most frequently targeted organs in this syndrome of liver transplantation are the GI tract, skin, and lungs *Signs/symptoms* 1. Frequent watery diarrhea, clay-colored stools, foul odor of stools most common manifestations 2. Enlarged and tender liver but may be mistaken for other complications 3. Skin thickened, pruritic, loses ability to sweat, likely to become infected
Lymphoproliferative disorders *Treatment:* antineoplastic therapy	*Signs/symptoms* 1. Lymphadenopathy 2. Extreme leukocytosis, including WBC blasts 3. Multisystem organ dysfunction
Discharge/home health	1. Multiple wound sites may require complex dressing changes 2. Arrange for home care nurses to assist with wound care 3. Teach patient and family T-tube care until internalization completed 4. Alert patient and family to signs and symptoms of rejection 5. Immunosuppression is for life

BP, blood pressure; GVHD, graft-versus-host disease.

Table 14.4 Kidney-Pancreas Transplantation

Feature	Specifics
Indications	1. End-stage pancreatic disease or trauma resulting in insulin-dependent diabetes 2. Chronic renal failure with evidence of other system involvement
Eligibility	1. Insulin-dependent diabetes 2. Complications of diabetes are more serious than risk of surgery and immunosuppression 3. Nephropathy (for combined pancreas-kidney transplant) 4. Uncontrolled hyperglycemia 5. Severe neuropathy

Table 14.4 *Continued*

Feature	Specifics
Contraindications	1. Presence of penetrating abdominal wounds 2. Burns >15% of body 3. Hypertension (unless in the presence of end-stage renal disease) 4. History of human immunodeficiency virus infection or metastasizing malignancy 5. Severe incapacitating neuropathies (eg, especially autonomic neuropathies causing dysrhythmias) 6. Inoperable peripheral vascular or cardiovascular disease

Process	1. Kidney-pancreas transplantation
	  a. Most common type of pancreas transplant
	  b. Both organs come from the same donor, or a kidney is transplanted within 6 months to a year following the pancreas transplant
	2. Human islet cell transplantation
	  a. Human islet cells are isolated from cadaver pancreas
	  b. Frequently requires multiple cadaver donors to obtain adequate number of islet cells
	  c. Islet cells are implanted through the portal vein of the patient
	  d. Problems include isolation of enough islet cells and greater risk of infectious complications in patients receiving immunosuppressive therapy from an earlier kidney transplant.
	3. Segmental pancreas transplantation
	  a. A living related donor provides the segmental pancreas
	  b. Remains under investigation regarding risk/benefit ratio
	4. Whole-organ pancreas transplantation
	  a. Indicated for nonuremic diabetics who have not previously received a kidney transplant
	  b. Remains under investigation regarding risk/benefit ratio
	5. The donor kidney is transplanted into the left iliac fossa and anastomosed to the recipient's bladder
	6. The donor pancreas is transplanted into the right iliac fossa and anastomosed via the pancreaticoduodenocystotomy approach; therefore, the exocrine secretions drain through the bladder. The existing pancreas of the host continues other exocrine functions via the GI tract.

Early complications
  Acute rejection
  Treatment: immunosuppressive agents
	Signs/symptoms: renal
	1. Increased creatinine
	2. Increased blood urea nitrogen
	3. Decreased urinary output
	4. Hypertension
	5. Increased weight
	6. Graft tenderness
	7. Fever
	8. Coagulopathies
	
	Signs/symptoms: pancreatic
	1. Decreased urinary amylase (precedes glucose changes)
	2. Graft tenderness
	3. Hyperglycemia
	4. Fever

Table 14.4 *Continued*

Feature	Specifics
Surgical complications *Treatment:* specific to problem	1. Pancreatitis due to surgical manipulation; manifested by epigastric discomfort, increased serum amylase and lipase, clay-colored stools, fatty-food intolerances 2. Dehydration due to hyperglycemic osmotic diuresis postoperatively until glucose normalizes
Infection of the graft *Treatment:* antimicrobial therapy	1. Nephritis heralded by flank or back discomfort, tenderness at incision site, fever 2. Urinary tract infection (eg, urethritis, cystitis) common occurrence with symptoms such as urinary urgency, urinary frequency, dysuria, hematuria
Graft thrombosis *Treatment:* Increase circulating blood volume or administer renal dose dopamine to increase glomerular filtration rate	Occlusion of graft vessels leads to acute graft pain, signs and symptoms of acute abdominal event, oliguria, hematuria
Late complications Chronic rejection *Treatment:* immunosuppressive agents	*Signs/symptoms* 1. Elevated temperature 2. Weight gain of 2–3 lb/d 3. Hypertension 4. Pain and tenderness over graft site 5. Hyperglycemia
Lymphoproliferative disorders *Treatment:* antineoplastic agents	*Signs/symptoms* 1. Lymphadenopathy 2. Extreme leukocytosis, including WBC blasts 3. Multisystem organ dysfunction
Discharge/home health	1. Return to normal diabetic precautions, because although hyperglycemia may be resolved with transplant, other effects of disease may still manifest 2. Advise patient to continue testing blood sugars several times a day for months after transplant; hyperglycemia may be an early symptom of rejection. If blood sugars are >200 mg/dL, patient is advised to call the health care team 3. Immunosuppression may be for life, although doses are tapered dramatically after several months without rejection symptoms 4. Patient should self-monitor for fluid retention and limit fluid intake if necessary 5. Advise patient to take bicarbonate tablets as ordered as replacement for normal kidney buffering

Table 14.5 Bone Marrow Transplantation

Feature	Specifics
Definition	Administration of very high doses of chemotherapy resulting in severe myelosuppression, which requires bone marrow transplantation as a "rescue" measure

Types	1. Autologous
	  a. Bone marrow that is "self-donated"
	  b. Only performed for malignant diseases while the patient is in remission
	  c. Diseases include lymphomas and solid tumors such as Ewing's sarcoma and Hodgkin's disease
	  d. Often performed with progenitor cells, which are generated by high-dose chemotherapy and obtained from the patient via pheresis prior to the bone marrow transplant
	  e. Some centers purge the marrow, ie, treat it with chemotherapy prior to retransplantation
	  f. Does not require HLA typing or mixed lymphocyte culture
	2. Allogeneic—bone marrow that is donated from another living donor
	  a. Requires HLA typing and mixed lymphocyte culture
	  b. Does not require ABO compatibility but is preferred
	  c. May be from either a related or unrelated donor
	  d. Performed for malignant and nonmalignant disorders such as acute myelogenous leukemia, acute lymphocytic leukemia, chronic myelogenous leukemia, aplastic anemia, myelodysplastic syndrome, or multiple myeloma
	3. Syngeneic
	  a. Bone marrow donated from a living identical twin
	  b. Usually allows for the closest match regarding HLA typing and mixed lymphocyte culture
	The type of bone marrow transplantation chosen depends on the type and extent of disease, HLA matching, donor availability, as well as the donor's meeting donation criteria

Indications	1. Hematologic malignancies—leukemia, lymphoma, multiple myeloma, Ewing's sarcoma 2. Nonhematologic malignancies (solid tumors) such as breast, small-cell, lung cancer, ovarian, and childhood brain tumors; testicular 3. Metabolic and genetic disorders such as severe combined immune deficiency syndrome, aplastic anemia
Eligibility	1. Defined indicator condition 2. Patient must be in remission 3. Adequate financial and social resources 4. Good organ function
Contraindications	1. Elevated creatinine 2. Decreased pulmonary function tests 3. Decreased myocardial ejection fraction 4. Age > 65 years 5. Increased transaminases 6. Contraindications are variable secondary to research protocols

Table 14.5 *Continued*

Feature	Specifics
Process	Autologous marrow transplantation For certain malignancies, a theorized dose–response relation states that very high doses of therapy will ablate the malignancy. During the life-threatening myelosuppression, the bone marrow is infused IV and seeds throughout the patient's body. This provides the patient with functioning bone marrow cells. The patient is required to be in remission for the bone marrow transplant. The most frequent chemotherapeutic agents used are alkylating agents 1. A double-lumen permanent venous access device (VAD), eg, Hickman, is placed 2. The patient receives high-dose chemotherapy and marrow-stimulating factors followed by pheresis of circulating marrow stem cells if indicated 3. Bone marrow harvest is performed 4. Bone marrow cells are purged and treated to destroy malignant cells if indicated 5. High-dose chemotherapy and/or TBI are administered 6. On day 0 the patient is reinfused with the bone marrow 7. The patient waits for the WBC count to return (>1000 with an ANC >500 cells/mm^3) Allogeneic marrow transplant This transplant requires total destruction of the host marrow with high-dose chemotherapy and/or radiation therapy and is followed with infusion of marrow that has been harvested from another person (the donor) during an operative procedure. The infused marrow migrates to the host bone marrow and engrafts 1. Bone marrow harvest and placement of a double-lumen Hickman 2. High-dose chemotherapy (TBI if indicated) 3. Bone marrow is purged from donor 4. High-dose chemotherapy is administered 5. On day 0 bone marrow reinfusion performed 6. Patient waits for the WBC count to return (>1000 with an ANC >500 cells/mm^3). Rationale: During the bone marrow transplant, the primary concern is engraftment of the bone marrow cells and prevention of infection

Early complications
  Acute rejection: acute GVHD
  Treatment:
  Immunosuppressive therapy
	1. Occurs primarily in allogeneic transplant, especially unrelated transplants; is minimal with syngeneic transplants
	2. Definition: T lymphocytes from the donor bone marrow recognize nonself surface antigens on various organs (frequently skin, GI tract, liver) in the recipient and mount an immune destruction of those organs. Acute GVHD occurs within the first 100 days following bone marrow transplant
	3. Signs/symptoms
	  a. Maculopapular rash varying in involvement from $<25\%$ of body to generalized erythroderma with bullous formation and desquamation; rash often begins on soles of feet, arms, shoulders, or trunk
	  b. GVHD of the liver appears as an elevated alkaline phosphatase, elevated bilirubin, jaundice, hepatomegaly, right upper quadrant tenderness

Table 14.5 *Continued*

Feature	Specifics
Early complications *(cont.)*	c. GVHD of the intestinal tract usually includes diarrhea > 500 mL/d, severe abdominal pain with or without paralytic ileus, GI bleeding, and negative stool cultures 4. Diagnosis—skin, liver, or GI tract biopsy is definitive diagnostic tool 5. Treatment—immunosuppressives
Mucositis *Treatment:* symptomatic support	1. Severe mucosal erosion is most severe on days 5–15 and is due to antineoplastic chemotherapy, radiotherapy, and some immunosuppressive regimens (antimetabolites) given to prevent rejection 2. Mucosal erosion may be severe (causing hemorrhage) and continuous within mouth to anus 3. Oral superinfection can occur unless meticulous mouth care is praticed and prophylactic antimicrobials are given
Hemorrhage *Treatment:* blood components, symptomatic support	1. Bone marrow suppression affects platelets almost immediately 2. Low platelet count exacerbates bleeding tendency from mucositis, or GVHD 3. Hepatic disease (GVHD or VOD) exacerbates tendency to bleed 4. Signs and symptoms—occult or overt bleeding, abnormal platelet count, and coagulation tests 5. Diagnosis—clinical symptoms and laboratory tests

Hepatic VOD *Treatment:* none known	1. Definition: fibrous granulation of vessels in the liver as a consequence of antineoplastic chemotherapy and radiation therapy. Causes compromised circulation through the liver and portal hypertension
	2. Signs/symptoms
	   a. Onset is between days 8 and 15 posttransplant. May be later in autologous bone marrow transplant, and may be earlier if patient was heavily pretreated with alkylating agents
	   b. First symptom usually right upper quadrant abdominal tenderness with hepatomegaly
	   c. Fluid retention and weight gain also occur early
	   d. Differentiated from GVHD of liver by the fact that isolated hyperbilirubinemia occurs first and transaminase elevation does not occur until later
	3. Diagnosis: liver biopsy confirms clinical suspicion

Failure to engraft *Treatment:* see "Specifics"	1. Definition: if engraftment with bone marrow recovery has not occurred by approximately 6–10 weeks (depends on institutional norm that is based on conditioning drugs used and method of preparing marrow prior to reinfusion); failure to engraft bone marrow results in functional aplastic anemia 2. Signs/symptoms: All marrow components are suppressed (WBCs, RBCs, platelets), so patient has signs and symptoms of anemia, bleeding, and infection 3. Diagnosis—bone marrow biopsy 4. Treatment a. Marrow stimulation with synthetic erythropoietin to enhance RBC growth; granulocyte colony stimulating factor (filgrastim) to enhance WBC growth; and folate, B_{12}, steroids to enhance platelet growth

Table 14.5 *Continued*

Feature	Specifics
Early complications (*cont.*)	b. Supportive care with blood component transfusions c. If autologous marrow transplant, a back-up marrow has usually been frozen but not treated as extensively; reinfusion of back-up marrow may have increased risk of malignancy recurrence d. Another matched transplant is performed as soon as possible; if none is available, HLA-unmatched transplant may be performed

Late complications
Chronic GVHD
	1. Process similar to acute disease but produces collagen substance with fibrosis
	2. Organs involved usually include skin, GI tract, and liver
	  a. Chronic thickened skin, poor sweating, tearing, or other normal excretions
	  b. Diarrhea with or without GI bleeding may occur
	  c. Elevated transaminases occur to signal liver involvement
	3. Bronchiolitis obliterans in setting of posttransplant is thought to be manifestation of chronic GVHD of lung
	  a. Obstructive symptoms on pulmonary function test (decreased functional residual capacity, increased diffusing lung capacity of CO_2)
	  b. Pulmonary hypertension may accompany respiratory symptoms
	  c. Rapidly progressive lung failure occurs despite corticosteroid therapy

Discharge/home health considerations	1. Most patients do not have normal immune function despite return of WBC count; infection prevention precautions are essential 2. Blood product support is often required for several months after discharge 3. All immune memory is eliminated with allogeneic bone marrow transplant; patients must later (after 2 years) be reimmunized against childhood illnesses, hepatitis, and pneumococcus; therefore, patients should avoid exposure during that time period 4. After allogeneic bone marrow transplant, a second drop in blood count occurs between days 50 and 70 5. Immunosuppressive agents will be tapered and discontinued after several years without rejection symptoms 6. Frequent blood counts, chemistry tests, and bone marrow biopsies are performed to evaluate success of the BMT and adequacy of engrafted marrow

HLA, human leukocyte antigen; ANC, absolute neutrophil count; TBI, total body irradiation; GVHD, graft-versus-host disease; VOD, venoocclusive disease; WBC, white blood cell; RBC, red blood cell.

Agents	Actions	Nursing Implications
Anti-inflammatory drugs—steroids: prednisone, prednisolone, methylprednisolone	Stabilizes cell membranes, suppressing monocytic activity, thereby decreasing sensitivity of host to antigen and reducing lymphocyte sensitization Slows T-lymphocytic recognition of foreign tissue (eg, transplanted organ, malignant cells) Used in prevention and treatment of rejection	*General* Infection prevention precautions (see Chap. 9) Special wound assessment and care with sterile dressing changes Assessment for wound healing complications—poor approximation, dehiscence, evisceration Frequent temperature monitoring Assess blood glucose levels and administer insulin as ordered Limit sodium and fluid intake if fluid retention becomes problematic Frequent weight, central venous pressures, and intake/output measurements to detect fluid retention Administer histamine H$_2$ blocker agents or sucralfate as ordered to prevent gastric ulceration Administer oral doses with food or milk Discuss possible increase in facial and body hair; advise patient that this may decrease as the dose is reduced Provide meticulous skin care, especially of the face; advise patient that acne occurs due to increased activity of the surface glands in the skin; common sites are the face and back Provide frequent bathing if increased sweating occurs *Long-term use* Advise patient of anticipated change in body image—hair growth, acne, sweating tendency, changes in fat distribution, edema Monitor appetite and dietary intake to avoid excessive weight gain from steroid use; referral to nutrition consult may be advisable Supplement calcium to counteract osteoporosis Encourage mobility to reduce long-term risk of osteoporosis Assess visual acuity periodically for cataract formation

Table 14.6 *Continued*

Agents	Actions	Nursing Implications
Antimetabolites: azathioprine (Immuran), 6-mercaptopurine, methotrexate	Interferes with cell nutrition or enzyme activity Interferes with nucleic acid synthesis in T lymphocytes resulting in cell death Suppresses T-lymphocyte reaction to antigens These agents used to *prevent* rejection only (especially renal and cardiac transplantation)	*General* Assess for bleeding symptoms due to thrombocytopenia—petechiae, ecchymoses; occult blood in urine, emesis, or feces; gum bleeding Bleeding precautions (see Chap. 8) Administer topical hemostatic agents as ordered Assess for infection (see Chap. 9) Infection prevention precautions (see Chap. 9) Frequent oral care with oxidizing agents (eg, sodium bicarbonate or quarter-strength peroxide solution), anesthetic agents, for management of oral stomatitis from agents Culture oral lesions to rule out infectious etiologies *Long-term use* Assess for altered tissue oxygenation due to anemia—paleness, hypothermia, low oxygen saturation Administer erythropoietin (Pro-crit) as ordered Administer blood components (platelets, RBCs) as ordered Monitor bilirubin, transaminase levels for hepatotoxicity If jaundiced, provide lotions and antipruritic agents (eg, diphenhydramine)
Cytotoxic agents: cyclophosphamide (Cytoxan), chlorambucil, lymphoid irradiation	Interferes with DNA synthesis of lymphocytes, reducing circulating number Interferes with T-lymphocyte cytokine release, which controls B- and T-cell responses against foreign tissue Used as a preventive and as treatment of transplant rejection	*General* Bleeding, infection, and anemia precautions as outlined previously Monitor for jaundice; persistent decrease in hematocrit and hemoglobin; enlarged spleen; and elevated reticulocyte count, which signals hemolytic anemia Monitor patient closely for hypersensitivity reactions during drug administration Monitor temperature and administer acetaminophen as ordered for relief of fever and discomfort from flulike syndrome Provide frequent rest periods to counteract fatigue and malaise Administer antiemetics as needed for nausea and vomiting Monitor oral intake and supplement nutrition as needed Administer antidiarrheals as ordered Careful intake and output, electrolyte monitoring if diarrhea is present

Monitor for abdominal pain, fatty-food intolerances, lipase and amylase to detect pancreatitis

Perform frequent heart sound, pulse, and jugular venous pulsation assessments 6–12 days after cyclophosphamide administration to detect drug-induced cardiomyopathy

Monitor urine for occult or overt blood, which can signal hemorrhagic cystitis that may occur within 5–15 days of cyclophosphamide administration

Long-term use

Advise the patient that partial hair loss is common but diminishes as dose is reduced

Monitor renal function for toxicity

Encourage fluids to reduce renal and bladder toxicity

Continue antiemetic therapy if needed

Polyclonal antibodies—anti-lymphocyte globulins: antithymocyte globulin (ATG), antilymphocyte serum (ALS)	Destroys lymphoid cells Used to treat rejection symptoms	*General* Intradermal test dose usually given to assist in predicting hypersensitivity Premedicate patient with acetaminophen and diphenhydramine about 30 min prior to drug administration to reduce severity of hypersensitivity reactions Have emergency equipment readily available during drug administration First dose of medication given more slowly (about 6 h), then over 4 h Large-volume infusion (about 1 L), which may require monitoring for heart failure and/or diuretics Monitor temperature and administer acetaminophen for relief of discomfort from fever and flulike symptoms Infection prevention precautions (see Chap. 9) Take extra care not to expose patient to viral pathogens when on this medication
Monoclonal antibodies: muromonab-CD3 (Orthoklone OKT3), OKT4, Xomazyme	Block immunologic function of lymphocytes Used to treat rejection symptoms	*General* No test dose required Premedicate patient with acetaminophen and diphenhydramine about 30 min prior to drug administration to reduce severity of hypersensitivity reactions Hypersensitivity most likely to occur within 45–60 min of administration Have emergency equipment readily available during drug administration May give peripherally or centrally Use filtered needle to withdraw medication from vial Usually administered intravenous push over 1–3 min

Table 14.6 *Continued*

Agents	Actions	Nursing Implications
Monoclonal antibodies (*cont.*)		Monitor temperature and administer acetaminophen for relief of discomfort from fever and flulike syndrome
		Concomitant steroids may be given with the first few doses to abrogate severe flulike syndrome
		Infection prevention precautions (see Chap. 9)
Polypeptide antibiotics: cyclosporine (Sandimmune)	Similar to antibiotics, but target specific proteins found on lymphoid cells called cyclophilines and block activation and mediator release by T cells, but without myelosuppression Used to prevent rejection, with possible dose escalations to treat rejection symptoms	*General*
		Monitor the patient closely for hypersensitivity reactions during initial drug administration
		Have emergency equipment readily available during drug administration
		Monitor blood pressure frequently; administer antihypertensive agents as ordered
		Assess for headache, dizziness, vomiting, altered mental status, reflex bradycardia, or other symptoms of hypertension
		Avoid fluid overload, which will worsen hypertension
		Monitor for common electrolyte disturbances—hyperkalemia and hypomagnesemia
		Weigh patient daily
		Perform mental status exams and routinely assess for confusion or inappropriate behavior indicative of neurotoxicity
		Assist with activities of daily living, particularly if drug-related tremors are present
		Monitor drug levels for possible toxicity, particularly with renal insufficiency or medications known to enhance toxicities (eg, busulfan decreases seizure threshold and may enhance neurotoxicity; aminoglycoside antibiotics or amphotericin B enhance renal toxicity)
		Risk of cyclosporine toxicity increased with histamine H_2 blockers, anabolic steroids, oral contraceptives, erythromycin, oral antifungals, calcium channel blockers
		Be aware of medications known to interfere with cyclosporine activity: rifampicin, phenytoin, barbiturates
		Cyclosporine increases risk of digoxin toxicity, possibly requiring lower doses

		Long-term use Instruct patient to monitor fluid intake Instruct patient to obtain and monitor blood pressure, reporting hypertension as defined by the physician Advise patient that tremors diminish as the dose is decreased Advise patient to maintain oral health and see the dentist at least every 6 months
Tacrolimas (Prograf, FK506)	Used in place of cyclo-sporine when renal dysfunction is present	*General* Monitor neurologic status while taking this medication Take with food to reduce GI distress Use cautiously with renal disease, hepatic disease Monitor hematology, chemistry, and hepatic transaminase studies

Reference

1. Danovitch G. *Handbook of Kidney Transplantation.* Boston: Little, Brown, 1992. p. 324.

Appendixes

Modalities Used in Critical Care

Mary Clark Robinson

I. Chest tubes

A. Indications
1. Pneumothorax.
2. Tension pneumothorax.
3. Pleural effusion.
4. Hemothorax.
5. Empyema.
6. Following cardiotomy.

B. Setup
1. Obtain the drainage system of choice; usually a closed drainage system or chest-tube bottle is used.
2. Unwrap the closed drainage system or bottle, and set it upright.
3. Fill the water seal by pouring sterile fluid through the latex suction tubing or top of the bottle.
4. If suction is desired, obtain wall suction or suction device.
5. Many closed drainage systems require that the suction control chamber be filled to the 20-cm H_2O mark. Other closed drainage systems may require as little as 15 mL of sterile water or none, according to manufacturer recommendations.
6. With sterile technique, connect the latex tubing from the collection chamber to the chest tube.
7. Connect the latex suction tubing to the suction source, and turn on suction. Remember that the amount of suction from the wall does not determine the amount of suction as ordered. Preset the wall suction between 20–25 cm H_2O.
8. Secure with tape all connections from chest drainage device to patient. Cross-bridging or using tape in opposite directions is helpful to prevent slippage of the connections.

C. Nursing care
1. Initiate actions to ensure assessment and promotion of respiratory function.
2. Auscultate breath sounds every 4 hours until stable and then every 8 hours. Assess breathing pattern (eg, rate, rhythm, and chest expansion).
3. Provide oxygen as ordered by the physician.

4. Monitor vital signs every hour until stable and then every 2 hours.
5. Assist patient into position of maximum ventilation and comfort (eg, elevate head of bed, upright position, support of body with pillows).
6. If postcardiotomy, assess chest tube drainage at least every hour until bleeding is decreased. If generous bleeding suddenly stops, immediately assess for cardiac tamponade (see Chap. 5) and notify physician.
7. Consult with respiratory therapist in regard to delivery, timeliness, effectiveness, and outcomes of respiratory procedures.
8. Initiate actions to ensure promotion of proper functioning of chest-tube drainage system.
9. Maintain a sterile closed drainage system. Protect chest-tube collection chambers. Keep chest-tube collection system below the chest level.
10. Monitor gentle bubbling action of chest-tube collection system if connected to suction.
11. Check water level in chamber every 8 hours and document. (After several days of suction use, water may need to be added to maintain the proper amount of suction).
12. Monitor quantity and character of drainage and/or air leaks every 4 hours.
13. Mark fluid level in collection chamber with date and time every 8 hours.
14. Assess chest tubes every 4 hours for obstruction, and gently massage tubes only if indicated (eg, blood clots).
15. Assess patient for chest pain, intercostal indentation, inspiration pain, shortness of breath, breath sounds absent over drainage area, and unequal chest expansion. Notify physician of any changes.
16. Monitor tracheal deviation, indicating mediastinal shift, and report any deviation immediately.
17. Initiate actions for prevention of infection.
18. Observe chest-tube insertion site for signs and symptoms of infection (eg, redness, tenderness, purulent drainage, and temperature) every shift. Reinforce dressing around chest tube insertion site if necessary.
19. Inspect respiratory secretions every shift for signs and symptoms of change in color, consistency, amount, and frequency. Obtain cultures for respiratory secretions if ordered.
20. Initiate actions to ensure education of patient and family or friends.

D. Complications
1. Continuously observe the patient for signs and symptoms of pneumothorax and pleural effusion because a disruption in the drainage system can cause these to recur.
2. If the patient pulls out the chest tube, evaluate whether an air leak was present. If no air leak, apply an occlusive dressing, and notify the physician. If there is an air leak, apply a dressing but release it periodically so air can escape or at any signs of respiratory distress.
3. If there is a lack of drainage, evaluate the patient's condition and disease process. Has the drainage tapered off over the past few shifts? Is the patient's condition deteriorating rapidly? If so, attempts should be made to gently massage or strip the tubing to dislodge clots. If the patient is stable, evaluate the system, and determine if there are kinks in the system or if gravity is not assisting the system to drain.

4. The collection chambers are full. Obtain a new system. Change the system out; maintain sterility at the chest-tube/chest-drainage connection.

II. Autotransfusion

A. Indications
   1. Trauma with thoracic bleeding injury.
   2. Hemothorax.
   3. Following open heart surgery.
   4. Significant bleeding in patients who have religious objections to transfusions.
   5. Contraindicated for patients with pericardial, mediastinal, pulmonary, or systemic infections; malignant neoplasms in the thorax; coagulopathies; and those with enteric contamination of the pleural space.
B. Setup
   1. Set up the autotransfer per manufacturer's instructions.
   2. Ensure that all clamps are open and all connections are tight.
   3. Mark the autotransfusion bag with the patient's name, date, and time of the start of blood collection.
   4. Blood collection and autotransfusion must be completed in less than 4 hours total.
C. Nursing care
   1. When a significant amount of blood has collected in the autotransfusion bag, clamp chest drainage tube and the tube attached to the chest drainage system. Disconnect autotransfusion setup from the patient. Reattach replacement autotransfusion bag. If further autotransfusion is needed, attach connector provided by the manufacturer between patient tubing and chest drainage tube. Unclamp tubes and continue with chest suction or autotransfusion.
   2. Measure and record the amount of blood in the autotransfusion system, and then remove and discard metal frame.
   3. Invert the autotransfusion bag so that the spike points upward, and remove the protective bag.
   4. Keeping the bag inverted, open the roller clamp of the transfusion set, and squeeze air out of the bag.
   5. Fill drip chamber to half full, adding an additional filter if mandated by hospital protocol.
   6. Turn the bag upright, and prime the remainder of the infusion set.
   7. Anticoagulation may or may not be used. If ordered, citrate–phosphate–dextrose (CPD) or heparin may be added to the autotransfusion bag, with an 18-gauge needle, via the latex port on the top of the bag. The usual dose of CPD is 30 mL per 300 mL of blood.
   8. Confirm that the blood is the patient's blood, and administer the blood to the patient. The autotransfusion procedure must be completed within 4 hours.
D. Complications
   1. Coagulopathies.
   2. Infection.
   3. Particulate or air embolism.
   4. Citrate toxicity if CPD used.

III. Hemodynamic monitoring

A. Indications
  1. Arterial pressure monitoring.
  2. Central venous pressure (CVP) monitoring.
  3. Pulmonary artery (PA) pressure monitoring.
  4. Left atrial pressure monitoring.
B. Setup
  1. Obtain equipment including: 500-mL bag of 0.9 normal saline or 5% dextrose in water, heparin additive per hospital policy, pressure bag, pressure tubing system with flush device and transducer, manifold for holding transducer, pressure cables, and IV pole.
  2. Prepare heparinized solution, mix thoroughly with IV solution, and label bag.
  3. Attach pressure tubing and transducer setup to IV bag. Place IV bag into the pressure bag, but do not inflate.
  4. Hang pressure bag, and tighten all connections.
  5. Prime the pressure tubing and entire system. Open stopcocks, remove all air, and recap with nonvented caps.
  6. Remove air from IV solution bag per hospital policy.
  7. Inflate the pressure bag to 300 mm Hg in order to provide for continuous flush of heparinized solution at 3 mL/h.
  8. Connect transducer to pressure monitor via cable following setup of the monitor for the mode of choice. Program pertinent patient information into the computer, and set alarms.
  9. Level the transducer, and complete zero and calibration measurements per manufacturer specifications. Ensure that the catheter is open to air via stopcock and closed to the patient for this procedure. Reopen stopcock to patient following procedure.
  10. The system is now ready to be attached to the arterial line, PA line, central venous pressure (CVP) line, or left ventricular line.
C. Nursing care
  1. Attach the pressure tubing to the monitoring catheter.
  2. Equalize the transducer's level with that of the right atrium or the phlebostatic axis (fifth intercostal space midaxillary line).
  3. Rezero and recalibrate if necessary. Ensure that stopcocks are in the proper position for monitoring.
  4. Rezero after each change in bed position and per policy.
  5. Document waveform and record values.
  6. Monitor values, adjust care, and interventions per physician orders.
D. Arterial pressure monitoring
  1. Check and compare cuff blood pressure with arterial pressure for baseline information.
  2. Assess the arterial waveform for evidence of a dicrotic notch, indicating closure of the aortic and pulmonic valves seen at the end of ventricular systole.
  3. Assess the color, pulse, and sensation distal to the arterial insertion site every 2 hours and document.

4. Notify the physician of any changes in circulation or signs of infection.
5. Change the dressing with sterile technique per hospital policy.
6. If the waveform dampens, check pressure bag inflated to 300 mm Hg, IV fluids in bag, position of extremity; flush line and evaluate patency. Notify the physician if unable to resolve.
7. On removal, hold pressure 5–10 minutes to ensure hemostasis.

E. Complications
   1. Infection.
   2. Sepsis.
   3. Loss of arterial circulation in the affected extremity.

F. Central venous pressure monitoring
   1. Attach the pressure tubing to the distal port of the triple- or double-lumen catheter for monitoring. If CVP monitoring is obtained via a thermodilution catheter, the proximal port or cardiac output port is attached to the pressure tubing.
   2. Obtain all readings with the transducer set at the level of the right atrium.
   3. Assess the waveform and values. The mean value should be determined at the end of expiration if the patient is breathing spontaneously.
   4. If the patient is ventilated, the CVP should be measured just before the inspiration cycle.
   5. Normal CVP values range from 4 to 12 mm Hg.

G. Complications
   1. If subclavian vein is used, pneumothorax, hemothorax, and air embolus all are potential complications during insertion.
   2. Infiltration of fluid into the pleural space.
   3. Dysrhythmias.
   4. Infection and sepsis.

H. PA pressure monitoring
   1. Attach the pressure tubing to the distal port (yellow) of the thermodilution catheter. The distal port should be positioned in the pulmonary artery and reflect these pressures.
   2. Obtain PA pressure readings continuously, and adjust care and interventions per physician order.
   3. Obtain readings with the transducer leveled (air–fluid interface to the phlebostatic axis).
   4. Measure all pressures at end-expiration.
   5. Analyze waveform for adequacy and document pressure readings.
   6. Place the patient supine with head of bed elevated no higher than 60 degrees.
   7. Do not use the distal port for any medications or IV fluids.
   8. Normal PA pressure values range from 20 to 30 mm Hg systolic and from 8 to 12 mm Hg diastolic.
   9. Mixed venous blood samples are obtained from this port.
   10. Change dressing per hospital policy.
   11. Continuously monitor the PA waveform for dampening, wedging, or backward migration to the right ventricle.

I. Complications
   1. Pneumothorax and hemothorax on insertion.

2. Ventricular dysrhythmias, particularly on insertion.
3. Thromboembolism.
4. Infection.
5. Clot formation.
6. Air embolism with wedging.
7. Pulmonary infarction.
8. Aortic rupture.

J. **Left atrial pressure monitoring.** The pulmonary artery wedge pressure (PAWP) is obtained by inflating the balloon port on the pulmonary artery catheter. The purpose of this reading is to provide information about the patient's left atrial pressure, which indirectly reflects the preload of the left side of the heart. Accurate measurement is affected by increased airway pressure such as that created with positive end-expiratory pressure (PEEP) and continuous positive airway pressure (CPAP).

1. Indication
   a. Left atrial pressure monitoring.
2. Setup
   a. The procedure for obtaining the PCWP involves inflating the balloon on the PA catheter with just enough air to obtain a wedge waveform, which is similar to a ventricular fibrillation pattern on the ECG. Never administer more than 1.5 mL of air to achieve this pattern.
   b. Normal values for the PCWP are 4–12 mm Hg.
3. Nursing care
   a. Allow the balloon to passively deflate following the measurement of the PCWP, and ensure the return of a pulmonary artery waveform on the monitor.
4. Complications
   a. Balloon rupture.
   b. Damage to the PA.
   c. Air embolism.
   d. Inadvertent wedging. If inadvertent wedging occurs or if a waveform is lost, request that the patient cough, turn the patient on side, move patient's arm, or flush catheter. Notify the physician if the wedging of the catheter continues.

IV. Cardiac output. Intermittent cardiac output (CO) determination involves the use of fluid bolus for determination of CO.

A. Indications
   1. Myocardial infarction with complications.
   2. Shock states.
   3. Multiple trauma with hemodynamic compromise.
   4. Cardiac tamponade.
   5. Sepsis.
B. Setup
   1. Obtain CO module.
   2. Turn on CO module and set parameters according to manufacturer's instructions and the computation constant of the thermodilution catheter used.

3. Connect the thermistor port with the CO module cable.
4. Obtain or access the closed system for delivery of injectate; obtain injectate solution (5% dextrose in water is typically used, however normal saline is acceptable). Iced or room-temperature injectate may be used as determined by physician.
5. Connect the injectate tubing to the proximal port (blue) using a three-way stopcock.
6. Attach the in-line temperature probe to the side port of the stopcock, on the side of the proximal lumen, in order for the machine to accurately determine CO values.

C. Nursing care
1. Begin the injection by turning the stopcock off to the proximal lumen, and withdrawing into the attached 10-mL syringe 10 mL of injectate solution from the IV bag. Purge all air bubbles prior to injection of solution into the proximal port.
2. Ensure that the PA catheter is properly placed by verifying the waveform.
3. Activate the CO computer and wait for the monitor to indicate that the computer is ready.
4. When the computer is ready, turn the stopcock off to the solution and open it between the filled syringe and the proximal port; press the start button on the computer.
5. Immediately inject the injectate solution into the proximal port. This should be done very quickly and be completed smoothly in less than 4 seconds.
6. Observe the thermodilution injection curve on the monitor to ensure adequate and consistent performance. An even injection is evidenced by a smooth and rapid upstroke on the curve.
7. At least three injections (repeating same process) are necessary to obtain an accurate calculation of CO. (If iced injectate is used, the injections must be spaced apart by at least one minute.
8. Once the process is completed, it will be necessary to restart the drip, or monitor that the proximal port was being used, or the port will need to be heparinized to maintain patency.
9. Normal CO value is considered 4 to 8 L/min.
   Note: Continuous CO monitoring via a specialized thermodilution catheter is available in some clinical settings. This catheter uses a thermal method for continuous CO measurement. A small amount of heat is generated in a pseudorandom binary sequence, and the distal thermistor detects the temperature changes and calculates the CO. No user intervention is required to obtain these continuous CO readings.

D. Complications
1. Inaccurate readings.
2. Arrhythmias.
3. Fluid volume overload is a rare complication if frequent CO is ordered for patients at risk for CHF.

V. Coronary artery bypass graft

A. Indications
   1. Treatment of severe angina pectoris when medical therapy or percutaneous transluminal coronary angioplasty (PTCA) has failed.
   2. Treatment of significant left main coronary atherosclerosis.
   3. Severe triple-vessel coronary artery disease.

B. Setup
   1. Secure an acute care intensive care bed for the recovery of the patient following coronary artery bypass graft (CABG).
   2. Prepare bedside for hemodynamic monitoring, ventilation, multiple IV drips, and possible use of hypothermia/hyperthermia unit.

C. Nursing care
   1. On the patient arrival to the ICU, establish monitoring of ECG, arterial line, pulmonary artery line, temperature, respirations, and arterial oxygen saturation (SaO_2).
   2. Assess breath sounds on admission and at least every 2 hours or on change in the patient's condition.
   3. Attach endotracheal tube to the ventilator. Set parameters per physician order.
   4. Evaluate the adequacy of ventilation through SaO_2 values, arterial blood gas (ABG) analysis, and patient's appearance. Ensure alarms are set.
   5. Validate adequacy of waveforms and BP cardiac output status.
   6. Record heart rate, BP, respiratory rate, pulmonary artery pressures on admission and every 15 minutes for 1 hour, then every 30 minutes until condition is stable, and then every hour for the first postoperative day.
   7. Monitor pulmonary wedge pressure, cardiac output, and systemic vascular resistance on admission and every 4 hours while PA catheter is in place.
   8. Monitor patient's temperature for symptoms of hypothermia/hyperthermia or infection.
   9. Monitor, document, and evaluate the patient's ECG on an ongoing basis for the presence of dysrhythmias and conduction defects. Notify the physician of pertinent changes in rhythm or rate.
   10. Assess mediastinal chest tube drainage on arrival and every hour for the first 8 hours. Attach to suction, if ordered, to promote patency and tape connections. Gentle stripping may be used for tubes that are not attached to suction. Notify the physician if blood loss is excessive or if bleeding suddenly stops.
   11. Promote adequate deep breathing, coughing, and/or suction every 2 hours to prevent pulmonary complications.
   12. Observe for abdominal distention on admission to the ICU and continuously while the patient is intubated. Consider insertion of a nasogastric tube if distention occurs.
   13. Place antiembolism/TED stockings on patient per physician order.
   14. Provide adequate pain assessment and relief in order to increase patient comfort as well as promote mobility and pulmonary function.
   15. Turn the patient every 2 hours as soon as condition is stable.

16. Assess the patient's readiness for weaning and extubation as evidenced by the following: patient response to verbal stimuli and ability to follow commands, Sao_2 maintained greater than 94%, spontaneous tidal volume of at least 5 mL/kg of patient weight, spontaneous respiratory rate greater than 8 breaths/minute and stable BP.

17. Monitor hourly intake and output, and correlate to hemodynamic parameters such as PA pressure, pulse rate, and arterial pressure.

18. Intervene per physician's orders with fluids, blood, volume expanders, and pharmacologic therapy.

19. Notify the physician of urine output less than 30 mL/hour.

20. Assess laboratory data for abnormal values, and report to the physician.

21. Monitor neurologic status, and notify the physician of any new deficits.

22. Promote early mobility to enhance pulmonary function and to prevent venous stasis.

23. Assess peripheral pulses, temperature, and color of extremities every hour for the first 8 hours.

24. Use sterile technique with dressing changes, endotracheal suctioning, urinary catheters, chest tubes, and IV lines to prevent infection.

25. Ensure support to the sternal incision during coughing or mobility activities.

26. Provide information and educate the patient and family as appropriate.

D. Complications
  1. Sternal wound infection.
  2. Development of dysrhythmias: atrial, ventricular, and heart blocks.
  3. Myocardial infarction.
  4. Stroke.
  5. Congestive heart failure.
  6. Cardiogenic shock.
  7. Cardiac tamponade.
  8. Pneumonia, atelectasis, pneumothorax, pulmonary embolism.
  9. Stress ulcer.
  10. Disseminated intravascular coagulation.
  11. Renal failure.

VI. Coronary stents

A. Indications
  1. Acute or threatened closure of a coronary artery.
  2. Acute or threatened closure of a coronary artery bypass graft (CABG).
B. Setup
  1. The patient considered for a stent must be adequately anticoagulated to reduce risks of thrombus.
  2. Any patient who might be considered for a stent following unsuccessful PTCA therapy should begin receiving aspirin, dipyridamole, and a calcium channel blocker prior to the procedure.
  3. Once the decision has been made to implant a stent, administration of heparin and dextran should be started.
  4. Nitroglycerin may be ordered prior to procedure to reduce the risk of coronary artery spasm.

C. Nursing care
   1. On arrival of the patient after stent placement, evaluate patient's hemo-dynamic status, groin access site, and comfort level.
   2. Prepare for continuous monitoring of the patient's hemodynamic status.
   3. Attach cable to transducer, and begin monitoring arterial pressures. Evaluate adequacy of arterial waveform. Monitor BP closely.
   4. Assess the affected groin area for bleeding or hematoma.
   5. Assess pulse, sensation, temperature, and color in affected extremity every 15–30 minutes.
   6. Unexplained hypotension should be assumed to be retroperitoneal bleeding until proven otherwise.
   7. Instruct the patient to notify the nurse of any symptoms of chest pain or discomfort, and emphasize the importance of this notification.
   8. Medicate patient to alleviate any chest pain, and immediately notify the physician of patient's condition.
   9. Obtain ECG immediately if the chest pain is cardiac in nature.
   10. IV drips should include heparin and dextran.
   11. Adjust heparin drip to maintain partial thromboplastin time (PTT) and activated clotting time (ACT) in therapeutic ranges. Heparin doses usually follow standard percutaneous transluminal coronary angioplasty (PTCA) protocols for the institution.
   12. The PTT should be checked at least every 6 hours while the patient is receiving heparin to ensure adequate anticoagulation.
   13. Monitor intake and output closely. Intervene to correct fluid deficits or fluid overload.
   14. Instruct the patient to lie supine and keep affected leg immobile while the sheath or sheaths are in place and for 24 hours following removal of the sheath.
   15. Over the next 24–48 hours, bed rest should be maintained with a gradual increase in activities.
   16. Do not elevate head of bed more than 30 degrees.
   17. Assist the patient in repositioning at least every 2 hours.
   18. Commonly ordered medications include warfarin, calcium channel blockers, and dipyridamole. These should be started as soon as they can be tolerated by the patient.
   19. It takes 4–7 days to adjust warfarin doses in stent patients. Once therapeutic prothrombin time (PT) is achieved, the heparin can be discontinued.
   20. Warfarin therapy will continue for 2 months poststenting.
   21. Heparin drip is discontinued temporarily to prepare for sheath removal. Monitor PTT or ACT results, and check prior to sheath removal.
   22. Remove sheath per unit protocol.
   23. Following sheath removal, it is important to promote adequate stasis without the development of hematoma or pseudoaneurysm. It is recommended that direct pressure be held a minimum of 60 minutes.
   24. Following sheath removal, monitor patient closely for bleeding from groin site and possible hematoma.
   25. Assess circulation to affected leg following removal of the sheath and periodically over the next 6 hours.

26. Instruct the patient to notify the nurse of any sensations of warmth in the affected area and/or back pain.
27. Following sheath removal, monitor the patient's hemodynamic status closely, and evaluate the need for possible fluid replacement.
28. Teach the patient about groin care, notification of physician about chest pain, medications, and the continued health threat of coronary artery disease.

D. Complications
1. Acute myocardial infarction (MI).
2. Tear of the coronary artery under manipulation.
3. Anaphylactic reaction to the stent.
4. Bleeding or hematoma at the site of insertion.
5. Damage to the circulation of the affected extremity.
6. Fragmentation of atherosclerotic plaque and possible embolism.
7. Emergency CABG surgery.

VII. Intra-aortic balloon pumps

A. Indications
1. Left ventricular failure with or without cardiogenic shock.
2. Left ventricular dysfunction with an ejection fraction less than 30% or a cardiac index of 1.8 or less.
3. Patients with heart failure who are awaiting transplantation.
4. Preoperatively for coronary artery disease with left coronary artery obstruction.
5. Intraoperatively for patients who demonstrate an inability to wean from the heart–lung bypass machine.
6. Acute MI.
7. Ventricular septal defects.
8. Unstable angina refractory to treatment.

B. Setup
1. Obtain baseline hemodynamics (arterial BP, pulse, respirations, and PA pressure) prior to insertion if possible.
2. If assisting with insertion, obtain the balloon catheter, percutaneous insertion kit, the balloon pump console, sterile gowns, gloves, and drapes, 4 × 4 in. sponges, povidone-iodine solution, lidocaine, suture, syringes, and needles.
3. Confirm that consent form has been signed, and assist with patient education as appropriate.
4. Begin monitoring the ECG. This may be accomplished by a monitor on the balloon console or through a slave cable from the bedside to the console. It is important to monitor in a lead that provides an adequate R wave and QRS complex, since this is used to trigger the pump to inflate and deflate.
5. Arterial monitoring is necessary and can be obtained via a radial artery catheter or through the central lumen of the intra-aortic balloon. The arterial line waveform is necessary for timing of inflation and deflation.
6. Thermodilution catheters are often used to assist in monitoring hemodynamic status.
7. Set up the balloon pump per manufacturer specifications.

8. Evaluate gas supply, ensure canister is full, and turn supply on.
9. Select trigger control.
10. Prepare the catheter for insertion via manufacturer specifications.
11. Prepare and drape patient, and provide sterile field; gowns, caps, and masks should be worn.
12. The physician should have training prior to insertion. The trained physician inserts the balloon catheter.
13. Typically the femoral site is used. Pulses should be checked prior to insertion and the site chosen based on this assessment.
14. When the catheter is correctly placed, the balloon–lumen connection tubing is then attached to the pump console by the nurse and counterpulsation is initiated.
15. The catheter is sutured at the insertion site.
16. Following insertion, check the pulses distal to the insertion site.

C. Nursing care
1. Following insertion, place a sterile dressing over insertion site, and keep clean and dry.
2. Assess balloon waveform for appropriate timing of inflation and deflation.
3. Set pump alarms on the console.
4. On the nursing record, place a tracing of the arterial line with intra-aortic balloon pump augmentation of 1:2 to document optimal timing. Document this at least once every 8 hours.
5. Observe the insertion site for bleeding or signs of hematoma formation. Check pulses distal to the site every 15 minutes for the first hour following insertion, then every 30 minutes for the next hour, and then every hour.
6. A daily chest x-ray should be ordered and evaluated for correct placement of the intra-aortic balloon pump catheter. The radiopaque square should be visible between the second and third intercostal space.
7. In an effort to maintain proper alignment, the patient should be instructed to keep the hip and leg of the affected extremity straight. This may require use of a soft restraint or sedation.
8. Do not elevate the head of the bed more than 30 degrees.
9. Monitor the left radial/brachial pulses hourly to ensure that the catheter has not migrated upward and occluded the left subclavian artery.
10. Hourly outputs should be recorded and the physician notified if urine output drops below 30 mL/hour for 2 hours and for sudden onset of anuria. These symptoms could indicate that the intra-aortic balloon pump catheter has migrated and occluded the renal arteries.
11. Assess neurologic status at least every 4 hours.
12. Evaluate for anxiety and education needs for the patient and family.
13. Evaluate the patient's tolerance to the pump; assess the arterial waveform for appropriateness of timing of inflation and deflation.
14. Adjust timing as necessary, and evaluate effectiveness of changes.
15. The physician is responsible for removal of the intra-aortic balloon pump catheter.

D. Complications
1. Early inflation will result in the balloon inflating during systole, which will increase the workload or afterload of the heart.

2. Late inflation causes decreased perfusion of the coronary arteries.
3. Early deflation can create a vacuum and result in decreased coronary artery perfusion.
4. Late deflation increases the pressure in the aorta and, therefore, increases afterload.
5. Balloon rupture, as evidenced by blood in the catheter or the high leak alarm.
6. Infection.
7. Skin breakdown.
8. Loss of circulation in the affected extremity.

VIII. Balloon valvuloplasty

A. Indication
1. Alternative treatment for mitral or aortic stenosis.
B. Setup
1. Set up pressure bag, IV pole, and manifold for monitoring of arterial pressure if continued monitoring is ordered.
2. Zero and calibrate equipment on patient arrival from the cardiac catheterization laboratory.
C. Nursing care
1. Prepare for continuous monitoring of hemodynamic status.
2. Attach cable to transducer, and begin monitoring arterial pressures. Evaluate adequacy of arterial waveform.
3. On patient arrival at the intensive care unit (ICU), assess the affected groin area for bleeding or hematoma.
4. Assess pulse distal to insertion site.
5. Assess pulse, sensation, temperature, and color in affected extremity every 15–30 minutes.
6. Instruct the patient to notify the nurse of any symptoms of chest pain or discomfort, and emphasize the importance of this notification.
7. Medicate to alleviate pain.
8. Monitor ECG closely for the development of atrial arrhythmias or heart blocks.
9. Notify the physician promptly if arrhythmias develop.
10. Evaluate adequacy of cardiac output, and monitor intake and output closely.
11. Intervene to correct fluid deficits or fluid overload.
12. Instruct the patient to lie supine and keep affected leg immobile while the sheath or sheaths are in place and for several hours following removal of the sheath.
13. Do not elevate the head of bed more than 30 degrees.
14. Assist the patient in repositioning at least every 2 hours.
15. Commonly ordered medications include heparin and positive inotropic agents.
16. Monitor PTT or ACT results, and check prior to sheath removal.
17. Remove sheath per ICU protocol.
18. Following sheath removal, monitor patient closely for bleeding from groin site and possible hematoma.
19. Assess circulation to affected leg following removal of the sheath and periodically over the next 6 hours.

20. Instruct the patient to notify the nurse of any sensations of warmth in the affected area and/or back pain.
21. Following sheath removal, monitor hemodynamic status closely, and evaluate the need for possible fluid replacement.
22. Educate the patient about groin care, medications, and activity level.

D. Complications
1. Infection.
2. Decreased cardiac output.
3. Development of atrial or ventricular dysrhythmias and/or heart block.
4. Bleeding or hematoma at the site of insertion.
5. Damage to the circulation of the affected extremity.

IX. Biventricular assist device

A. Indications
1. Following acute myocardial infarction with cardiogenic shock that is unresponsive to pharmacologic interventions and intra-aortic balloon pump.
2. Post-cardiotomy ventricular dysfunction that is unresponsive to pharmacologic interventions and intra-aortic balloon support.

B. Setup
1. Obtain biventricular assist device console, and once inserted transport to surgical area to prepare for attachment to surgical cannulas.
2. Power up the console prior to priming level to allow for automated self-testing.
3. While surgical cannulization is being completed, prime the sterile blood pumps, purge of air, and connect to console.
4. Position the pumps at the level of the patient's atria, usually no lower than 25 cm below the patient's atria.
5. After connection of the blood pump tubing to the surgically implanted cannula, pumping is initiated.
6. The console automatically adjusts beat rate and systolic/diastolic ratios to optimize outflows.
7. The console is powered by electricity and air; however, if fully charged, an internal battery is available for 1 hour of operation.

C. Nursing care
1. Monitor electrocardiogram (ECG), arterial pressures, and filling pressures of the blood pump.
2. Observe blood pump flow and rate.
3. Observe arterial pressures for native contribution indications. The pump produces a pyramidlike arterial waveform; if native contributions are present, a variation resembling a dicrotic notch will appear in the waveform.
4. Laboratory protocols include hematologic studies for red cell damage, coagulation studies, blood chemistry analysis, urinalysis, and ABG analysis.
5. Key assessments include neurologic status, hemodynamics, hypothermia, oxygen status, and dysrhythmias. The presence of refractory rhythms will not decrease the cardiac output; however, they do increase the workload of the heart.
6. Assess and plan care to meet patient's psychosocial needs.

7. Adequate fluid volumes must be maintained, since this modality is volume sensitive and preload dependent.
8. Maintain ACTs between 180 and 200 seconds.
9. Adjust pump height for optimal flow. Other adjustments that affect output are provided by the machine.
10. Monitor patient's temperature continuously.
11. Heat loss is a potential problem with this treatment modality. Therefore, it is important to cover the connecting tubing with the thermal sleeves provided.
12. Infection is a potential risk, and patients should be placed on antibiotic therapy for 3 days following initial insertion.
13. Place sheepskin (wool side down) under the connecting tubing to prevent skin breakdown.
14. Implement nutritional support as soon as possible.
15. In the event of cardiac arrest, do not perform external cardiac massage because of risk of structural damage due to the presence of the cannulas in the myocardium.

D. Complications
1. Neurologic deficits related to embolism or decreased perfusion.
2. Infection.
3. Renal failure.
4. Bleeding.
5. Respiratory failure.
6. Failure to wean from assist device due to irreversible myocardial failure.

X. Automatic implantable cardioverter–defibrillator

A. Indications
1. Treatment of ventricular tachyarrhythmias in patients who have a high risk of sudden cardiac death. These patients have had one episode of cardiac arrest, not associated with a myocardial infarction (MI), which they survived.
2. Treatment of ventricular tachyarrhythmias that are inducible; treatment of a sustained hypotensive ventricular tachycardia or fibrillation that does not respond to conventional antiarrhythmic drug therapy.

B. Setup
1. All patients who are candidates for this treatment should undergo extensive cardiac evaluation, including angiography, electrophysiology testing, exercise stress testing, and serial drug testing.
2. Prior to insertion of the automatic implantable cardioverter–defibrillator (AICD), information must be gathered about the patient's normal rhythm, maximum heart rate, and types of ventricular and atrial rhythms that occur.
3. Before beginning implantation, it is important to verify the operational status of the equipment.
4. Obtain a standard external defibrillator for backup use during insertion and programming.

5. Implantation is the physician's responsibility and a procedure that is usually reserved for a cardiologist. This procedure is performed in the operating room.

C. Nursing care

1. On the patient's arrival at the unit, establish monitoring of ECG, arterial line, PA line, temperature, respirations, and Sao_2.
2. Assess breath sounds on admission and at least every 2 hours or on change in the patient's condition.
3. Attach endotracheal tube to the ventilator-set parameters per physician's order.
4. Evaluate the adequacy of ventilation through Sao_2 values, ABGs, and patient's appearance. Ensure that alarms are set.
5. Validate adequacy of waveforms and blood pressure (BP)/cardiac output status.
6. Record heart rate, BP, respiratory rate, and PA pressures on admission; continue to record every 15 minutes for 1 hour, then every 30 minutes until the patient's condition is stable, and then every hour for the first postoperative day.
7. Monitor patient's temperature for symptoms of hypothermia or hyperthermia or infection.
8. Monitor, document, and evaluate the patient's ECG on an ongoing basis for the presence of arrhythmias and conduction defects. Notify the physician of pertinent changes in rhythm.
9. Assess mediastinal tube drainage on arrival and every hour for the first 8 hours. Attach to suction, if ordered, to promote patency. Tape and secure all connections. Gentle stripping may be used for tubes that are not attached to suction. Notify the physician if blood loss is excessive.
10. Promote adequate deep breathing, coughing, and/or suction every 2 hours to prevent pulmonary complications.
11. Observe for abdominal distention on admission to the ICU and continuously while the patient is intubated. Consider insertion of a nasogastric (NG) tube if distention occurs.
12. Provide adequate pain assessment and relief to increase patient comfort, mobility, and pulmonary function. Use an objective pain scale to monitor discomfort.
13. Turn the patient every 2 hours as soon as condition is stable.
14. Assess the patient's readiness for weaning and extubation as evidenced by the following: patient response to verbal stimuli and ability to follow commands, Sao_2 maintained greater than 94%, spontaneous tidal volume of at least 5 mL/kg of patient weight, spontaneous respiratory rate greater than 8 breaths/minute, and stable BP.
15. Monitor hourly intake and output and correlate to hemodynamic parameters such as PA pressure, heart rate, and arterial pressure.
16. Intervene per physician's orders with fluids, blood, volume expanders, and pharmacologic therapy.
17. Notify the physician of urine output less than 30 mL/hour.
18. Assess laboratory data for abnormal values, and report to the physician.

19. Monitor neurologic status and document any deficits. Notify the physician of any new deficits.
20. Promote early mobility to enhance pulmonary function and to prevent venous stasis.
21. Assess peripheral pulses, temperature, and color of extremities every hour for the first 8 hours.
22. Prevent infection through the use of sterile technique with dressing changes, endotracheal (ET) suctioning, urinary catheters, chest tubes, and intravenous (IV) lines.
23. Ensure support to the sternal incision during coughing or mobility activities.
24. Observe cardiac rhythm for the development of ventricular tachycardia, and intervene with external defibrillation if the internal defibrillator fails and the patient loses consciousness.
25. Provide information and educate the patient and family as appropriate.

D. Complications
1. Infection.
2. Bleeding.
3. Thromboemboli.
4. Myocardial damage.
5. Potential mortality due to inability to defibrillate.
6. Acceleration of arrhythmias.
7. Fluid accumulation or formation of hematomas, cysts, or fibrotic tissue.
8. Psychological effects that include imagined shocking, fear of shocking, fear of loss of shocking capability, and dependency on mechanical device.

XI. Noninvasive temporary pacemakers

A. Indications
1. For the management of symptomatic second-degree atrioventricular block type I or Mobitz II and third-degree atrioventricular block.
2. To sustain the patient's rhythm until the conduction system returns to normal function.
3. May be used in an effort to treat atropine resistant bradycardias or for asystole unresponsive to pharmacologic interventions.

B. Setup
1. Place ECG monitoring electrodes on the chest to monitor ECG and attach to cable in the ECG input connection port.
2. A rhythm should appear on the screen. Adjust the gain to obtain a QRS with adequate R-wave height, and set alarms.
3. Prepare the skin prior to application to ensure good contact. Never shave hair under the electrodes; only clip hair if necessary.
4. Apply the electrode labeled "Back" to the back of the patient, on the left side, just below the scapula and beside the spine.
5. Apply the electrode labeled "Front," remove the covering over gel, and position on the left side of the precordium until the best waveform is achieved. Once this position is established, remove outer covering of

adhesive and press onto skin. Press on adhesive portion only to prevent gel displacement.

6. The heart should be centered anteriorly and posteriorly between the two electrodes.

C. Nursing care

1. Evaluate the patient's anxiety and need for education if possible.
2. If time is available, consider sedation and educate and reassure as the process continues.
3. Prior to activating the unit, inform the patient that he or she might experience twitching and discomfort when the pacemaker discharges.
4. Offer sedation and medication for pain as ordered.
5. Set the electrical current, measured in milliamperes (mA), to 0 before connecting the electrode cable to the monitor output cable. Ensure that the R wave is of adequate height to be sensed so that inappropriate discharge does not result.
6. Inform the patient, and turn the pacemaker on.
7. Turn the pacing rate dial to 10 beats beyond the patient's intrinsic rhythm and observe for pacemaker spikes.
8. Once spikes are observed, increase the mA output until capture is obtained. Capture is evidenced by each pacing spike being followed by a QRS complex. Once this is visualized, pacing threshold has been achieved. The mA should then be increased by 10% to ensure consistent capture.
9. Select the pacing mode in collaboration with physician. Demand mode should be chosen if ECG sensing is available. Fixed mode generates impulses that may compete with the patient's intrinsic rhythm.
10. Document the paced rhythm, mA mode, and rate during each shift and with any change in patient's condition.
11. Check the patient's vital signs, and evaluate whether or not the paced rhythm is contributing to an adequate cardiac output. Palpate pulse with every captured beat.

D. Complications

1. Anxiety and pain.
2. Competing dysrhythmias.
3. Burns and skin reactions in the area of electrode placement.
4. Inappropriate discharge and development of ventricular tachycardia or ventricular fibrillation.

XII. Temporary pacemakers: Transvenous and epicardial

A. Indications

1. Following open heart surgery, to prevent loss of cardiac output from bradyarrhythmias, atrial arrhythmias, or rhythms that may require overdrive pacing.
2. Following a myocardial infarction in which damage to the conduction system has occurred as evidenced by Mobitz II or third-degree heart block.
3. Symptomatic bradycardia caused by atrioventricular block, drug toxicity, and/or electrolyte imbalance.

B. Pacemaker setup

1. Obtain necessary equipment including the pacing catheter, the introducer kit, alligator clips, the pacing generator, pacing cables, sterile gowns, gloves, towels and drapes, povidone-iodine solution, syringes, gauze, and lidocaine; the exact equipment will depend on whether epicardial or transvenous pacing will be used.

2. Test pulse generator and check that battery is charged and functional. Press the "battery test" button to determine how much battery life remains.

3. Attach ECG monitor to patient, and assure that a peripheral IV is available and patent.

4. Prepare site chosen by the physician. The subclavian, jugular, antecubital, and femoral sites are typically used.

5. Transvenous catheter may be placed by an ECG-guided method or with the assistance of fluoroscopy per physician choice and availability of fluoroscopy.

C. Nursing care

1. The pacing wires can be inserted into the pulse generator or attached with a connecting cable.

2. Set the pacemaker rate to 10 beats above patient's intrinsic rate or at a rate determined by the physician.

3. Set the mA output to 0.

4. Turn the pacemaker on, and observe for a pacing spike and any evidence of capture as the mA output is slowly increased.

5. The pace indicator light should flash each time a pacing spike is noted on the ECG monitor.

6. Consult with physician to determine the sensitivity parameters and mode. Set threshold based on these parameters.

7. Use the lowest energy level needed for one-to-one capture.

8. Once satisfactory pacing is achieved, cover the catheter insertion site with povidone-iodine ointment and a sterile dressing.

9. Obtain an ECG recording, and document paced rhythm.

10. Provide continuous monitoring, and obtain a 12-lead ECG following placement.

11. Assess the pacing wires, generator, and connections every 8 hours.

12. Keep the patient on bed rest while the temporary catheter is in place.

13. Change the pacemaker dressing daily with sterile technique to prevent infection. Assess the insertion site for any signs of infection.

14. Change the battery for every 2–3 days of continuous use.

15. Wear rubber gloves when manipulating the wires or pacemaker to prevent electrical injury.

16. Check pacing parameters frequently, and keep clear plastic cover over pacing controls to prevent accidental changes in pacing settings.

17. Document rhythm and pacing parameters each shift and if the patient's status changes.

18. Notify the physician of rhythm disturbances or problems with failure to capture and misfiring.

D. Complications

1. Failure to pace. Check cable connections, and ensure that they are intact. Evaluate the position of the pacing wires by current or most recent x-ray.

Ensure that the generator is on, and replace the battery. Check the settings, adjust mA output and rate in an effort to correct problem. If available, change to another generator.

2. Failure to capture. Check to be sure that the settings on the pacemaker have not been changed. Check all connections, and increase the mA output slowly. Turn the patient on left side and then on right, if ineffective. Switch the electrodes from positive to negative terminal and vice versa.

3. Failure to sense patient's intrinsic beats. If pacemaker is undersensing, turn up sensitivity; if it is oversensing, turn down sensitivity. Determine if pacemaker is sensing an external stimulus. Remove all sources of electrical interference from the room, and ensure that the ground is intact. If unable to stop misfiring, turn pacemaker off, provided the patient's underlying rate will support an adequate cardiac output. Notify the physician.

4. Infection.

5. Inappropriate discharge and the development of life-threatening arrhythmias.

6. Punctured lung or heart.

XIII. Permanent pacemakers

A. Indications
   1. Symptomatic bradycardias.
   2. Unresolved second-degree heart block type II or third-degree heart block.

B. Setup
   1. Permanent pacemakers are placed surgically either in the operating room or a cardiac catheterization laboratory.
   2. Patient needs to be educated preoperatively about the pacemaker, the procedure, and postimplantation care.
   3. The pacing generator is usually placed on the left or right side of the patient's chest at the level of the pectoral fascia.
   4. Once the pacing lead is in place, the physician will connect the lead to a pacing systems analyzer, and stimulation and pacing thresholds will be set.
   5. The lead is then connected to the patient's pacing generator, and the ECG is observed for adequate capture and function.
   6. The pacing generator is then sutured in place, and the patient is transferred to a stepdown or telemetry unit for observation.

C. Nursing care
   1. On return to the ICU, the patient's vital signs need to be checked, the dressing evaluated, and pain assessed.
   2. Bed rest may be required or the patient may be asked not to use his or her arm for the day.
   3. Obtain a 12-lead ECG if ordered.
   4. Observe BP and rhythm closely to ensure that pacemaker is functioning adequately and cardiac output is optimal.
   5. Document rhythm and vital signs.
   6. Prior to discharge, educate patient and family about monitoring patient's pulse and periodic transmission of ECG by telephone if applicable.

7. Educate about signs and symptoms of decreased cardiac output and situations requiring physician notification.
8. Discuss the pacer identification card and the importance of patient carrying it at all times.

D. Complications
1. Infection.
2. Failure to capture or inappropriate discharge; the permanent pacemaker can be readjusted and set by the patient's cardiologist.
3. Competitive dysrhythmias.

XIV. Percutaneous transluminal angioplasty (PCTA)

A. Indications
1. Symptomatic single- or multiple-vessel coronary artery disease that is amenable to dilation.
2. Acute evolving myocardial infarction (MI) with or without thrombolytic therapy.
3. Partially occluded CABGs.

B. Setup
1. Set up pressure bag, IV pole, and manifold for monitoring of arterial pressure if continued monitoring is ordered.
2. Zero transducer and calibrate equipment on patient's arrival from the cardiac catheterization laboratory.

C. Nursing care
1. Prepare for continuous monitoring of patient's hemodynamic status.
2. Attach cable to transducer, and begin monitoring arterial pressures. Evaluate adequacy of arterial waveform.
3. On patient's arrival to the ICU, assess the affected groin area for bleeding or hematoma.
4. Assess the pulse distal to the insertion site, sensation, temperature, and color in affected extremity, every 15–30 minutes per ICU protocol and document.
5. Instruct the patient to notify the nurse of any symptoms of chest pain or discomfort, and emphasize the importance of this notification.
6. Medicate to alleviate any chest pain, and notify the physician immediately of change in patient's condition.
7. Obtain a stat ECG if patient's chest pain is cardiac in nature.
8. Monitor intake and output closely. Increased fluid intake is necessary for dye removal. Intervene to correct fluid deficits or fluid overload.
9. Instruct the patient to lie flat, and keep affected leg immobile while the sheath or sheaths are in place and for several hours following removal of the sheath.
10. Do not elevate the head of bed more than 30 degrees.
11. Assist the patient with repositioning at least once every 2 hours.
12. Commonly ordered medications include nitroglycerin, heparin, calcium channel blockers, and dipyridamole.
13. Discontinue heparin infusion prior to sheath removal as ordered.
14. Monitor PTT or ACT results, and check prior to sheath removal.
15. Remove sheath per ICU protocol.

16. Following sheath removal, monitor patient closely for bleeding from groin site and for possible hematoma formation. Instruct the patient to notify nurse immediately of any wet sensation around the removal site or leg.

17. Assess circulation to affected leg, following removal of the sheath and periodically over the next 6 hours.

18. Instruct the patient to notify the nurse of any sensations of warmth in the affected area and/or back pain.

19. Following sheath removal, monitor the patient's hemodynamic status closely, and evaluate need for possible fluid replacement.

20. Teach patient about groin care, medications, continued risk of death related to coronary artery disease, and how to notify the physician for follow-up.

D. Complications

1. Partial or total occlusion of recently opened coronary artery(ies).
2. Acute myocardial infarction.
3. Tear of the coronary artery under manipulation.
4. Dissection of the coronary artery.
5. Bleeding or hematoma at the site of insertion.
6. Damage to the circulation of the affected extremity.
7. Fragmentation of atherosclerotic plaque and possible embolism requiring emergency CABG surgery.

XV. Intracranial pressure monitoring

A. Indications

1. Space-occupying lesions in the brain.
2. Severe head trauma.
3. Subarachnoid bleeding, resulting in a decrease in level of consciousness.
4. Clinical conditions, resulting in intracranial hypertension, in which knowledge of intracranial pressure (ICP) will assist in patient management.

B. Setup

1. Ensure consent and educate the patient about the procedure.
2. Obtain the ICP monitor, and attach monitor cable to bedside monitor.
3. Set up the ICP monitor per manufacturer instructions.
4. Prepare the insertion site with povidone-iodine scrub.
5. Assist the physician with insertion by instructing the patient to lie supine with head immobilized.
6. Sterile conditions must be maintained during insertion.
7. Attach the preamplifier connector from the ICP monitor to the sterile transducer connection. Zero the monitor. If the monitor does not zero, the physician may adjust the zero setting with a tool from the catheter kit. The monitor must be zeroed before insertion of the catheter.

C. Nursing care

1. Obtain baseline neurologic assessment.
2. Obtain baseline ICP reading.
3. Assess ICP every hour for the first 24 hours and then every 2 hours if the patient is stable.
4. Notify physician if ICP reading exceeds 20 mm Hg for 30 minutes.
5. Assess waveform, and document every shift.

6. Notify physician if waveform becomes dampened or is lost.
7. Maintain adequate oxygenation, and use caution when suctioning.
8. Prevent straining at stool.
9. Maintain the patient's neck in midline position.
10. Maintain quiet nonstressful environment.
11. Elevate head of bed 30–45 degrees.
12. Avoid positive pressure ventilation.
13. Maintain normothermia, and monitor temperature continuously.
14. Secure the ICP catheter, and use caution when moving the patient.
15. Observe the insertion site closely for signs and symptoms of infection.
16. Change the dressing every 72 hours using sterile techniques.
17. Provide pain management measures.
18. Restrain the patient, if necessary, to prevent pulling at the ICP catheter.
19. Perform neurologic assessment every 2 hours.
20. If the patient needs to be transported to the operating room or for computerized axial tomographic scan, the ICP catheter can be disconnected from the ICP monitor and reconnected with no problem.

D. Complications
1. Infection.
2. Kinking or bending of the catheter.
3. Dampening or loss of the ICP waveform.

XVI. Gastrointestinal intubation

A. Indications
1. Gastrointestinal bleeding.
2. Prevention of aspiration in intubated patients.
3. Administration of feedings and medications.
4. Abdominal surgery.
5. Continuous unrelieved nausea and vomiting.

B. Setup
1. Obtain and validate order for nasogastric tube insertion.
2. Measure the patient for the length of tube needed by measuring from the earlobe to the tip of the nose and down to the xiphoid process.
3. Position patient in a semi-Fowler's position if possible.
4. Obtain water soluble lubricant, and apply liberally to the end of the nasogastric tube.
5. Insert the tube through the nose, and gently pass down the back of the throat. If possible, request that the patient swallow, and offer sips of water to help advance the tube.
6. In the intubated patient, it may be helpful to flex the patient's head forward to advance the tube.
7. Insert the tube to the premeasured length.
8. Monitor closely for episodes of vomiting on insertion and signs and symptoms of respiratory distress. Remove the nasogastric tube at once if respiratory distress is noted.
9. Following placement, verify position by inserting 10–20 mL of air into tube and auscultating over stomach for air bubbling, or through aspiration of gastric contents.

10. Further verification may be documented by x-ray per physician order or per hospital policy. The more flexible feeding tube, such as the Entriflex (Sherwood Medical, St. Louis, MO), requires a chest x-ray to verify placement. Gastric contents are not always obtained with aspiration. These tubes may migrate into the lungs with violent coughing. Ensure proper position with tape markings.
11. Secure the nasogastric tube when proper placement is confirmed.
12. If unable to insert the nasogastric tube through the nasal passage, another option is to insert into the stomach via the mouth.

C. Nursing care
1. Confirm placement of the tube every shift and when the nasogastric tube is used for nutrition and medications.
2. When administering medications through the feeding tube, use liquid preparations whenever possible.
3. Document amount, color, and consistency of drainage if suction is in use.
4. Flush the feeding tube or irrigate every 4–6 hours with 60 mL of water.
5. Flush the feeding tube with at least 30 mL of water before and after administration of medications, and clamp for 30 minutes following administration.
6. Observe for signs and symptoms of aspiration.
7. Monitor bowel sounds every 8 hours.
8. In patients who have undergone gastric or esophageal surgery, manipulation of the tube should never occur without the appropriate order from the physician.
9. To promote tissue integrity, remove and replace the tape securing the tube daily.

D. Complications
1. On insertion, it is possible that the tube will go into the trachea instead of the esophagus. Patients must be monitored closely for respiratory distress, and placement must be documented.
2. Perforation of the pleural cavity or the occurrence of a pneumothorax are potential complications seen on insertion.
3. Aspiration pneumonia following aspiration of tube feedings or medications.
4. Nasal trauma following difficulty with insertion.

XVII. **Continuous arteriovenous hemofiltration–dialysis**

A. Indication
1. Treatment of patient who requires dialysis but whose condition becomes hemodynamically unstable with hemodialysis, or patient for whom peritoneal dialysis is contraindicated.

B. Setup
1. Obtain permits for continuous arteriovenous hemofiltration–dialysis (CAVH-D).
2. Obtain filter and tubing. Prime tubing and cap prior to connection.
3. Hang a 2-liter bag of dialysate on pump.
4. Mix heparin drip per hospital protocol, and hang drip on a second pump.
5. Hang filtration replacement fluid as ordered on a third pump. Prime, cap, and have ready.

6. Determine that all baseline data such as laboratory work, weight, and vital signs are complete and available prior to initiation of treatment.
7. Give loading dose of heparin as ordered 3 minutes prior to opening arterial and venous ports of the CAVH-D filter.
8. Place clamps at the bedside, and maintain at bedside throughout the treatment.

C. Nursing care
1. Complete setup, and prepare the patient for treatment.
2. Three minutes after loading dose of heparin, connect the dialysate to "in" end of dialysate side of filter, and set pump to run per physician's order.
3. Connect the heparin drip to the special port that appears thinner and longer on arterial access side of the filter, and set the pump to run per order.
4. Connect the filter replacement fluid to the pigtail on the venous return side of the filter, and set to run per physician's order and per calculations reflective of input and output and patient's positive or negative balance.
5. Place filter and maintain at the level of the heart at all times. Unclamp the lines to begin flow of blood through the filter.
6. Keep the lines from being compressed or kinked.
7. Flow rate is adjusted and affected by the position of the ultrafiltration bag, BP, and volume overload. The patient should have a systolic BP of at least 80–90 mm Hg and, for better results, preferably a systolic reading of 100 mm Hg.
8. Lowering the bag will increase negative pressure and increase the ultrafiltration rate. Never raise the ultrafiltration bag above the level of the filter.
9. Monitor the ultrafiltration bag carefully to ensure compliance with ranges specified by the physician.
10. Determine filtration replacement fluids based on previous hour's intake and output.
11. Monitor laboratory work and complete as ordered.
12. Monitor lines for equal warmth and no separation of blood in the line.
13. Assess pulse in the extremity used for cannulization at least every 4 hours.
14. Notify the physician of any vascular access problems, volume status problems, low systolic BP (< 60 mm Hg), and separation of the blood in the tubing.

D. Complications
1. Infiltration: Leakage, hematoma, or drainage at access site; patient arrest: clamp off arterial port.
2. Filter clots off: Decrease in hemoglobin and hematocrit.

XVIII. Slow and continuous ultrafiltration/continuous arteriovenous hemofiltration

A. Indications
1. Patient having acute renal failure, who require dialysis, but whose condition becomes hemodynamically unstable with hemodialysis, or patient for whom peritoneal dialysis is contraindicated.
2. Patient who has chronic renal failure and fluid overload.

B. Setup
1. Obtain hemofilter and tubing. Prime tubing and cap prior to connection using sterile technique.
2. Hang a 1000-liter bag of normal saline with 5000 U of heparin. Hang a 1000-liter bag of normal saline with 12.5 g of human albumin.
3. Attach a Y-type IV tubing setup to both bags, and prime the IV line with the albumin solution. Leave the second bag clamped.
4. Attach a three-way stopcock to the venous and arterial sides of the tubing on the filter.
5. Clamp the ultrafiltrate port, and attach the ultrafiltrate collection bag to the port.
6. Prime the filter and tubing.
7. Hang filtration replacement fluid as ordered on a third pump. Prime, cap, and have ready.
8. Determine that all baseline data such as laboratory work, weight, and vital signs are complete and available prior to initiation of treatment.
9. Place clamps at the bedside, and maintain at bedside throughout the treatment.

C. Nursing care
1. Complete setup, and prepare patient for treatment.
2. Attach the heparin drip of 12,500 U of heparin in 500 mL of 5% dextrose in water to the special port that appears on the arterial-access side of filter, and set pump to run per order.
3. Administer heparin bolus if ordered.
4. Connect the filter replacement fluid to the venous-return side of the filter, and set to run per physician order and per calculations reflective of input and output and patient's positive or negative balance.
5. Connect blood filter tubing to shunt connections, arterial side to arterial side and venous side to venous side.
6. Turn on the heparin drip as ordered, and unclamp arterial and venous tubing.
7. To begin hemofiltration, unclamp ultrafiltration port after 5 minutes of adequate blood flow through the filter.
8. Place the filter at the level of the heart at all times. Unclamp the lines to begin flow of blood through the filter.
9. Keep the lines from being compressed or kinked.
10. Flow rate is adjusted and affected by the position of the ultrafiltration bag, BP, and volume overload.
11. Lowering the bag will increase negative pressure and increase the ultrafiltration rate. Never raise the ultrafiltration bag above the level of the filter.
12. Monitor the ultrafiltration bag carefully to ensure compliance with ranges specified by the physician.
13. Determine filtration replacement fluids based on previous intake and output.
14. Monitor laboratory work, and complete as ordered.
15. Monitor lines for equal warmth and no separation of blood in the line.
16. Assess pulses in the extremity used for cannulization at least every 4 hours.
17. Notify the physician of any vascular access problems, volume status problems, low systolic BP (< 60 mm Hg), and separation of the blood in the tubing.

D. Complications
1. Infiltration.
2. Leakage, hematoma, or drainage at access site.
3. Patient arrest: Clamp off arterial port, and reinfuse blood and fluid replacement therapy as needed.
4. Clotting of filter.
5. Decrease in hemoglobin and hematocrit.
6. Infection.
7. Shock.

XIX. Peritoneal dialysis

A. Indications
1. Acute renal failure.
2. Chronic renal failure.
3. Fluid overload.
B. Setup
1. Obtain necessary equipment: Warmed dialysate, tubing administration set, syringes and needles, drainage bag, mask and sterile gloves, povidone-iodine solution, 4 × 4 in. gauze, and tape.
2. Obtain all predialysis laboratory work, and weigh the patient.
3. Wash hands, and use sterile technique throughout the procedure.
C. Nursing care
1. Evaluate the dialysate bag. Ensure that solution is warmed and clear and that bag is without leaks.
2. Check for added medications per physician's order, or prepare to add medications. Heparin and potassium are commonly added.
3. Add medications to bag under sterile conditions.
4. Prepare the medication port on the dialysis bag with povidone-iodine, and add each medicine with a separate needle.
5. Label the bag with names of medications, amount added, date, and time.
6. Prepare the patient for the procedure by answering questions and allaying concerns.
7. Spike the dialysate bag with the dialysis administration tubing, and prime the tubing with the dialysate solution.
8. Clean the end of the peritoneal catheter with povidone-iodine, and allow to dry.
9. Apply mask, and don sterile gloves.
10. Attach the dialysis administration tubing to the peritoneal catheter.
11. Begin instillation of the dialysate by gravity; usually a volume of 500–2000 mL is ordered and infused over a period of 10–20 minutes.
12. Observe the patient closely for any changes in vital signs, nausea, development of diarrhea, or respiratory compromise that could indicate malposition.
13. Following the infusion of the dialysate, clamp the tubing, and allow the dialysate to dwell in the peritoneal cavity 20–30 minutes.
14. After the dwell time is complete, open the clamp on the administration set, lower the dialysate bag, and allow the fluid to flow out.
15. Document the amount of drainage, its appearance, and clarity. The return

dialysate should appear clear and be either colorless or resemble the color of urine, unless this is one of the first few times the catheter has been used.

16. Calculate fluid balances accurately; the balance should be zero or negative.

17. Change the peritoneal dressing daily following sterile technique.

18. Assess the site frequently for signs of infection.

19. Monitor glucose levels to ensure tolerance of dialysate.

D. Complications

    1. Hypotension can result from hemodialysis. BP should be closely monitored; fluids and medications may be needed to counteract hypotension.

    2. Malpositioning of the peritoneal catheter.

    3. Perforation of the bowel or bladder.

    4. Infection and/or sepsis.

    5. Peritonitis.

    6. Fluid overload or dehydration.

XX. Mechanical ventilation

A. Indications

    1. Apnea

        a. Hypoxemia.

        b. Acute respiratory acidosis.

        c. Relieve respiratory distress.

        d. Prevent or reverse atelectasis.

        e. Stabilize the chest wall.

        f. Permit sedation.

        g. Decrease systemic or myocardial oxygen consumption.

    2. Acute respiratory distress syndrome (ARDS).

    3. Respiratory failure, defined as an ABG with arterial oxygen tension of less than 50 mm Hg, arterial carbon dioxide tension greater than 50 mm Hg in a patient without chronic lung disease, and a pH less than 7.25.

    4. Neurologic disorders such as amniotropic lateral sclerosis and Guillain-Barré syndrome.

    5. Neurologic injury that results in inadequate respiration.

B. Setup

The decision to use a ventilator is made by the physician. The type of ventilator and settings are usually predetermined.

    1. Ensure that the airway is supported by either an endotracheal or tracheostomy tube.

    2. Support ventilation via bag-valve mask device until ventilator is set up and values are obtained.

    3. Mechanical ventilation may occur via negative-pressure or positive-pressure ventilators. Negative-pressure ventilation is rarely used.

    4. Select the desired mode of ventilation: Assist control, synchronized intermittent mandatory ventilation, continuous positive airway pressure, pressure support ventilation, high-frequency jet ventilation, and positive end-expiratory pressure.

    5. Set the ventilator to the desired settings, which should include the fraction of inspired oxygen, tidal volume, respiratory rate, alarm limits, and sensitivity.

6. Begin ventilation.
7. Immediately evaluate effectiveness of ventilation via auscultation of breath sounds, pulse oximeter readings, vital signs, and cardiac monitor.
8. ABGs may be ordered after 30 minutes to evaluate patient response to mechanical ventilation and as needed throughout the period of artificial ventilatory need.

C. Nursing care
1. Assess respiratory rate, rhythm, and quality through auscultation and observation before mechanical ventilation and at least every 2 hours during mechanical ventilation.
2. Monitor for bilateral, full expansion of the lungs every 2 hours.
3. Evaluate vital signs and level of consciousness every 2 hours and laboratory values as ordered.
4. If the patient experiences signs and symptoms of respiratory distress and failure, notify the physician of changes.
5. Assess the position and patency of the artificial airway. Keep the skin clean and dry under the tracheostomy tube.
6. Note and record landmarks on the endotracheal tube every shift, and evaluate position on chest x-ray if available.
7. Suction the airway and mouth as needed based on assessment findings.
8. Provide education to patient, family, and significant others.
9. Ensure adequate ventilator function.
10. Identify ordered settings and confirm these settings and alarm parameters every 2 hours. Document all changes.
11. Maintain a bag-valve mask and oral airway at the bedside at all times.
12. Evaluate current nutritional status, and refer to dietitian for assistance in evaluating and maintaining patient's nutritional needs.
13. Ensure skin and tissue integrity during mechanical ventilation.
14. Change the position of the endotracheal tube daily from one side of the mouth to the other.
15. Check the cuff pressure of the artificial airway every shift to ensure pressure is less than 21 cm H_2O.
16. Secure the airway with tape or ties.
17. Initiate actions to minimize the risk of infection.
18. Use universal precautions.
19. Monitor secretions for appearance, consistency, and amount.
20. Turn the patient every 2 hours as appropriate.
21. Initiate actions to alleviate patient and family anxiety during the course of mechanical ventilation.
22. Educate the patient and family about equipment and monitors.
23. Provide an alternate means of communication and encourage communication.
24. Provide comfort measures.
25. Inform the patient of status and changes in condition.

D. Complications
1. Tube misplacement or dislocation.
2. Changes in breath sounds may forewarn of complications; thorough assessment is warranted.

3. If the patient is "bucking" the ventilator, assess for possible causes such as alteration in respiratory status, increased secretions or a mucous plug, oxygen disconnection, kinked tubing, inadequate ventilator settings, pneumothorax, alcohol or drug withdrawal, anxiety, or pain.

4. If the high-pressure alarm is activated, check for contributing causes, including secretions in the respiratory tract, water in the tubing, kinked tubing, biting of the tube, agitation, or pneumothorax.

5. If the low-pressure alarm is activated, evaluate for tubing disconnection or cuff leak.

6. Provide 100% oxygen via bag-valve mask if the source of the problem cannot be located and quickly corrected.

7. Cardiac arrest.

8. Barotrauma with positive-pressure ventilation.

9. Tracheal erosion.

XXI. Continuous positive airway pressure

This mode of ventilation is designed to increase lung volume and oxygenation by elevating end-expiratory pressure to levels above atmospheric pressure. It is proposed to reduce the pressure gradient between the mouth and the alveoli in patients with air trapping. This mode of ventilation is designed to assist spontaneously breathing patients and therefore requires an intact respiratory drive. It is useful in patients who have hypoxemia in part secondary to decreased lung volume. This mode of ventilation may be used in intubated as well as nonintubated patients.

A. Indications
1. Alveolar hypoventilation.
2. Persistent hypoxemia and/or hypercapnia.
3. Ventilatory muscle dysfunction.
4. Difficulty following extubation.
5. Upper-airway obstruction.
6. Refractory hypoxemia.

B. Setup
1. Two types of systems are available: (1) systems that use a ventilator and a demand valve and (2) systems that work on the principle of continuous high flow of pressurized gas in an external circuit from which the patient can breathe spontaneously.
2. Determine set-up parameters, which include pressure level and sensitivity. If using the demand-valve system, set the level of negative pressure. Flow threshold and basal flow rate are determined and set for continuous flow systems.

C. Nursing care
1. Auscultate respiratory rate, rhythm, and quality before mechanical ventilation and at least every 2 hours during mechanical ventilation.
2. Monitor for bilateral, full expansion of the lungs every 2 hours.
3. Evaluate breathing pattern, vital signs, and level of consciousness every 2 hours and laboratory values as needed.
4. Use pulse oximeter for continuous SaO_2 monitoring.
5. Mask ventilation does not guarantee either a patent or protected airway.

Special care should be taken when applying mask ventilation to patients who are obtunded or unconscious.

6. Monitor for compliance.
7. If the patient experiences signs and symptoms of respiratory distress and failure, notify the physician of changes.
8. Identify ordered settings, and confirm these settings and alarm parameters every 2 hours. Document all changes.
9. Maintain a bag-valve mask and oral airway at the bedside at all times.
10. Evaluate current nutritional status, and refer to dietitian for assistance in evaluating and maintaining patient's nutritional needs.
11. All patients with endotracheal tubes should have nasogastric tubes to prevent aspiration.
12. Ensure that disconnect alarms are set and functional.
13. Initiate actions to alleviate patient and family anxiety during the course of mechanical ventilation.
14. Educate the patient and family about equipment and monitors.
15. Provide comfort measures.
16. Inform the patient of status and changes in condition.

D. Complications
1. Cardiac/respiratory arrest.
2. Pneumothorax.
3. Pneumomediastinum.
4. Shortness of breath.
5. Tachycardia or severe bradycardia.
6. Gastric aspiration.
7. Hypotension.
8. Nausea.
9. Shakiness, dizziness.

XXII. Pressure-controlled inverse-ratio ventilation

Pressure-controlled inverse-ratio ventilation (PC-IRV) is a ventilatory mode in which the conventional inspiratory to expiratory ratio is inverse and mechanical breaths are pressure limited. In this mode of ventilation, the ventilator generates a servo-controlled square wave of pressure to the airways via a decelerating inspiratory flow. Flow profiles of appropriate length and inspiratory "holds" or "pauses" are applied as necessary for the desired inspiration-expiration (I:E) ratio. This mode may be desirable because it increases contact time between air and blood and increases mean airway pressure.

A. Indications: ARDS.
B. Setup. See Mechanical ventilation setup, p. 453.
C. Nursing care
1. Deep sedation or paralysis is nearly always required for this mode of ventilation, to avoid dyssynchrony with the ventilator.
2. Hemodynamic status may be adversely affected by this mode of ventilation; therefore, PA pressure monitoring and arterial pressure lines should be in place and assessed when PC-IRV is implemented.

3. Careful monitoring of minute ventilation is required during PC-IRV because tidal volume is markedly dependent on respiratory mechanics, especially compliance.
4. The auto-PEEP level, which may develop as the I:E ratio increases, should be measured at regular intervals.
5. Provide additional nursing care as delineated in the ventilation section of this addendum.

D. Complications
1. Pulmonary barotrauma.
2. Hemodynamic deterioration.

XXIII. Pressure support ventilation. Pressure support ventilation (PSV) is used to augment the patient's spontaneous tidal volume and decrease the work of breathing. As a breath is initiated, the ventilator delivers flow to the patient in proportion to patient's inspiratory effort while maintaining a preset inspiratory pressure. The patient must be capable of initiating a tidal volume to use this mode.

A. Indication
1. To augment patient's spontaneous tidal volume and decrease the work of breathing.

B. Setup
1. Obtain a ventilator that is functionally capable of providing pressure support.
2. Pressure support is started at the level that provides minute ventilation or tidal volume similar to conventional ventilation (10–12 mL/kg).
3. Set inspiratory pressure level.
4. There is no set tidal volume in pressure control ventilation unless it is used in conjunction with synchronized intermittent mandatory ventilation.

C. Nursing care
1. PSV reduces the work of breathing for most patients; therefore, patient comfort and tolerance of the ventilator may be enhanced by this mode.
2. Assess respiratory rate, rhythm, and quality through auscultation and observation before mechanical ventilation and at least every 2 hours during mechanical ventilation and as needed.
3. Ensure adequate humidity.
4. Monitor every 2 hours for bilateral, full expansion of the lungs.
5. Evaluate breathing pattern, vital signs, and level of consciousness every 2 hours and laboratory values as needed.
6. Evaluate for leaks around the cuff that may be due to the pressure-support gas flow.
7. If the patient experiences signs and symptoms of respiratory distress or failure, notify the physician of changes.
8. Assess the position and patency of the artificial airway.
9. Note and record landmarks on the endotracheal tube every shift, and evaluate position on chest x-ray if available.
10. Suction the airway and mouth as needed.
11. Provide education to patient, family, and significant others.
12. Ensure adequate ventilator function.

13. Identify ordered settings, and confirm these settings and alarm parameters every 2 hours. Document all changes.
14. Maintain a bag-valve mask and oral airway at the bedside at all times.
15. Evaluate pulmonary artery pressure, heart rate, BP, cardiac output, and mixed venous oxygen tension ($S\bar{v}o_2$) to determine tolerance to ventilation mode as ordered.
16. Evaluate current nutritional status and refer to dietitian for assistance in evaluating and maintaining patient's nutritional needs.
17. Take steps to ensure skin and tissue integrity during mechanical ventilation.
18. Change the position of the endotracheal tube daily from one side of the mouth to the other.
19. Check the cuff pressure of the artificial airway every shift to ensure pressure is less than 21 cm H_2O.
20. Secure the airway with tape or ties.
21. Initiate actions to minimize the risk of infection.
22. Monitor vital signs every 2 hours.
23. Monitor secretions for consistency, amount, and color.
24. Evaluate the need to suction every 2 hours and as needed.
25. Turn the patient every 2 hours as appropriate.
26. Initiate actions to alleviate patient and family anxiety during the course of mechanical ventilation.
27. Educate the patient and family about equipment and monitors.
28. Provide an alternate means of communication and encourage communication.
29. Provide comfort.
30. Inform the patient of status and changes in condition.

D. Complications
1. This technique may be poorly tolerated by patients with high airway resistance. Remember to monitor chest x-rays, breath sounds, chest excursion, mean airway pressure, and vital signs.
2. May cause alterations in cardiac output and patient's hemodynamic status.

XXIV. High-frequency jet ventilation

A. Indications
1. Critically ill patients with acute respiratory failure.
2. Anesthesia.
3. Adult respiratory distress syndrome (ARDS).
B. Setup
1. Clinicians must be very familiar with ventilatory settings, types of injection, and humidification.
2. Obtain a ventilator that is mechanically able to provide small tidal volumes at high frequencies.
3. Set frequency at 100–600 cycles per minute.
C. Nursing care
1. Assess respiratory rate, rhythm, and quality through auscultation and observation before mechanical ventilation and at least every 2 hours during mechanical ventilation.

2. Monitor for bilateral, full expansion of the lungs every 2 hours.
3. Evaluate breathing pattern, vital signs, and level of consciousness every 2 hours and laboratory values as needed.
4. Frequent suctioning may be required initially and to ensure open airway.
5. If the patient experiences signs and symptoms of respiratory distress and failure, notify the physician of changes.
6. Assess the position and patency of the artificial airway.
7. Note and record landmarks on the endotracheal tube every shift, and evaluate position on chest x-ray if available.
8. Suction the airway and mouth every 2 hours and as needed.
9. Ensure adequate humidification of delivered gases throughout period of high-frequency jet ventilation.
10. Provide patient education to families, patients, and significant others.
11. Ensure adequate ventilator function.
12. Identify ordered settings, and validate these settings and alarm parameters every 2 hours. Document all changes.
13. Maintain a bag-valve mask and oral airway at the bedside at all times.
14. Monitor mean airway pressure using an intratracheal catheter located at least 5 cm below the injection site.
15. Evaluate cardiac status and ensure that cardiac output and venous return are not compromised through the use of this treatment modality.
16. Evaluate current nutritional status and refer to dietitian for assistance in evaluating and maintaining patient's nutritional needs.
17. Take steps to ensure skin and tissue integrity during mechanical ventilation.
18. Change the position of the endotracheal tube from one side of the mouth to the other on a daily basis.
19. Check the cuff pressure of the artificial airway every shift to ensure pressure is less than 21 cm H_2O.
20. Secure the airway with tape or ties.
21. Initiate actions to minimize the risk of infection.
22. Monitor vital signs every hour.
23. Monitor secretions for consistency, amount, and color.
24. Turn the patient every 2 hours as appropriate.
25. Initiate actions to alleviate patient and family anxiety during the course of mechanical ventilation.
26. Educate the patient and family about equipment and monitors.
27. Provide an alternate means of communication and encourage communication.

D. Complications
1. Obstruction; if total obstruction occurs, extubation and reintubation must be rapidly initiated.
2. Hemodynamic compromise.
3. Barotrauma.
4. Necrotizing tracheobronchitis.
5. Tension pneumothorax.
6. Pneumothorax.

XXV. Intravascular oxygenator

This investigational device provides supplemental gas exchange for failing lungs.

A. Indications

1. For temporary ventilatory support in patients with acute reversible respiratory insufficiency such as ARDS.
2. Respiratory insufficiency is defined as the presence of interstitial infiltrates on x-ray, pulmonary capillary pressure less than 16 mm Hg, and arterial hypoxia evidenced by O_2 delivery at greater than 50% with deteriorating ABGs.
3. The patient must be ventilated on positive pressure ventilation and has one of the following: positive end-expiratory pressure (PEEP) greater than 10 cm H_2O, mean airway pressure greater than 30 cm H_2O, peak inspiratory pressure greater than 45 cm H_2O, or minute volume greater than 150 mL/minute/kg body weight.
4. May also be used for those patients who cannot tolerate the cuffed endotracheal tube or mechanical ventilation, lung transplants, trauma, or pulmonary reactions that damage lung tissue.

B. Setup

1. Obtain intravascular oxygenator (IVOX) device and gas controller unit, which serves as the oxygen source, and capnography machine.
2. Obtain baseline vital signs including cardiac output, cardiac index, CVP, pulmonary capillary wedge pressure, systemic vascular resistance, mean arterial pressure, arterial pressure, peripheral vascular resistance, arterial and mixed venous blood gases, and Sao_2 (by pulse oximetry) values.
3. The IVOX device is inserted in the operating room; it is placed at the vena cava via the femoral vein. Assessment of the circulation at the potential site of insertion must be ascertained prior to the procedure.
4. Setup and test the circuit in the operating room prior to insertion of the IVOX.

C. Nursing care

1. On arrival at the ICU, patient assessment should include assessment of lung sounds, adequacy of oxygenation, arterial BP, level of consciousness, respiratory rate, urine output, circulation to affected extremity, and integrity of IVOX dressing.
2. Assess lung sounds and ensure proper placement of the endotracheal tube at least every 2 hours and with changes in the patient's condition.
3. Sedate the patient, and consider use of paralytic agents to decrease respiratory effort.
4. Suction frequently, and support maximum pulmonary function with chest physiotherapy and movement of the patient from side to side as tolerated.
5. Monitor pulse oximeter readings continuously, and obtain mixed venous saturation values every 12 hours unless an oximetric pulmonary artery catheter is in place.
6. Arterial and mixed venous blood gases should be obtained immediately following implantation of the IVOX device.

7. Monitor blood gases as needed to evaluate ventilator changes or deteriorations in the patient's condition.
8. Monitor vital signs and cardiac output every hour until the patient has stabilized, then once every 2–4 hours.
9. Turn the patient every 2 hours when stable, and elevate the head of the bed no higher than 30 degrees.
10. Evaluate nutritional status, and provide parenteral or enteral support of nutritional needs based on the patient's condition and the physician's orders.
11. Provide anticoagulation therapy as ordered, and monitor ACT or PTT every hour until the ACT is 180–200 seconds or the PTT is 1.5–1.6 times the control value.
12. Replace blood loss incurred during catheter insertion, and monitor intake and output continuously.
13. Report any changes in hemodynamic values or vital signs that are indicative of low cardiac output or blood loss.
14. Decrease risk for infection through the use of sterile technique for catheter changes, dressing changes, and suctioning.
15. IV and monitoring lines should be changed every 4 days; however, the PA catheter should not be changed while the IVOX is in place, since this may cause damage to some of its hollow fibers.
16. Keep the affected leg straight, and evaluate circulation, temperature, discoloration, and pulses every hour.
17. Pneumatic compression stockings should be used following insertion of the IVOX.
18. Monitor the skin closely for signs of breakdown.
19. Provide psychosocial support and educate patient and family about the device and patient's status following insertion and removal of the device.
20. Document gas inflow rate, amount of vacuum, and percentage of CO_2 in the exhaust gas on the ICU flow record.

D. Complications
1. Bleeding.
2. Infection and sepsis.
3. Platelet loss.
4. Deep vein thrombosis.
5. Impairment of venous return.

XXVI. Weaning patient from ventilatory support

A. Indications

Weaning the patient from the ventilatory assist device is indicated when the patient's physiologic status has improved in a manner that reflects adequate alveolar and tissue oxygenation. The parameters that are typically used to identify the effectiveness of the patient's inherent breathing abilities are fraction of inspired oxygen, vital capacity of at least 10 mL/kg, maximum inspiratory pressure of at least 20 cm H_2O, tidal volume of at least 5 mL/kg, minute ventilation no more than 10 liters/minute, and voluntary ventilation more than twice the value of the patient's minute ventilation; respiratory rate, $S\bar{v}O_2$ values, and arterial blood gas values are individualized. A study by Tahvanainen [1] reports that low urine output, positive blood culture, and low respiratory quotient values are better correlates with unsuccessful extubation than the standard weaning parameters.

B. Setup

1. Identify patient's ability to maintain an acceptable respiratory status with baseline arterial blood gases, spontaneous tidal volume, vital capacity, and work of breathing.
2. Obtain a ventilator that provides SIMV as a mode for weaning. However, mode selection is often driven by the availability of various modes and the physician's preference.
3. Access a T-bar setup for use once the patient has been weaned from the ventilator and for use prior to extubation.
4. Adequate nutrition is a prerequisite to successful patient weaning.
5. $S\bar{v}O_2$ monitoring is necessary to evaluate the ongoing effects of the weaning process on the patient in conjunction with other parameters.

C. Nursing care

1. Never begin the weaning process unless there is evidence that the patient may have success in this process.
2. Record respiratory parameters prior to initiating weaning.
3. Inform the patient about the process in advance.
4. Inform the patient about mechanisms for communication during this process.
5. Assess the patient's breath sounds and cardiovascular status for baseline information.
6. Set the machine at the established parameters to begin weaning.
7. Monitor the patient's respiratory rate, heart rate, work of breathing, anxiety level, level of discomfort or pain, tidal volume, $S\bar{v}O_2$, SaO_2, minute ventilation, and other established parameters.
8. The pace of ventilator withdrawal must be based on these parameters. For a patient who is weak or has left ventricular dysfunction, weaning may take longer.
9. As the patient tolerates the process, ventilation rates are decreased at an individualized level. The weaning process may need to be stopped or discontinued when the patient shows signs or symptoms of fatigue, discomfort, or respiratory distress.
10. Weaning efforts are most successful when a standard plan is adopted by the members of the team caring for the patient. Guidelines and parameters for measuring success in a particular patient should be established and clear prior to the initiation of weaning.
11. Once the patient has been successfully weaned from the ventilator, the endotracheal or tracheotomy tube is left in place and attached to a T bar to ensure the patient's ability to breathe without the ventilator circuit for a period of 1–4 hours.
12. If, during that time, the patient demonstrates the ability to oxygenate and cough adequately, then the endotracheal cuff is deflated, the endotracheal tube is suctioned, and the tube is removed.
13. Provide the patient with an alternate source of oxygen support once the tube is removed.

14. Continue to monitor patient's ventilatory status closely for the next 24 hours to ensure weaning success.

D. Complications

1. Respiratory distress.
2. Respiratory failure.
3. Anxiety.
4. Failure to wean.

Reference

1. Tahvanainen, J. Extubation criteria after weaning from intermittent mandatory ventilation and continuous positive airway pressure. *Crit. Care Med.* 11:702–707, 1983.

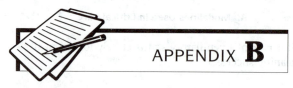

APPENDIX **B**

Dysrhythmias

Mary Clark Robinson

I. Sinus rhythms

A. Rhythm: Sinus rhythm (Fig. B.1).
   1. Electrocardiographic (ECG) criteria: P waves are upright and precede each QRS complex. The P-R interval is consistent and within normal limits (0.12–0.20 second). The QRS complex is consistent and its duration within normal limits (0.06–0.10 second). The ventricular (R-R) and atrial (P-P) rates occur at essentially regular intervals. The rate ranges from 60 to 100 beats/minute.
   2. Physiologic explanation: Impulses arise at regular and timely intervals from the sinus node and conduct through to the ventricles.
   3. Clinical significance: Normal rhythm.
   4. Nursing and/or medical intervention: Identify and document rhythm in appropriate charting mechanism.
B. Rhythm: Sinus bradycardia (Fig. B.2).
   1. ECG criteria: P waves are upright and precede each QRS complex. The P-R interval is consistent and within normal limits (0.12–0.20 second). The QRS complex is consistent and within normal limits (0.06–0.10 second). The ventricular rate (R-R) and atrial rate (P-P) occur at regular and predictable intervals. The rate is less than 60 beats/minute and is usually 40–60 beats/minute.
   2. Physiologic explanation: The hallmark of this rhythm is the decrease in the rate of firing of the sinus node that results in a rate less than 60 beats/minute. This may be due to increased parasympathetic tone or

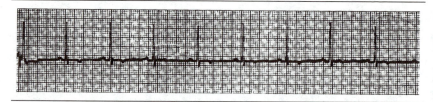

Figure B.1 Sinus rhythm. (From *Manual of Electrocardiography* (2nd ed.). Mudge, G. H., Jr. Boston: Little, Brown and Company, 1986. P. 240.)

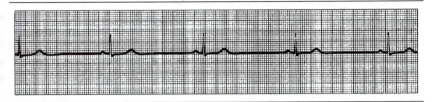

Figure B.2 Sinus bradycardia.

increased vagal influences, or a diseased sinus node, or the effects of various drugs such as calcium channel blockers, beta blockers, and digitalis.

3. Clinical significance: The clinical significance of this rhythm is related to patient response. This rhythm can cause significant alterations in hemodynamic status for some individuals, depending on cardiovascular status and rate of bradycardia. This rhythm may cause a decrease in cardiac output and may potentiate ventricular arrhythmias due to decreased tissue perfusion. It should be noted that a slower heart rate can be beneficial for some individuals, because it decreases myocardial oxygen demands and enhances diastolic filling, thereby enhancing preload.

4. Nursing and/or medical intervention: Identify and document the rhythm. Assess patient for response to rhythm (blood pressure, level of consciousness, new onset of chest pain). If patient is symptomatic and compromised, initiate protocol for bradycardia management. Atropine is the first-line drug recommended for the treatment of bradycardia. Evaluate the patient for contributing causes such as drugs and increased vagal stimulation. Access transcutaneous pacemaker and determine possible need for transvenous pacemaker.

C. Rhythm: Sinus tachycardia (Fig. B.3).

1. ECG criteria: P waves are upright and precede each QRS complex. The P-R interval is consistent and within normal limits (0.12–0.20 second). The QRS complex is consistent and within normal limits (0.06–0.10 second). The ventricular rate (R-R) and atrial rate (P-P) occur at regular and predictable intervals. The rate is usually 100–150 beats/minute.

2. Physiologic explanation: This rhythm is characterized by an increased rate of firing from the sinus node. This enhanced automaticity is due to either an increase in circulating catecholamines or a vagal withdrawal. This may be secondary to multiple factors such as fever, exercise, anxiety,

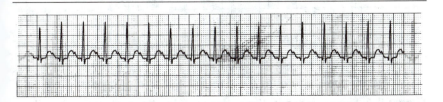

Figure B.3 Sinus tachycardia.

stress, pain, heart failure, hypovolemia, hypotension, and drugs. Sinus tachycardia is generally a response of the body to an increased demand for cardiac output.

3. Clinical significance: May cause decreased filling time for coronary arteries as well as an increase in myocardial oxygen demand. The combination of these two factors in patients with coronary artery disease may cause a myocardial infarction (MI) or an extension of an MI.

4. Nursing and/or medical intervention: Identify and document the rhythm. Evaluate the patient for hemodynamic response to the rhythm. Identify potential causative factors. It is important to treat the cause and not the rhythm.

D. Rhythm: Sinus arrhythmia (Fig. B.4).

1. ECG criteria: P waves are upright and precede each QRS complex. The P-R interval is consistent and within normal limits (0.12–0.20 second). The QRS complex is consistent and within normal limits (0.06–0.10 second). The rhythm is irregular but presents a pattern that often fluctuates with respirations. The R-R interval decreases with inspiration and increases with expiration. The hallmark for diagnosis of this rhythm is the fact that the difference between the shortest and longest R-R cycle should measure more than 0.12 second. The rate is usually 60–100 beats/minute.

2. Physiologic explanation: The vagus nerve innervates both the sinus node and the lungs, which results in fluctuations in heart rate in coordination with respirations in some individuals.

3. Clinical significance: This rhythm is a normal variation in many people, especially the young.

4. Nursing and/or medical intervention: Identify and document the rhythm. No intervention is necessary for this, because it is considered a normal rhythm.

E. Rhythm: Sinus arrest (Fig. B.5).

1. ECG criteria: P waves are positive and precede each QRS complex. The underlying rhythm is regular but is interrupted by one or more dropped P-QRS-T complexes. The P-R interval is consistent and regular prior to the event. The pause is of no predictable length and is not a multiple of the original or underlying P-P interval. The rate is usually 60–100 beats/ minute. The rhythm is regular except for the event.

2. Physiologic explanation: The automaticity of the sinus node is depressed

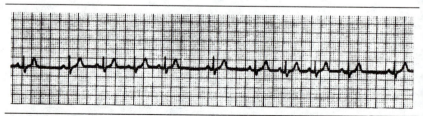

Figure B.4 Sinus arrhythmia. (From *Manual of Electrocardiography* (2nd ed.). Mudge, G. H., Jr. Boston: Little, Brown and Company, 1986. P. 103.)

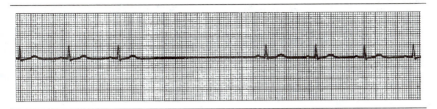

Figure B.5 Sinus arrest.

and fails to initiate an impulse for one or more beats. There are multiple causes of this depressed automaticity, and these may include incidence of MI, digitalis toxicity, and rheumatic fever.

3. Clinical significance: The clinical significance is related to the number and length of pauses and patient response to these pauses. Patients may become symptomatic with slow rates.

4. Nursing and/or medical intervention: Identify and document the rhythm. If arrests are prolonged and cause the patient to become symptomatic, it may be necessary to treat the patient with atropine to decrease vagal effects that may be contributing to the arrhythmia. If the patient continues to be symptomatic, transcutaneous or transvenous pacing may be required. If the patient is receiving digitalis or quinidine, consider holding the drug, and notify the physician. The duration of pauses should be trended and the physician notified if the pauses increase in length.

F. Rhythm: Sinus exit block (Fig. B.6).

1. ECG criteria: P waves are positive and precede each QRS complex. The underlying rhythm is regular but is interrupted by one or more dropped P-QRS-T complexes. The duration of the QRS complex is 0.06–0.10 second. Usually only one P-QRS-T complex is missing. The P-R interval is consistent and regular prior to the event. The pause is exactly two R-R intervals, and P waves can be plotted through the event with the exception of the dropped complexes. This characteristic distinguishes this from a sinus pause or sinus arrest. The rate is usually 60–100 beats/minute. The rhythm is regular except for the event.

2. Physiologic explanation: The sinus node fires and is not conducted; therefore, it is a "perfectly" dropped beat because the sinus node fires again as it should. There are multiple causative factors that include ischemia to the

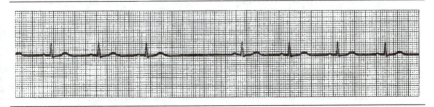

Figure B.6 Sinus exit block.

sinus node, infection, conduction defects, digitalis toxicity, and myocardial disease.

3. Clinical significance: The clinical significance is related to the number and length of pauses and patient response to these pauses. Patients may become symptomatic with slow rates.

4. Nursing and/or medical intervention: Identify and document the rhythm. If arrests are prolonged and cause the patient to become symptomatic, it may be necessary to treat the patient with atropine to decrease vagal effects that may be contributing to the arrhythmia. If the patient continues to be symptomatic, transcutaneous or transvenous pacing may be required. If the patient is receiving digitalis or quinidine, consider holding the drug, and notify the physician.

II. Atrial dysrhythmias

A. Rhythm: Premature atrial contraction (PAC) (Fig. B.7).

1. ECG criteria: Rhythm is regular with the exception of an early beat. The P wave of the premature complex may be different from the normal sinus P wave. It may be inverted, or it may be concealed in the T wave of the preceding beat. The P-R interval is usually within normal limits (0.12–0.20 second). If there is aberrant conduction, the QRS complex can be wide.

2. Physiologic explanation: The PAC is one of the most common reasons for a pause on the ECG. An ectopic focus in the atrium takes over as pacemaker intermittently and initiates atrial depolarization. This alternate pacemaker site is attributed to changing the appearance of the P wave. This may be due to electrolyte imbalances; hypoxia; congestive heart failure; atrial enlargement; fever; infection; emotion; fatigue; digitalis toxicity; or excessive use of coffee, tea, alcohol, and cigarettes.

3. Clinical significance: Significance depends on the frequency of the PACs. This may indicate atrial irritability or act as a precursor of more significant atrial arrhythmias such as atrial flutter, atrial fibrillation, and atrial tachycardias.

4. Nursing and/or medical intervention: Identify and document the rhythm. If this is a new occurrence or is an increase in frequency, the physician should be notified. PACs are monitored for frequency and often are not treated unless they are very frequent. Due to the potential for causation from medications, it is important to review the patient's medications as

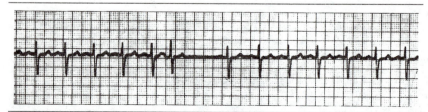

Figure B.7 Premature atrial contraction. (From *Manual of Electrocardiography* (2nd ed.). Mudge, G. H., Jr. Boston: Little, Brown and Company, 1986. P. 103.)

well as possibilities for other underlying causes. Mild sedation may be helpful in some situations.

B. Rhythm: Nonconducted PACs (Fig. B.8).

1. ECG criteria: P wave is present within the T wave; no QRS complex follows in the affected beats. The T wave will appear distorted, and a pause will follow.

2. Physiologic explanation: A premature atrial depolarization finds the atrioventricular (AV) junction refractory to the stimulus because the conduction system has not repolarized, and, therefore, the impulse is not conducted. No QRS complex is formed.

3. Clinical significance: Significance depends on the frequency of the nonconducted PACs. This may indicate atrial irritability or act as a precursor to more significant atrial arrhythmias such as atrial flutter, atrial fibrillation, and atrial tachycardias.

4. Nursing and/or medical intervention: Identify and document the rhythm. If these are new occurrences or have increased in frequency, the physician should be notified. Nonconducted PACs are monitored for frequency and often are not treated. Due to the probability that the rhythm is caused by medications, it is important to review the patient's medications as well as possibilities for other underlying causes.

C. Rhythm: Paroxysmal atrial tachycardia (PAT) (Fig. B.9).

1. ECG criteria: The atrial rate for this rhythm is 150–250 beats/minute. P waves are present but may or may not be recognized due to the rate and the fact that they may be buried in the T wave. The P-R interval is normal if P waves are seen. The P waves may differ in appearance from the sinus P. The QRS is of normal duration (0.06–0.12 second) as ventricular conduction is not usually affected by these changes within the atria. The rhythm is usually regular. The term "paroxysmal" refers to the characteristic of this rhythm to start and stop abruptly. This rhythm is sometimes referred to as supraventricular tachycardia (SVT), especially if the onset is not seen.

2. Physiological explanation: PAT can result from the creation of a reentry circuit, or it can be due to an irritable focus in the atria that takes over as pacemaker, firing at very rapid rates, causing a tachycardia. Causes may include enhanced automaticity or reentry mechanisms as well as hyperventilation, emotional stress, excessive caffeine, MI, hypoxia, mitral valve

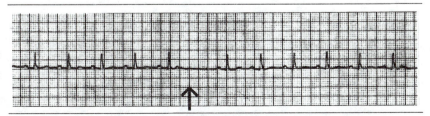

Figure B.8 Nonconducted premature atrial contraction. (From *Manual of Electrocardiography* (2nd ed.). Mudge, G. H., Jr. Boston: Little, Brown and Company, 1986. P. 104.)

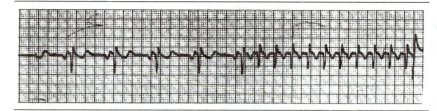

Figure B.9 Paroxysmal atrial tachycardia. (From *Manual of Electrocardiography* (2nd ed.). Mudge, G. H., Jr. Boston: Little, Brown and Company, 1986. P. 105.)

disease, chronic obstructive pulmonary disease (COPD), hyperventilation, and Wolff-Parkinson-White syndrome.

3. Clinical significance: This rhythm may result in a decrease in cardiac output due to the loss of atrial contribution and decreased ventricular filling time. Patients may report syncope and general feelings of malaise. In addition, the fast rate increases the myocardial oxygen demands and may increase infarct size.

4. Nursing and/or medication intervention: Identify and document the rhythm. Assess the patient for symptoms and any hemodynamic consequences. Treat underlying cause if possible. It may be necessary to elicit a vagal response in order to identify P waves or in an attempt to convert the rhythm to a sinus rhythm. Pharmacologic interventions include adenosine, verapamil, digitalis, and quinidine. Cardioversion may be necessary in some cases. Overdrive pacing may be used as well.

D. Rhythm: Atrial tachycardia with a block (Fig. B.10).

1. ECG criteria: The atrial rate is 150–250 beats/minute. The ventricular rate is regular but slower than the atrial rate. P waves are present without QRS complexes. The duration of the QRS complex is within normal limits (0.06–0.10 second). The P waves are often difficult to recognize because they are hidden in the T wave of the preceding QRS.

2. Physiologic explanation: An irritable focus in the atria takes over as pacemaker, firing at very rapid rates, causing an atrial tachycardia. However, the AV node acts to protect the ventricle from fast atrial rates by blocking some of the impulses. Causes may include enhanced automaticity or

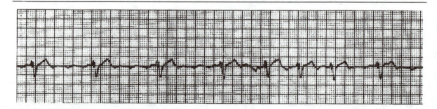

Figure B.10 Atrial tachycardia with a block. (From *Manual of Electrocardiography* (2nd ed.). Mudge, G. H., Jr. Boston: Little, Brown and Company, 1986. P. 123.)

reentry mechanisms as well as hyperventilation, emotional stress, excessive caffeine, MI, hypoxia, mitral valve disease, COPD, hyperventilation, and Wolff-Parkinson-White syndrome.

3. Clinical significance: Patients may report syncope and general feelings of malaise. However, this rhythm usually benefits the patient, and there is no perception of a change.

4. Nursing and/or medical intervention: The block that occurs in this rhythm is considered a physiologic block and is beneficial to the patient. Identify and document the rhythm. Assess the patient for symptoms and any hemodynamic consequences. Treat underlying cause if possible. Pharmacologic interventions include adenosine, verapamil, digitalis, and quinidine.

E. Rhythm: Atrial flutter (Fig. B.11).

1. ECG criteria: P waves are present but are identified as flutter waves that present as a sawtooth baseline due to the rapid depolarization within the atria. The atrial rate is regular at 250–350 beats/minute. The R-R interval can be regular or irregular depending on conduction through the AV node. The ratio of atrial beats to ventricular beats can be very stable or can vary as a result of conduction through the AV node.

2. Physiologic explanation: This rhythm is often initiated by a PAC. An irritable focus in the atrial wall stimulates the atria to contract at a rate of 250–350 beats/minute. The AV node will act to block many of these impulses because of its refractoriness but does allow some of them to conduct through. This rhythm can be the result of a reentry circuit, mitral or tricuspid valve disease, congestive heart failure, or coronary artery disease.

3. Clinical significance: Identify and document the rhythm. Assess the patient for hemodynamic consequences. The loss of atrial contribution may contribute to a significant loss in cardiac output. Patients may experience palpitations, angina and dyspnea, and infarct size may be increased.

4. Nursing and/or medical intervention: If the patient is severely symptomatic, cardioversion is the treatment of choice for this rhythm. For a mildly symptomatic patient, the pharmacologic treatments include verapamil, digitalis, beta-blockers, or diltiazem to slow the ventricular response. Quinidine and procainamide are the antiarrhythmics of choice once rate control has been achieved. Cardioversion may be necessary in those patients who do not respond to pharmacologic therapy.

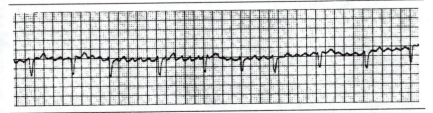

Figure B.11 Atrial flutter. (From *Manual of Electrocardiography* (2nd ed.). Mudge, G. H., Jr. Boston: Little, Brown and Company, 1986. P. 107.)

F. Rhythm: Atrial fibrillation (Fig. B.12).

1. ECG criteria: The atrial rate in this rhythm cannot be measured. P waves are unidentifiable. Chaotic electrical activity is present in the atria and is identified as fibrillatory waves in the baseline. It is reported that the atria fire at a rate greater than 350 beats/minute. The R-R interval is irregular, and the rate can reach 160–180 beats/minute. The QRS duration is normal, and the amplitudes of the R waves may vary.

2. Physiologic explanation: This rhythm may be the result of multiple areas of irritability within the atrial walls or from multiple areas of reentry. The rate of impulse firing results in very rapid electrical activity, causing depolarization of small areas throughout the myocardium. As a result, the atria twitches, and no uniform depolarization occurs, and, thus, no P wave is formed. Only a select few of these impulses travel to the AV node, resulting in a random irregular rhythm. This dysrhythmia is associated with hypoxia, sick sinus syndrome, increased atrial pressure, pericarditis, postoperative cardiac surgery, MI, or underlying heart disease. In addition, this is very often due to increased atrial wall tension caused by congestive heart failure or pulmonary edema (fluid overload). This rhythm can occur in healthy people in times of stress or fatigue or from excessive coffee, tea, or alcohol intake, or cigarettes.

3. Clinical significance: Identify and document the rhythm. Assess the patient for hemodynamic consequences. The loss of atrial contribution may be responsible for a significant loss in cardiac output. Patients may experience rate-related palpitations, angina, and dyspnea, and infarct size may be increased. Patients with enlarged atria, mitral stenosis, and cardiomyopathy have the potential of developing mural thrombi and run the risk of throwing emboli and stroke.

4. Nursing and/or medical intervention: Identify and document the rhythm. Assess the patient's blood pressure and any signs of clinical distress. Cardioversion is the treatment of choice for severely symptomatic patients. Pharmacologic approaches to treatment include the use of digitalis, verapamil, or beta-blocking agents. Success in cardioverting and control of atrial fibrillation depends on the atrial size and the length of time in atrial fibrillation. Anticoagulation should be considered for all patients with atrial fibrillation prior to cardioversion or pharmacologic treatment. Diltiazem is used to control rate.

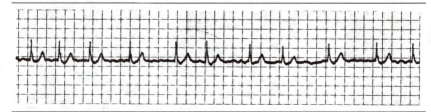

Figure B.12 Atrial fibrillation. (From *Manual of Electrocardiography* (2nd ed.). Mudge, G. H., Jr. Boston: Little, Brown and Company, 1986. P. 107.)

G. Rhythm: Wandering atrial pacemaker (Fig. B.13).

    1. ECG criteria: P waves appear different on a beat-to-beat basis. The P-P interval will vary, and the R-R interval also may vary. The QRS complex is of normal duration (0.06–0.10 second). The P wave may disappear or become inverted if the impulse is initiated close to or in the AV junction. Usually at least three different P-wave configurations are identified as a wandering atrial pacemaker rhythm.

    2. Physiologic explanation: The pacemaker for the heart changes from the sinus node to other supraventricular foci on a beat-to-beat basis. This may be related to enhanced vagal influences on the sinus node.

    3. Clinical significance: This is not considered a serious arrhythmia and can be a normal occurrence in the very young or the very old. It may indicate atrial irritability or forewarn of more serious arrhythmias in some patient populations.

    4. Nursing and/or medical intervention: Identify and document the rhythm. Physician notification is necessary but not urgent. This rhythm is frequently not treated, but continued monitoring is warranted in those patients prone to having more serious atrial arrhythmias.

III. Junctional dysrhythmias

A. Rhythm: Premature junctional contraction (PJC) (Fig. B.14).

    1. ECG criteria: This complex is identified as an electrical impulse that originates from the AV junction and occurs before the next expected beat. The QRS complex of the early beat is not altered in configuration because conduction is not affected. The P wave of the early beat may precede, coincide with, or follow the QRS complex. In complexes in which the P wave precedes the QRS, the P-R interval is less than 0.12 second and typically is inverted.

    2. Physiologic explanation: A PJC occurs as the result of an electrical impulse arising in the AV junction; this impulse thus assumes pacing function for one beat. It commonly is due to increased automaticity in the AV node.

    3. Clinical significance: This rhythm is not usually clinically significant.

    4. Nursing and/or medical intervention: Identify and document the rhythm. Treatment of this rhythm is not usually warranted.

B. Rhythm: Accelerated junctional rhythm (Fig. B.15).

    1. ECG criteria: This rhythm originates from the AV junction. The QRS complex is usually normal, and the rhythm is regular. P waves may precede, coincide with, or follow the QRS complex. In those complexes where the P

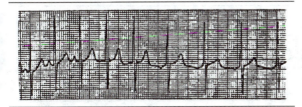

Figure B.13 Wandering atrial pacemaker.

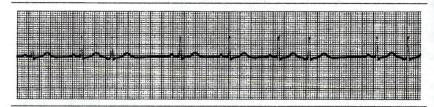

Figure B.14 Premature junctional contraction.

wave precedes the QRS, the P-R interval is less than 0.12 second and is typically inverted. The ventricular rate is 60–100 beats/minute.

2. Physiologic explanation: An irritable focus in the AV junction fires repeatedly and assumes pacemaker function for the heart. Most often, arrhythmias associated with the AV node are the result of enhanced automaticity or digitalis toxicity. This can be seen following an MI, after open heart surgery, or in association with heart disease.

3. Clinical significance: This rhythm is not usually clinically significant unless the rate is not effective in maintaining an adequate cardiac output.

4. Nursing and/or medical intervention: Identify and document the rhythm. This rhythm often is not treated unless the patient is symptomatic in terms of cardiac output or if digitalis toxicity is suspected. May need to look for causative factors. Notify the physician for possible digitalis level or change in medications. The serum potassium level should be checked and potassium given if levels are low.

C. Rhythm: Junctional tachycardia (Fig. B.16).

1. ECG criteria: This rhythm is identified as a series of complexes with electrical impulses that originate from the AV junction. The QRS complex is usually normal. The rhythm is regular. P waves may precede, coincide with, or follow the QRS complex. In complexes in which the P wave precedes the QRS, the P-R interval is less than 0.12 second. The ventricular rate is greater than 100 beats/minute.

2. Physiologic explanation: An irritable focus in the AV junction fires repeatedly and assumes pacemaker function for the heart. Most often arrhythmias associated with the AV node are the result of enhanced automaticity or digitalis toxicity. This can be seen after an MI, after open heart surgery, or in association with heart disease.

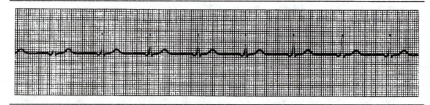

Figure B.15 Accelerated junctional rhythm.

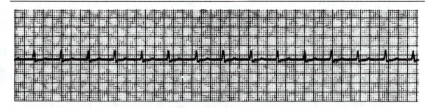

Figure B.16 Junctional tachycardia. (From *Manual of Electrocardiography* (2nd ed.). Mudge, G. H., Jr. Boston: Little, Brown and Company, 1986. P. 125.)

   3. Clinical significance: Rapid rhythms may cause decreases in cardiac output, and some patients may become symptomatic with the loss of atrial kick.
   4. Nursing and/or medical intervention: Identify and document the rhythm. Assess the patient's blood pressure and investigate for contributing causes such as digitalis toxicity. Notify the physician for possible digitalis level or change in medications. The serum potassium level should be checked and potassium given if levels are low.
D. Rhythm: Junctional rhythm (Fig. B.17).
   1. ECG criteria: The QRS complex is normal unless there is a ventricular conduction problem. The rhythm is regular. P waves may precede, coincide with, or follow the QRS complex. In those complexes where the P wave precedes the QRS, the P-R interval is less than 0.12 second. The ventricular rate is 40–60 beats/minute.
   2. Physiologic explanation: This rhythm represents a protective mechanism of the AV node. Typically, the sinus node is the primary pacemaker of the heart. However, in those instances when the sinus impulse does not arrive at the AV node within approximately 1.0–1.5 seconds, the AV node will initiate this rhythm.
   3. Clinical significance: Significance is dependent on rate and the patient's tolerance of decreased cardiac output. In addition, slow rates may allow for breakthrough ventricular arrhythmias. This rhythm is due to upper pacemaker failure and can be unreliable as a primary pacemaker.
   4. Nursing and/or medical intervention: Identify and document the rhythm. Evaluate the patient's hemodynamic response to the rhythm. Atropine,

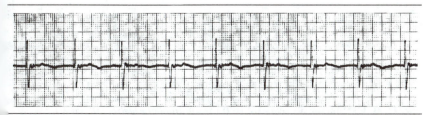

Figure B.17 Junctional rhythm. (From *Manual of Electrocardiography* (2nd ed.). Mudge, G. H., Jr. Boston: Little, Brown and Company, 1986. P. 109.)

isoproterenol, or a pacemaker may be necessary for symptomatic brady-cardias. Evaluate for any causative factors such as digitalis and quinidine. Avoid any vagal stimulation.

E. Rhythm: Junctional escape beats (Fig. B.18).

1. ECG criteria: A junctional escape beat is an electrical impulse that occurs after the expected sinus impulse. The QRS of the late complex is normal unless there is a ventricular conduction problem. The rhythm is irregular. P waves of this escape beat may precede, coincide with, or follow the QRS complex. In those complexes where the P wave precedes the QRS and the P-R interval is less than 0.12 second, a junctional escape beat can be identified. The P wave is often inverted because of retrograde conduction away from the positive pole in which patients are monitored.

2. Physiologic explanation: This complex represents a protective mecha-nism of the AV node. Typically, the sinus node is the primary pacemaker of the heart. However, in those instances when the sinus impulse does not arrive at the AV node within approximately 1.0–1.5 seconds, the AV node will initiate a junctional escape beat. This occurs because of the failed initiation of a sinus beat or because of a conduction problem between the sinus node and the AV node.

3. Clinical significance: Junctional escape beats are considered an "escape mechanism" and an attempt to maintain an adequate cardiac output.

4. Nursing and/or medical interventions: Identify and document the rhythm. Physician notification may be necessary to evaluate the mecha-nisms and causes of sinus failure. Continue to monitor for further prob-lems with the sinus node.

IV. Heart blocks

A. Rhythm: First-degree AV block or sinus rhythm with prolonged AV conduc-tion (Fig. B.19).

1. ECG criteria: The appearance and duration of the QRS complex are nor-mal. The rhythm is regular. P waves are normal in appearance, and precede each QRS complex. Although the P-R interval is prolonged (> 0.20 second), this interval is constant.

2. Physiologic explanation: This rhythm represents a delay in conduction of the impulse from the sinus node to the AV node. All impulses are then conducted through to the ventricles. Digitalis can be a causative factor for this conduction delay.

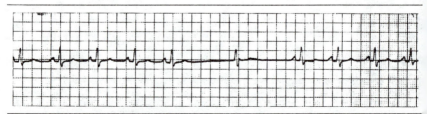

Figure B.18 Junctional escape beats. (From *Manual of Electrocardiography* (2nd ed.). Mudge, G. H., Jr. Boston: Little, Brown and Company, 1986. P. 109.)

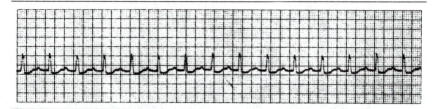

Figure B.19 First-degree AV block or sinus rhythm with prolonged AV conduction. (From *Manual of Electrocardiography* (2nd ed.). Mudge, G. H., Jr. Boston: Little, Brown and Company, 1986. P. 120.)

    3. Clinical significance: In general, patients are not symptomatic with this rhythm. However, monitor for worsening of heart block.

    4. Nursing and/or medical intervention: Identify and document the rhythm. In general, this rhythm causes no symptoms, and there is no need to intervene.

B. Rhythm: Second-degree AV block, Mobitz type 1 (Wenckebach) (Fig. B.20).

    1. ECG criteria: The atrial rhythm is regular; the ventricular rhythm is irregular with progressive lengthening of the P-R interval, followed by a dropped QRS complex. The R-R interval will progressively lengthen prior to the blocked impulse. P waves will appear normal, and all will be followed by a QRS with the exception of the dropped beat. Usually only a single impulse is dropped, and the pattern is repeated. The conduction ratio that reflects this pattern (4:3) should be documented. The QRS is of normal duration.

    2. Physiologic explanation: This block occurs at the AV level and is often due to increased parasympathetic tone or from the effect of drugs such as digitalis, propranolol hydrochloride, and verapamil. With each conduction, AV nodal repolarization is delayed until finally, the electrical impulse is blocked because the AV node has not yet recovered. After the blocked beat (QRS), the AV node has had the opportunity to fully repolarize, and the cycle begins again.

    3. Clinical significance: Patients do not generally experience symptoms related to this rhythm unless the resulting rate is insufficient to meet cardiac output demands.

    4. Nursing and/or medical intervention: Identify and document the rhythm. Evaluate the patient's medications for possible causative factors. Rarely it

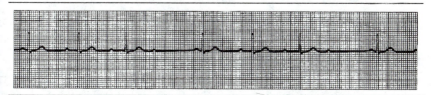

Figure B.20 Second-degree AV block, Mobitz type 1 (Wenckebach).

may be necessary to intervene with atropine if the patient experiences a symptomatic bradycardia.

C. Rhythm: Second-degree AV block, Mobitz type 2 (Fig. B.21).

1. ECG criteria: The overall rhythm is irregular. The atrial rhythm is usually regular, and the ventricular rhythm is irregular. Pauses are present and associated with the nonconducted atrial beats. P waves are present and normal; each is followed by a QRS with the exception of the blocked beat. The QRS complex is of normal duration if the block occurs at or above the bundle of His. The QRS may be widened if the bundle branches are involved. The P-R interval can be either normal or prolonged but remains constant.

2. Physiologic explanation: This block occurs below the level of the AV node and most often involves the bundle branches. Often this rhythm is attributed to an intermittent bundle branch block. The patient will experience a constant block involving two of the three fascicles and occasionally develops a block that involves the third fascicle. This is usually associated with an organic lesion in the conduction pathway and is frequently seen following the occurrence of an acute anterior MI. Due to the nature of the problem, this block is associated with a poorer prognosis.

3. Clinical significance: This rhythm may proceed the development of complete heart block and is considered an unreliable pacemaker for the heart. Patients may experience a decrease of cardiac output with this rhythm depending on the underlying rate and patient response.

4. Nursing and/or medical intervention: Identify and document the rhythm. Assess the patient for hemodynamic response. Notify the physician, and begin treatment with atropine if the patient is symptomatic. Access a transcutaneous pacemaker, and prepare for transvenous pacemaker insertion.

D. Rhythm: 2:1 AV block (Fig. B.22).

1. ECG criteria: P-P intervals are regular. Every other P wave is not followed by a QRS complex. P-R intervals of conducted beats are constant.

2. Physiologic explanation: This rhythm can be seen following the occurrence of a Mobitz type 1 (Wenckebach) or a Mobitz II block. The origin of this block is difficult to identify due to the frequency of dropped beats. In general, the QRS complex is a good indication of the source of the block. If the QRS complex is of normal duration, then the block occurs in the AV

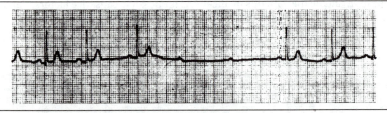

Figure B.21 Second-degree AV block, Mobitz type 2. (From *Manual of Electrocardiography* (2nd ed.). Mudge, G. H., Jr. Boston: Little, Brown and Company, 1986. P. 122.)

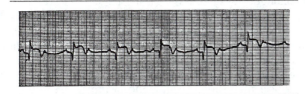

Figure B.22 2:1 AV block.

node. If the QRS is wide, then the rhythm is usually attributed to a disruption in the bundle of His or bundle branches. Therefore, if the QRS is of normal duration, then the AV block results from a Mobitz type 1 (Wenckebach) block. If the QRS is wide, it is probably due to a Mobitz type 2 heart block.

3. Clinical significance: It is important to determine the source of this rhythm due to the serious nature of a Mobitz type 2 block and the risk for development of third-degree block. The physician may perform vagal maneuvers in an effort to slow the rhythm down so that a differential diagnosis can be made.

4. Nursing and/or medical intervention: Identify and document the rhythm. Assess the patient for hemodynamic compromise. Notify the physician, and intervene with atropine and pacemaker if necessary.

E. Rhythm: Third-degree AV block (Fig. B.23).

1. ECG criteria: The atrial and ventricular rates are regular. The ventricular rate is slower than the atrial rate. P waves are present and appear normal. The QRS complex may be normal in duration or widened if a block is present on the bundle branch level. The P-R interval is variable due to the independent functioning of both an atrial and ventricular pacemaker.

2. Physiologic explanation: This rhythm is the result of a complete lack of conduction between the atria and the ventricles. As the result of this lack of communication, two independent pacemakers depolarize the atria and ventricles. If the block is associated with problems in the AV node, a junctional pacemaker will act to pace the heart. In general, this rhythm is the result of increased parasympathetic tone from an MI, or from toxic levels of drugs such as digitalis or propranolol. If the block occurs lower in

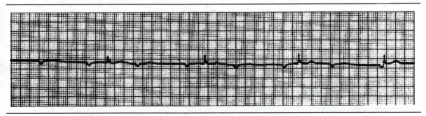

Figure B.23 Third-degree AV block. (From *Manual of Electrocardiography* (2nd ed.). Mudge, G. H., Jr. Boston: Little, Brown and Company, 1986. P. 122.)

the ventricular conduction system, this indicates the presence of infra-nodal conduction damage. This may be associated with anterior MIs or from the damage of atherosclerosis.

3. Clinical significance: This may result in a slow rhythm and inadequate cardiac output. The ventricular pacemaker is considered unreliable and may cease pacing at any time.

4. Nursing and/or medical intervention: Identify and document the rhythm. Evaluate the patient's hemodynamic status. Report the rhythm and findings to the physician. Traditional approaches to management include atropine, transcutaneous pacemaker, catecholamine infusions, and transvenous pacemaker.

F. Rhythm: Pulseless electrical activity.

1. ECG criteria: Any rhythm other than ventricular fibrillation (VF) or ventricular tachycardia (VT) that occurs without the presence of a pulse.

2. Physiologic explanation: A variety of conditions can occur that contribute to the presence of a functional conduction system without coordinated muscle contraction. These include hypovolemia, hypoxia, cardiac tamponade, tension pneumothorax, hypothermia, massive pulmonary embolism, drug overdose, hyperkalemia, and massive acute MI.

3. Clinical significance: No cardiac output and impending death unless interventions to correct the problem are effective in 3–5 minutes.

4. Nursing and/or medical intervention: Identify and document the rhythm and evaluate for pulselessness. Chest compressions must be started immediately to supply the patient with a cardiac output. Immediate steps must be taken to rule out treatable causes. Drug therapy includes epinephrine and atropine. Provide airway management, and hyperoxygenate the patient. A fluid challenge should be attempted to rule out causes from hypovolemia.

V. Ventricular dysrhythmias

A. Rhythm: Premature ventricular contraction (PVC) (Fig. B.24).

1. ECG criteria: The rhythm is irregular. The QRS complex is early, wide, and abnormal in configuration (greater than 0.12 second). There are no associated P waves, and the T wave is of opposite polarity to the QRS complex.

2. Physiologic explanation: This rhythm disturbance is attributed to impulses that originate from the ventricular conduction system and occur

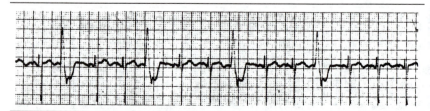

Figure B.24 Premature ventricular contraction. (From *Manual of Electrocardiography* (2nd ed.). Mudge, G. H., Jr. Boston: Little, Brown and Company, 1986. P. 111.)

before the next expected sinus beat. The QRS is widened due to the impulse formation in the ventricular conduction system and the altered depolarization that follows. The ventricles may depolarize separately, and conduction occurs more slowly outside of the normal conduction pathways. PVCs may be attributed to hypoxia, ischemia, MI, catecholamines, metabolic imbalance, hypokalemia, hypercalcemia, digitalis toxicity, and caffeine.

3. Clinical significance: PVCs can occur as unifocal impulses, or they may reflect a variety of sites of depolarization and, therefore, may indicate ventricular irritability. The significance depends on the frequency, where they fall in the cardiac cycle, and the clinical status of the patient. PVCs that fall on the T wave may precipitate VF or VT.

4. Nursing and/or medical intervention: Identify and document the rhythm. Assess the patient's status and hemodynamic response. The treatment of isolated PVCs is rarely needed. Physicians should be notified of incidence and occurrence. In the setting following an acute MI, the patient needs to be treated to alleviate ischemia or MI and underlying pathology. In instances where symptomatic treatment is needed, lidocaine is the drug of choice.

B. Rhythm: VT (Fig. B.25).

1. ECG criteria: VT is identified as a series of broad, rapid QRS complexes. The rhythm is usually regular. The ventricular rate is greater than 100 beats per minute. P waves are not associated with the QRS, but the P wave may be seen in part of the QRS or T wave. The ST segment and T wave are of opposite polarity to the QRS.

2. Physiologic explanation: The primary pacing site shifts to the ventricles for three or more consecutive beats. AV dissociation is usually present but may not be visible, because conduction from the atria to ventricles is overriden by the rapid ventricular activity and the refractoriness of the ventricles. Causes include increased automaticity, MI, ischemia, hypoxia, hypokalemia, hypotension, and digitalis toxicity.

3. Clinical significance: Individual responses to this rhythm vary. Some patients may experience no symptoms; others may suffer life-threatening hemodynamic compromise. The response is strongly associated with the presence or absence of myocardial dysfunction and the rate of the VT. Atrial contribution is usually lost, which accounts for a decrease in 20–30% of the cardiac output. This rhythm may deteriorate into VF.

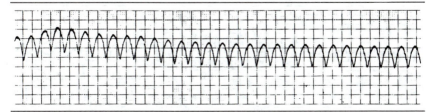

Figure B.25 Ventricular tachycardia. (From *Manual of Electrocardiography* (2nd ed.). Mudge, G. H., Jr. Boston: Little, Brown and Company, 1986. P. 112.)

4. Nursing and/or medical intervention: Identify and document the rhythm. Evaluate the patient's hemodynamic status and level of consciousness. Pulseless VT should be treated as VF. If the patient is stable, drug treatment with lidocaine, procainamide, or bretylium is recommended. Electrical cardioversion may be necessary for those patients who have serious signs and symptoms and a heart rate greater than 140 beats/minute.

C. Rhythm: Torsades de pointes (Fig. B.26).

1. ECG criteria: This rhythm is described as a multifocal irregular VT in which the polarity of the QRS complex shifts from negative to positive or vice versa over a series of beats. This characteristic gives it the French name, which means "turning of the points." The QRS is wide, and P waves are not often identifiable. The rhythm is regular, and the rate is greater than 100 beats/minute. The Q-T interval is usually greater than 0.40 second.

2. Physiologic explanation: This form of VT is often attributed to drug toxicity or a reaction to antiarrhythmics. These include quinidine, procainamide, disopyramide, or any agent that can prolong the Q-T interval. This rhythm is associated with the presence of a prolonged Q-T interval. It is often seen with hypokalemia, hypomagnesemia, and bradycardia.

3. Clinical significance: This rhythm is considered a lethal arrhythmia. Patients may experience a decrease in cardiac output and present with or report an episode of syncope.

4. Nursing and/or medical intervention: Assess the patient's hemodynamic status. If the patient is unstable, treat per American Heart Association advanced cardiac life support protocol for VT, or if pulseless, treat as VF; however, avoid the use of procainamide. Identify and document the rhythm. Measure the Q-T interval of the rhythm that preceded the occurrence of this rhythm. Evaluate for the use of antiarrhythmic drugs that may contribute to this rhythm and discontinue. Treatment protocols include magnesium sulfate, overdrive pacing, and occasionally isoproterenol to increase the heart rate, which results in a shortened Q-T interval, thus possibly breaking the torsades de pointes rhythm.

D. Rhythm: VF (Fig. B.27).

1. ECG criteria: This rhythm is identified as a severe derangement of the heart beat. There are no identifiable P waves or QRS complexes. Irregular waves and complexes are visible and vary from fine to coarse depending on the level of electrical energy.

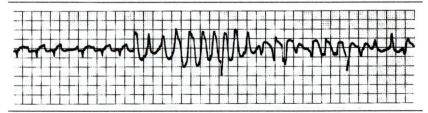

Figure B.26 Torsades de pointes. (From *Manual of Electrocardiography* (2nd ed.). Mudge, G. H., Jr. Boston: Little, Brown and Company, 1986. P. 176.)

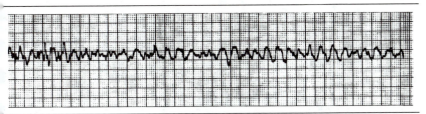

Figure B.27 Ventricular fibrillation. (From *Manual of Electrocardiography* (2nd ed.). Mudge, G. H., Jr. Boston: Little, Brown and Company, 1986. P. 113.)

2. Physiologic explanation: This rhythm is the result of multiple areas of rapid chaotic ventricular activity that represents depolarization and repolarization without coordinated heart muscle contraction. The myocardium quivers as a result of this unorganized electrical activity. This is most often seen with coronary artery disease, with acute MI, or following advanced heart block. Other causative agents include inadequate cardiac pacing, anesthesia, cardioversion, electrocution, and the R-on-T phenomenon.

3. Clinical significance: This rhythm is usually fatal within 3–5 minutes unless treatment is initiated to correct the rhythm. This generates no cardiac output.

4. Nursing and/or medical intervention: Identify and document the rhythm. Ensure that the patient is pulseless. Perform cardiopulmonary resuscitation (CPR) until defibrillator available. Defibrillation is the definitive therapy and should be initiated as soon as possible. Drugs include epinephrine, lidocaine, bretylium, magnesium sulfate, and procainamide.

E. Rhythm: Idioventricular rhythm (Fig. B.28).

1. ECG criteria: The R-R interval is usually regular. The QRS is wide and abnormal in configuration with no associated P waves. The ventricular rate is less than 40 beats/minute.

2. Physiologic explanation: The pacemaker function shifts to the ventricles due to sinus, atrioventricular, or nodal failure or conduction defects.

3. Clinical significance: The significance is generally related to the rate. Some patients may experience an appreciable decrease in cardiac output and become symptomatic as a result. This rhythm is not usually fast enough to maintain an adequate cardiac output. The ventricular pacing site is unreliable and may stop functioning at any time.

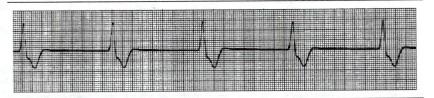

Figure B.28 Idioventricular rhythm.

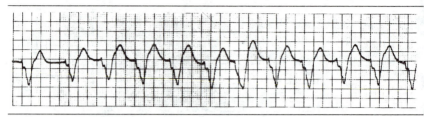

Figure B.29 Accelerated idioventricular rhythm. (From *Manual of Electrocardiography* (2nd ed.). Mudge, G. H., Jr. Boston: Little, Brown and Company, 1986. P. 114.)

4. Medical and/or nursing intervention: Identify and document the rhythm. Evaluate patient's hemodynamic status and any symptoms that may be rate related. Intervene per bradycardia protocol if the patient is symptomatic. Drugs may include atropine, dopamine, and isoproterenol. A transcutaneous pacemaker or transvenous pacemaker may be used to support a regular rhythm.

F. Rhythm: Accelerated idioventricular rhythm (Fig. B.29).

1. ECG criteria: The R-R interval is usually regular. The QRS is wide and abnormal in configuration with no associated P waves. The ventricular rate is 40–100 beats/minute.

2. Physiologic explanation: This results from a failure of the upper pacemakers combined with an increased automaticity in the ventricles. This is usually related to digitalis toxicity or the occurrence of an acute MI.

3. Clinical significance: The significance of this rhythm depends on the rate and the patient's, hemodynamic response to that rate. The atrial contribution is usually lost with this rhythm, and therefore patients sustain a decrease in cardiac output of approximately 25%.

4. Nursing and/or medical intervention: Identify and document the rhythm. Evaluate the patient's hemodynamic status. If the rate is slow atropine may be used. Identify if digitalis is a causative factor and discontinue if necessary.

G. Rhythm: Agonal rhythm (Fig. B.30).

1. ECG criteria: The rhythm is very slow and may be regular or irregular. QRS complexes are present but are wide and abnormal in configuration. There are no P waves.

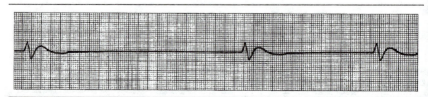

Figure B.30 Agonal rhythm.

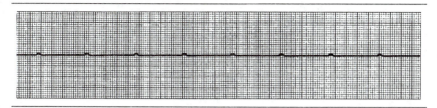

Figure B.31 Ventricular standstill.

2. Physiologic explanation: The conduction system has failed. There is no electrical activity in the atria and limited electrical response in the ventricles. This can be due to a variety of causes such as hypoxia, complete heart block, or unsuccessful resuscitation efforts.
3. Clinical significance: No cardiac output is associated with this rhythm. The patient is pulseless and apneic.
4. Nursing and/or medical intervention: Identify and document the rhythm. Assess hemodynamic status and begin CPR. Consider possible causes such as hypoxia, hyperkalemia, hypokalemia, or preexisting acidosis. Epinephrine, atropine, and a transcutaneous pacemaker may be used.

H. Rhythm: Ventricular standstill (Fig. B.31).
1. ECG criteria: P waves are visible with an absence of QRS complexes.
2. Physiologic explanation: Complete heart block exists with no lower pacemaker firing as a compensatory mechanism. No electrical activity is present within the ventricular region of the heart.
3. Clinical significance: Atrial activity exists; however, the absence of ventricular activity contributes to an absence of cardiac output. Death is imminent unless ventricular activity can be restored.
4. Nursing and/or medical intervention: Identify and document the rhythm. Verify that the patient is pulseless. Begin CPR and treat as asystole. Consider possible causes and attempt immediate transcutaneous pacing. Epinephrine and atropine may be used to increase electrical activity within the myocardium.

I. Rhythm: Asystole (Fig. B.32).
1. ECG criteria: Absence of P waves and QRS complexes. It is identified as a straight line on the ECG monitor.

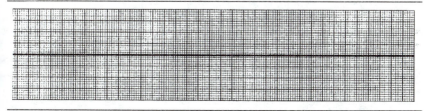

Figure B.32 Asystole.

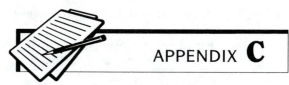

Advanced Cardiac Life Support Algorithms*

*From Emergency Cardiac Care Committee, Guidelines for cardiopulmonary resuscitation and emergency care. *JAMA* 268: 2216–2227. Copyright 1992, American Medical Association.

Figure C.1 Universal Algorithm for Adult
Emergency Cardiac Care

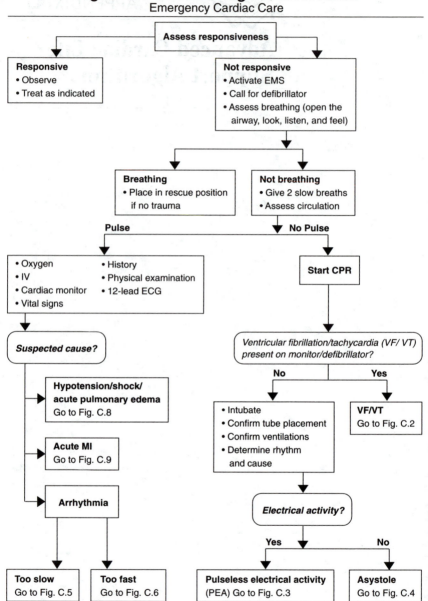

Figure C.2 Ventricular Fibrillation/ Pulseless Ventricular Tachycardia Algorithm (VF/VT)

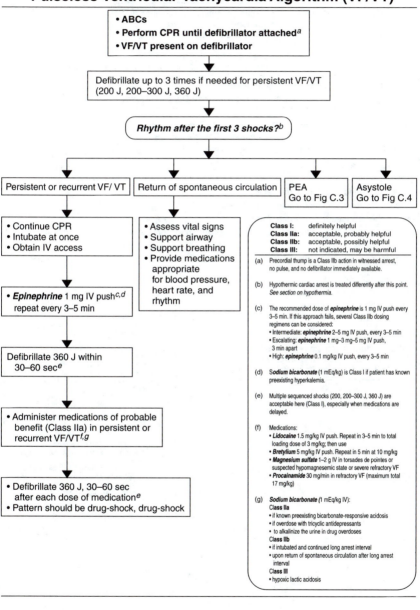

• ABCs
• Perform CPR until defibrillator attached[a]
• VF/VT present on defibrillator

Defibrillate up to 3 times if needed for persistent VF/VT (200 J, 200–300 J, 360 J)

Rhythm after the first 3 shocks?[b]

Persistent or recurrent VF/ VT | Return of spontaneous circulation | PEA Go to Fig C.3 | Asystole Go to Fig C.4

• Continue CPR
• Intubate at once
• Obtain IV access

• Assess vital signs
• Support airway
• Support breathing
• Provide medications appropriate for blood pressure, heart rate, and rhythm

• *Epinephrine* 1 mg IV push[c,d] repeat every 3–5 min

Defibrillate 360 J within 30–60 sec[e]

• Administer medications of probable benefit (Class IIa) in persistent or recurrent VF/VT[f,g]

• Defibrillate 360 J, 30–60 sec after each dose of medication[e]
• Pattern should be drug-shock, drug-shock

Class I: definitely helpful
Class IIa: acceptable, probably helpful
Class IIb: acceptable, possibly helpful
Class III: not indicated, may be harmful

(a) Precordial thump is a Class IIb action in witnessed arrest, no pulse, and no defibrillator immediately available.

(b) Hypothermic cardiac arrest is treated differently after this point. *See section on hypothermia.*

(c) The recommended dose of *epinephrine* is 1 mg IV push every 3–5 min. If this approach fails, several Class IIb dosing regimens can be considered:
• Intermediate: *epinephrine* 2–5 mg IV push, every 3–5 min
• Escalating: *epinephrine* 1 mg–3 mg–5 mg IV push, 3 min apart
• High: *epinephrine* 0.1 mg/kg IV push, every 3–5 min

(d) S*odium bicarbonate* (1 mEq/kg) is Class I if patient has known preexisting hyperkalemia.

(e) Multiple sequenced shocks (200, 200–300 J, 360 J) are acceptable here (Class I), especially when medications are delayed.

(f) Medications:
• *Lidocaine* 1.5 mg/kg IV push. Repeat in 3–5 min to total loading dose of 3 mg/kg; then use
• *Bretylium* 5 mg/kg IV push. Repeat in 5 min at 10 mg/kg
• *Magnesium sulfate* 1–2 g IV in torsades de pointes or suspected hypomagnesemic state or severe refractory VF
• *Procainamide* 30 mg/min in refractory VF (maximum total 17 mg/kg)

(g) *Sodium bicarbonate* (1 mEq/kg IV):
Class IIa
• if known preexisting bicarbonate-responsive acidosis
• if overdose with tricyclic antidepressants
• to alkalinize the urine in drug overdoses
Class IIb
• if intubated and continued long arrest interval
• upon return of spontaneous circulation after long arrest interval
Class III
• hypoxic lactic acidosis

Figure C.3 Pulseless Electrical Activity (PEA) Algorithm
(Electromechanical Dissociation [EMD])

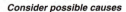

Includes: • Electromechanical dissociation (EMD)
• Pseudo-EMD
• Idioventricular rhythms
• Ventricular escape rhythms
• Bradyasystolic rhythms
• Postdefibrillation idioventricular rhythms

• Continue CPR   • Obtain IV access
• Intubate at once   • Assess blood flow using Doppler ultrasound

▼

Consider possible causes
(parentheses = possible therapies and treatment)

• Hypovolemia (volume infusion)
• Hypoxia (ventilation)
• Cardiac tamponade (pericardiocentesis)
• Tension pneumothorax (needle decompression)
• Hypothermia (see hypothermia algorithm)
• Massive pulmonary embolism (surgery, ***thrombolytics***)
(Fig. C.10)

• Drug overdoses such as tricyclics,
digitalis, beta-blockers, calcium
channel blockers
• Hyperkalemia[a]
• Acidosis[b]
• Massive acute myocardial infarction
(go to Fig C.9)

▼

• ***Epinephrine*** 1 mg IV push[a,c]
repeat every 3–5 min

▼

• If absolute bradycardia (< 60 beats/min) or
relative bradycardia, give ***atropine*** 1 mg IV
• Repeat every 3–5 min to a total of 0.04 mg/kg[d]

Class I:	definitely helpful
Class IIa:	acceptable, probably helpful
Class IIb:	acceptable, possibly helpful
Class III:	not indicated, may be harmful

(a) ***Sodium bicarbonate***
(1 mEq/kg) is Class I if patient has known preexisting
hyperkalemia.

(b) ***Sodium bicarbonate*** (1 mEq/kg)
Class IIa
• if known preexisting bicarbonate-responsive acidosis
• if overdose with tricyclic antidepressants
• to alkalinize the urine in drug overdoses
Class IIb
• if intubated and long arrest interval
• upon return of spontaneous circulation after long arrest
interval
Class III
• hypoxic lactic acidosis

(c) The recommended dose of ***epinephrine*** is 1 mg IV push
every 3–5 min. If this approach fails, several Class IIb dosing
regimens can be considered:
• Intermediate: ***epinephrine*** 2–5 mg IV push, every 3–5 min
• Escalating: ***epinephrine*** 1 mg–3 mg–5 mg IV push, 3 min
apart
• High: ***epinephrine*** 0.1 mg/kg IV push, every 3–5 min

(d) Shorter ***atropine*** dosing intervals are possibly helpful in
cardiac arrest (Class IIb).

Figure C.4 Asystole Treatment Algorithm

- **Continue CPR**
- **Intubate at once**
- **Obtain IV access**
- **Confirm asystole in more than one lead**

↓

Consider possible causes
- Hypoxia
- Hyperkalemia
- Hypokalemia
- Preexisting acidosis
- Drug overdose
- Hypothermia

↓

Consider immediate transcutaneous pacing (TCP)[a]

↓

- ***Epinephrine*** 1 mg IV push[b,c]
  repeat every 3–5 min

↓

- ***Atropine*** 1 mg IV
  repeat every 3–5 min up to a total of 0.04 mg/kg[d,e]

↓

Consider termination of efforts [f]

Class I: definitely helpful
Class IIa: acceptable, probably helpful
Class IIb: acceptable, possibly helpful
Class III: not indicated, may be harmful

(a) TCP is a Class IIb intervention. Lack of success may be due to delays in pacing. To be effective TCP must be performed early, simultaneously with drugs. Evidence does not support routine use of TCP for asystole.

(b) The recommended dose of ***epinephrine*** is 1 mg IV push every 3–5 min. If this approach fails, several Class IIb dosing regimens can be considered:
  - Intermediate: ***epinephrine*** 2–5 mg IV push, every 3–5 min
  - Escalating: ***epinephrine*** 1 mg–3 mg–5 mg IV push, 3 min apart
  - High: ***epinephrine*** 0.1 mg/kg IV push, every 3–5 min

(c) ***Sodium bicarbonate*** (1 mEq/kg) is Class I if patient has known preexisting hyperkalemia.

(d) Shorter ***atropine*** dosing intervals are Class IIb in asystolic arrest.

(e) ***Sodium bicarbonate*** 1 mEq/kg IV:
  Class IIa
  - if known preexisting bicarbonate-responsive acidosis
  - if overdose with tricyclic antidepressants
  - to alkalinize the urine in drug overdoses
  Class IIb
  - if intubated and continued long arrest interval
  - upon return of spontaneous circulation after long arrest interval
  Class III
  - hypoxic lactic acidosis

(f) If patient remains in asystole or other agonal rhythms after successful intubation and initial medications and no reversible causes are identified, consider termination of resuscitative efforts by a physician. Consider interval since arrest.

Figure C.5 Bradycardia Algorithm
(Patient is not in cardiac arrest)

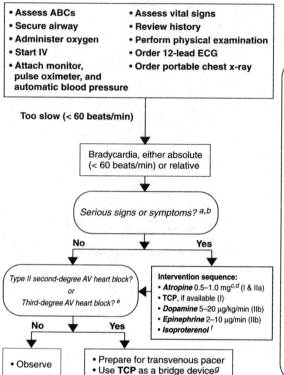

- **Assess ABCs**
- **Secure airway**
- **Administer oxygen**
- **Start IV**
- **Attach monitor, pulse oximeter, and automatic blood pressure**

- **Assess vital signs**
- **Review history**
- **Perform physical examination**
- **Order 12-lead ECG**
- **Order portable chest x-ray**

Too slow (< 60 beats/min)

Bradycardia, either absolute (< 60 beats/min) or relative

Serious signs or symptoms? a,b

No — **Yes**

Type II second-degree AV heart block?
or
Third-degree AV heart block? e

No — **Yes**

Intervention sequence:
- *Atropine* 0.5–1.0 mg c,d (I & IIa)
- **TCP**, if available (I)
- *Dopamine* 5–20 μg/kg/min (IIb)
- *Epinephrine* 2–10 μg/min (IIb)
- *Isoproterenol* f

- Observe

- Prepare for transvenous pacer
- Use **TCP** as a bridge device g

(a) Serious signs or symptoms must be related to the slow rate. Clinical manifestations include:
  - symptoms (chest pain, shortness of breath, decreased level of consciousness)
  - signs (low BP, shock, pulmonary congestion, CHF, acute MI)

(b) Do not delay TCP while awaiting IV access or for *atropine* to take effect if patient is symptomatic.

(c) Denervated transplanted hearts will not respond to *atropine*. Go at once to pacing, *catecholamine* infusion, or both.

(d) *Atropine* should be given in repeat doses in 3–5 min up to total of 0.04 mg/kg. Consider shorter dosing intervals in severe clinical conditions. It has been suggested that *atropine* should be used with caution in atrioventricular (AV) block at the His-Purkinje level (type II AV block and new third-degree block with wide QRS complexes) (Class IIb).

(e) Never treat third-degree heart block plus ventricular escape beats with *lidocaine*.

(f) *Isoproterenol* should be used, if at all, with extreme caution. At low doses it is Class IIb (possibly helpful); at higher doses it is Class III (harmful).

(g) Verify patient tolerance and mechanical capture. Use analgesia and sedation as needed.

Figure C.6 Tachycardia Algorithm

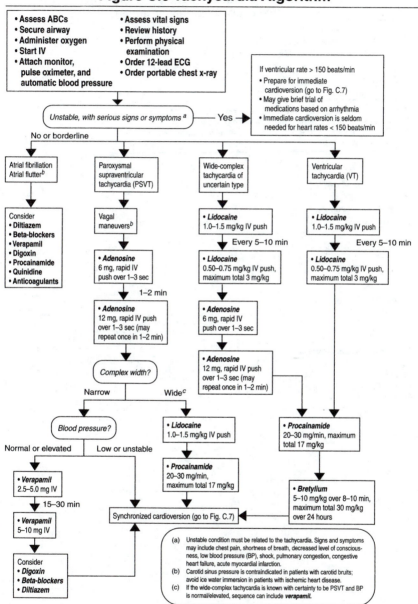

(a) Unstable condition must be related to the tachycardia. Signs and symptoms may include chest pain, shortness of breath, decreased level of consciousness, low blood pressure (BP), shock, pulmonary congestion, congestive heart failure, acute myocardial infarction.

(b) Carotid sinus pressure is contraindicated in patients with carotid bruits; avoid ice water immersion in patients with ischemic heart disease.

(c) If the wide-complex tachycardia is known with certainty to be PSVT and BP is normal/elevated, sequence can include *verapamil*.

Figure C.7 Electrical Cardioversion Algorithm
(Patient is not in cardiac arrest)

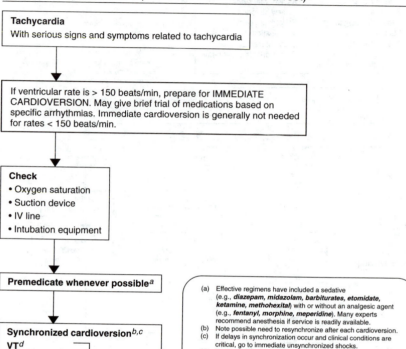

Tachycardia
With serious signs and symptoms related to tachycardia

↓

If ventricular rate is > 150 beats/min, prepare for IMMEDIATE CARDIOVERSION. May give brief trial of medications based on specific arrhythmias. Immediate cardioversion is generally not needed for rates < 150 beats/min.

↓

Check
• Oxygen saturation
• Suction device
• IV line
• Intubation equipment

↓

Premedicate whenever possible[a]

↓

Synchronized cardioversion[b,c]
VT[d]
PSVT[e]
Atrial fibrillation
Atrial flutter[e]
— 100 J, 200 J, 300 J, 360 J

(a) Effective regimens have included a sedative (e.g., *diazepam, midazolam, barbiturates, etomidate, ketamine, methohexital*) with or without an analgesic agent (e.g., *fentanyl, morphine, meperidine*). Many experts recommend anesthesia if service is readily available.
(b) Note possible need to resynchronize after each cardioversion.
(c) If delays in synchronization occur and clinical conditions are critical, go to immediate unsynchronized shocks.
(d) Treat polymorphic VT (irregular form and rate) like VF: 200 J, 200–300 J, 360 J.
(e) PSVT and atrial flutter often respond to lower energy levels (start with 50 J).

Figure C.8 Hypotension/Shock/Acute Pulmonary Edema Algorithm

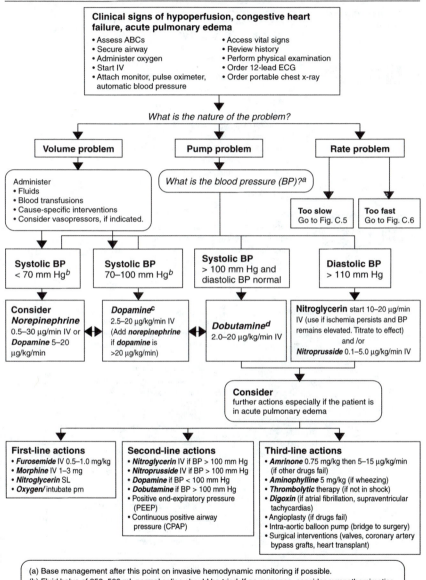

Clinical signs of hypoperfusion, congestive heart failure, acute pulmonary edema
- Assess ABCs
- Secure airway
- Administer oxygen
- Start IV
- Attach monitor, pulse oximeter, automatic blood pressure
- Access vital signs
- Review history
- Perform physical examination
- Order 12-lead ECG
- Order portable chest x-ray

What is the nature of the problem?

Volume problem | **Pump problem** | **Rate problem**

Administer
- Fluids
- Blood transfusions
- Cause-specific interventions
- Consider vasopressors, if indicated.

What is the blood pressure (BP)?[a]

Too slow Go to Fig. C.5

Too fast Go to Fig. C.6

Systolic BP < 70 mm Hg[b]

Systolic BP 70–100 mm Hg[b]

Systolic BP > 100 mm Hg and diastolic BP normal

Diastolic BP > 110 mm Hg

Consider *Norepinephrine* 0.5–30 µg/min IV or ***Dopamine*** 5–20 µg/kg/min

Dopamine[c] 2.5–20 µg/kg/min IV (Add *norepinephrine* if *dopamine* is >20 µg/kg/min)

Dobutamine[d] 2.0–20 µg/kg/min IV

Nitroglycerin start 10–20 µg/min IV (use if ischemia persists and BP remains elevated. Titrate to effect) and /or ***Nitroprusside*** 0.1–5.0 µg/kg/min IV

Consider further actions especially if the patient is in acute pulmonary edema

First-line actions
- ***Furosemide*** IV 0.5–1.0 mg/kg
- ***Morphine*** IV 1–3 mg
- ***Nitroglycerin*** SL
- ***Oxygen/*** intubate prn

Second-line actions
- ***Nitroglycerin*** IV if BP > 100 mm Hg
- ***Nitroprusside*** IV if BP > 100 mm Hg
- ***Dopamine*** if BP < 100 mm Hg
- ***Dobutamine*** if BP > 100 mm Hg
- Positive end-expiratory pressure (PEEP)
- Continuous positive airway pressure (CPAP)

Third-line actions
- ***Amrinone*** 0.75 mg/kg then 5–15 µg/kg/min (if other drugs fail)
- ***Aminophylline*** 5 mg/kg (if wheezing)
- ***Thrombolytic*** therapy (if not in shock)
- ***Digoxin*** (if atrial fibrillation, supraventricular tachycardias)
- Angioplasty (if drugs fail)
- Intra-aortic balloon pump (bridge to surgery)
- Surgical interventions (valves, coronary artery bypass grafts, heart transplant)

(a) Base management after this point on invasive hemodynamic monitoring if possible.
(b) Fluid bolus of 250–500 mL normal saline should be tried. If no response, consider sympathomimetics.
(c) Move to *dopamine* and stop *norepinephrine* when BP improves.
(d) Add *dopamine* when BP improves. Avoid *dobutamine* when systolic BP < 100 mm Hg.

Figure C.9 Acute Myocardial Infarction Algorithm

Recommendations for early management of patients with chest pain and possible AMI

 COMMUNITY

Community emphasis on "Call First, Call Fast, Call 911"

EMS SYSTEM

EMS system approach that should address
- Oxygen, IV, cardiac monitor, vital signs
- *Nitroglycerin*
- Pain relief with narcotics
- Notification of emergency department
- Rapid transport to emergency department
- Prehospital screen for *thrombolytic* therapy*
- 12-lead ECG, computer analysis, transmission to emergency department*
- Initiation of *thrombolytic* therapy*

EMERGENCY DEPARTMENT

"Door-to-drug" team protocol approach
- Rapid triage of patients with chest pain
- Clinical decision maker established (emergency physician, cardiologist, or other)

Time interval in emergency department

Assessment

Immediate:
- Vital signs with automatic BP
- Oxygen saturation
- Start IV
- 12-lead ECG (MD review)
- Brief, targeted history and physical
- Decide on eligibility for *thrombolytic* therapy (Fig. C.10)

Soon:
- Chest x-ray
- Blood studies (electrolytes, enzymes, coagulation studies)

*Optional guidelines

Treatments to consider if there is evidence of coronary thrombosis and no reasons for exclusion:
(some but not all may be appropriate)

- *Oxygen* at 4 L/min
- *Nitroglycerin* SL, paste or spray (if systolic blood pressure > 90 mm Hg)
- *Morphine* IV
- *Aspirin* PO
- *Thrombolytic* agents (Go to Fig. C.10)
- *Nitroglycerin* IV (limit systolic BP drop to 10% if normotensive; 30% drop if hypertensive; never drop below 90 mm Hg systolic)
- *Beta-blockers* IV
- *Heparin* IV
- Routine *lidocaine* administration is NOT recommended for all patients with **AMI**
- *Magnesium sulfate* IV
- Percutaneous transluminal coronary angioplasty

30–60 min to *thrombolytic* therapy

Figure C.10 Acute Myocardial Infarction/r-TPA Protocol

A. Inclusion criteria: Acute infarction irrespective of infarct location

B. Absolute contraindications
1. Active internal bleeding
2. Suspected aortic dissection
3. Recent head trauma or known intracranial neoplasm
4. Pregnancy
5. History of cerebrovascular accident known to be hemorrhagic
6. Severe uncontrolled hypertension

C. Relative contraindications
1. Recent trauma or surgery > 2 weeks; trauma or surgery more recent than 2 weeks, which could be a source of rebleeding, is an absolute contraindication
2. History of chronic severe hypertension with or without drug therapy
3. Active peptic ulcer
4. History of cerebrovascular accident
5. Known bleeding diathesis or current use of anticoagulants
6. Significant liver dysfunction
7. Prolonged or traumatic cardiopulmonary resuscitation
8. Recorded blood pressure > 200/120 mm Hg
9. Diabetic hemorrhagic retinopathy or other hemorrhagic opthalmic condition

D. Preparations before infusion
1. Establish 2–3 peripheral IV sites
2. If ABGs are required, select radial site for puncture
3. Initial lab work: CBC, CHEM 20, PT, PTT, cardiac enzymes, isoenzymes
4. Recommended: ASA 325 mg PO stat and daily

E. Rapid infusion guidelines
IV Bolus 15 mg over 1–2 minutes, then
        50 mg over 30 minutes,
        35 mg over 1 hour.
Total Infusion = 100 mg over 90 minutes.
Weight dosing should be considered for patients under 140 lbs.
NOTE: Avoid shaking vial to prevent foaming; drip should IMMEDIATELY follow bolus; r-TPA should run in a dedicated nonfiltered IV line. Once r-TPA bag/bottle is empty, add 20 mL D5W and use as "chaser" to complete infusion.

F. Concomitant heparin therapy
Begin heparin therapy as soon as possible following initiation of r-TPA. Bolus heparin 5,000 U IV followed by drip of 1000 U/hr. Adjust PTT to 1.5–2 times control.

Laboratory Values

Merrily A. Kuhn

Complete blood count

Hematocrit (Hct)	40–54% (male)
	37–47% (female)
Hemoglobin (Hgb)	13.5–17.5 g/dL (male)
	12–16 g/dL (female)
Red blood cells (RBCs)	4.25–5.50 million/mL (male)
	3.6–5.0 million/mL (female)
Reticulocytes	0.5–1.5% of total erythrocytes (adults)
White blood cells (WBCs)	5000–10,000/mL
Basophils	0.5–1.0% of total WBC
Eosinophils	1–4 of total WBC
Lymphocytes	20–40% of total WBC
Monocytes	2–6% of total WBC
Segmented neutrophils (segs) or Polymorphonuclear neutrophils (PMNs)	50–60% of WBC

Serum coagulation

Platelets	150,000–350,000/mL
Prothrombin time (PT)	10–14 sec
Partial thromboplastin time (PTT)	30–45 sec
Activated partial thromboplastin time (APTT)	16–25 sec
Activated clotting time (ACT)	92–128 sec
Factors	
I. Fibrinogen	0.15–0.35 g/mL
II. Prothrombin	60–140%
III. Tissue thromboplastin, tissue factor	—
IV. Calcium	4.5–5.5 mEq/L or 9–11 mg/dL
V. Proaccelerin labile factor (accelerator globulin)	60–140%
VI. Not assigned	—
VII. Proconvertin stable factor	70–130%
VIII. Antihemophilic factor (AHF)	50–200%
IX. Plasma thromboplastin (Christmas factor B)	60–140%
X. Stuart factor, Prower factor, thrombokinase	70–130%
XI. Plasma thromboplastin	60–140%
XII. Hageman factor	60–140%
XIII. Fibrin-stabilizing factor, Laki-Lorand factor, fibrinase	—
Fibrin degradation products (FDP)	2–10 μg/mL

Continued

Serum chemistry

Albumin	3.5–5.0 g/dL
Alkaline phosphatase	4–13 U (King-Armstrong)
Alanine aminotransferase (ALT) (serum glutamate pyruvate transaminase)	4–35 U/L
Ammonia	18–54 μmol/L (male)
	12–50 μmol/L (female)
Amylase	4–25 U/mL
Anion gap	8–16 mEq/L
Aspartate aminotransferase (AST) (serum glutamic oxaloacetic transaminase)	8–46 U/L
Bicarbonate	24–32 mEq/L
Bilirubin	
Total	0.2–1.0 mg/dL
Direct	0–0.2 mg/dL
Indirect	Total—direct (0.5–1.2 mg/dL)
Blood urea nitrogen (BUN)	10–20 mg/dL
BUN:creatinine ratio	10:1 to 15:1
Calcium	8.5–10.5 mg/dL
Cholesterol	120–200 mg/dL
High-density lipoprotein (HDL)	26–63 mg/dL (male)
	39–92 mg/dL (female)
Low-density lipoprotein (LDL)	70–180 mg/dL
	< 130 is desirable
LDL/HDL ratio	< 3.0
Cholesterol/HDL ratio	< 4.5
Chloride	98–106 mEq/L
Creatinine	0.7–1.3 mg/dL (male)
	0.6–1.2 mg/dL (female)
Glucose	70–110 mg/dL

Glucose tolerance test (GTT)   (adult)

Time	Serum (mg/dL)	Blood (mg/dL)
Fasting	70–110	60–100
0.5 hr	< 160	< 150
1 hr	< 170	< 160
2 hr	< 125	< 115
3 hr	Fasting level	Fasting level

Iron	50–150 μg/dL
Lactate	0.3–1.3 mmol/L
Lactate dehydrogenase (LDH)	70–250 IU/L
Lipase	4–24 IU/L
Magnesium	1.3–2.1 mEq/L

Continued

Serum chemistry (*cont.*)

Osmolality	275–295 mOsm/kg
Potassium	3.5–5.0 mEq/L
Phosphorus	2.5–4.5 mg/dL
Protein	6–8 g/dL
Sedimentation rate	0–10 mm/hr (male)
	0–15 mm/hr (female)
Sodium	135–145 mEq/L
Thyroxine (T_4)	4.5–11.5 μg/dL
Triglyceride	10–150 mg/dL (male, 20–40 yr)
	10–190 mg/dL (male, 40–60 yr)
	10–140 mg/dL (female, 20–40 yr)
	10–180 mg/dL (female, 40–60 yr)
Triiodothyronine (T_3)	0.8–1.1 μg/dL
Uric acid	3.5–8.0 mg/dL

Cardiac profile

AST	7–34 U/L (female)
	8–46 U/L (male)
With myocardial infarction	
Onset	12–18 hr
Peak	24–48 hr
Duration	3–4 days
Creatine kinase (CK)	96–140 U/L (female)
	38–174 U/L (male)
With myocardial infarction	
Onset	4–6 hr
Peak	12–24 hr
Duration	3–4 days
Creatine kinase MB isoenzyme (CK-MB)	0%
With myocardial infarction	
Onset	4–6 hr
Peak	12–20 hr
Duration	2–3 days
Lactate dehydrogenase (LDH)	70–180 mg/dL
With myocardial infarction	
Onset	12–24 hr
Peak	3–6 days
Duration	8–14 days
LDH_1	17.5–28.3% of total LDH
LDH_2	30.4–36.4% of total LDH
With myocardial infarction: $LDH_1 > LDH_2$	
Onset	12–24 hr
Peak	48 hr
Duration	Variable

Continued

Serology

Antinuclear antibodies (ANA)	Negative
Carcinoembryonic antigen (CEAA) (may be done by nuclear medicine)	<2.5 ng/mL
Cold agglutinins (CA)	1:8 antibody titer
Complement C3	80–180 mg/dL (white male)
	76–120 mg/dL (white female)
	16–66 mg/dL (black adult)
Complement C4	15–60 mg/dL (white male)
	15–52 mg/dL (white female)
	16–66 mg/dL (black adult)
C-reactive protein (CRP)	0
Febrile agglutinin titers	*Brucella* species <1:20
	Francisella tularensis <1:40
	Salmonella species <1:40
	Proteus species <1:40
Hepatitis B surface antigen (HBsAg) (by nuclear medicine)	Negative
Immunoglobulins (Ig)	
IgE	0.01–0.07 mg/dL
IgG	800–1800 mg/dL
IgA	100–400 mg/dL
IgM	50–150 mg/dL
IgD	0.5–3.0 mg/dL
Rheumatoid factor (RF)	<1:20 titer
Thyroid antibodies (TA) (may be done by nuclear medicine)	Negative or <1:20 titer

Urine

Amylase	35–260 Somogyi U/hr
	6.5–48.1 U/L (SI units)
	800–4200 Somogyi U/24 hr
Bence-Jones protein	Negative to trace
Bilirubin or bile	Negative to 0.02 mg/dL
Catecholamines	<100 μg/24 hr
Epinephrine	<100–230 μg/24 hr
Norepinephrine	<100–230 μg/24 hr
Creatinine clearance	100–180 L/24 hr
Creatinine	20–26 mg/kg per 24 hr; 0.18–0.23 mmol/kg per 24 hr (SI units) (male)
	14–22 mg/kg per 24 hr; 0.12–0.19 mmol/kg per 24 hr (SI units) (female)
Osmolality	50–1200 mOsm/kg per H_2O
	Average 200–800 mOsm/kg per H_2O
Porphyrins: coproporphyrins	Random 3–20 μg/dL

Continued

Urine (*cont.*)

Urinalysis	
pH	4.5–8.0
Specific gravity (SG)	1.005–1.030
Protein	Negative
Glucose	Negative
Ketones	Negative
RBC	Negative or rare
WBC	Negative or rare
Casts	Occasional hyaline
Urobilinogen	0.05–2.50 mg per 24 hr
Vanillylmandelic acid (VMA)	1.5–7.5 mg per 24 hr

Urine electrolytes

Sodium	40–220 mEq/day
Spot sodium	<20 mEq
Potassium	25–125 mEq/day
Chloride	110–250 mEq/day
Calcium	100–250 mg per 24 hr

Cerebral spinal fluid (CSF)

Pressure (initial)	70–180 mm H_2O
Albumin	11–48 mg/dL
Cells	0–5 mononuclear cells
Chloride	120–130 mEq/L
Glucose	50–75 mg/dL
IgG	0–8.6 mg/dL
Protein	15–45 mg/dL (lumbar)
Total cells	0–8 mm^3

Drug level

Digoxin	1–2 ng/mL
Phenytoin	10–20 mg/L
Theophylline	10–20 mg/L
Barbiturate	10 mg/dL (coma)
Gentamicin	
Trough	1–2 μg/mL
Peak	6–8 μg/mL
Lidocaine	1.5–5.0 μg/mL
Tobramycin	
Trough	1–2 μg/mL
Peak	6–8 μg/mL
Vancomycin	
Trough	5–10 μg/mL
Peak	30–40 μg/mL

Continued

Pulmonary function

Expiratory reserve volume (ERV)	Approximately 1200–1500 mL
Forced vital capacity (FVC) or forced expiratory volume (FEV)	Approximately 4800 mL
Functional residual capacity (FRC)	Approximately 2400–3000 mL
Peak expiratory flow rate (PEFR)	Average 300 L/min
Peak inspiratory flow rate (PIFR)	Average ≥ 300 L/min
Residual volume (RV)	1200–1500 mL
Total lung capacity (TLC)	Approximately 5500 mL
Vital capacity (VC)	4000–4800 mL

Blood gases

Arterial

Oxygen saturation (Sao_2)	95%
Oxygen tension (Pao_2)	80–100 mm Hg
Carbon dioxide tension ($PaCo_2$)	35–45 mm Hg
pH	7.35–7.45
Bicarbonate	22–26 mEq/L

Venous

Oxygen saturation ($S\bar{v}o_2$)	60–80%
Oxygen tension ($P\bar{v}o_2$)	35–45 mm Hg
Carbon dioxide tension ($P\bar{v}co_2$)	41–51 mm Hg
pH	7.31–7.41
Bicarbonate	22–26 mEq/L

Difference

Difference in O_2 content between arterial and mixed venous blood $C(a\text{-}\bar{v}o_2)$	3.5–5.0 mL/100 mL

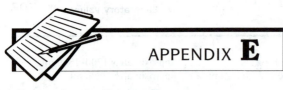

Scoring Systems

Merrily A. Kuhn

Table E.1 APACHE III Scoring Components

Age (yr)	Points
≤44	0
45–59	5
60–64	11
65–69	13
70–74	16
75–84	17
≥85	24
Chronic health	
Cirrhosis	4
Immunosuppression	10
Leukemia/multiple myeloma	10
Metastatic cancer	11
Lymphoma	13
Hepatic failure	16
AIDS	23

Source: From Jaysm, W., Wagberm, D. P., Draper, E. A., et al. APACHE III physiological scoring for vital signs and laboratory tests. *Chest* 102:1919–1920, 1992; as modified from Knaus, W. A., et al. The APACHE III prognostic system: Risk prediction of hospital mortality for critically ill hospitalized adults. *Chest* 100:1619–1636, 1991. With permission from the American College of Chest Physicians.

Figure E.1

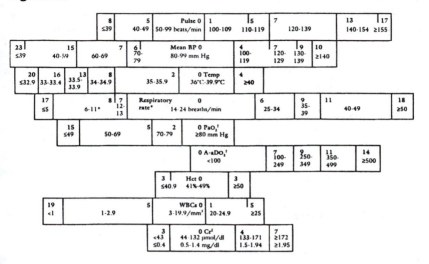

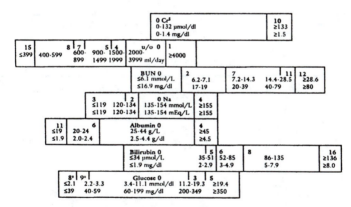

Modified from Knaus WA et al: The APACHE III prognostic system, Chest (in press).

BP, Blood pressure; *Temp*, temperature; *PaO₂*, arterial oxygen tension or partial pressure; A-aDO_2, alveolar-arterial oxygen gradient;

Hct, hematocrit; *WBCs*, white blood cells (count); *Cr*, creatinine; *u/o*, urine output; *BUN*, blood urea nitrogen; *Na*, sodium.

*For patients on mechanical ventilation, no points are given for respiratory rates 6–12.

†Only use A-aDO_2 for intubated patients with FiO₂ ≥0.5. Do not use PaO₂ weights for these patients.

‡Creatinine without acute renal failure (ARF). ARF is defined as creatinine ≥1.5 dl/day and urine output <410 ml/day and no chronic dialysis.

§Creatinine with ARF.

ǁGlucose ≤39 mg/dl is lower weight than 40–59.

With permission: American College of Chest Physicians. Jaysm, Wm, Wagberm, DP, Draper, EA, Zimmerman, JE., et. al. Apachee III Physiological Scoring for Vital Signs and Laboratory Tests. p. 696

Table E.2 Trauma Score

Assessment parameter		Trauma score
Glasgow coma scale score	14–15	5
	11–13	4
	8–10	3
	5–7	2
	3–4	1
Respiratory rate (breaths/min)	10–24	4
	25–35	3
	>35	2
	1–9	1
	0	0
Respiratory expansion	Normal	1
	Shallow	0
	Retractive	0
Systolic blood pressure (mm Hg)	>90	4
	70–90	3
	50–69	2
	1–49	1
No carotid pulse	0	0
Capillary refill	Normal	2
	Delayed	1
	None	0

Source: Champion, H. R., Gainer, P. S., Yackee, E. A progress report on the trauma score in predicting a fatal outcome. *J. Trauma* 26:927–931, 1988.

Table E.3 Projected Estimate of Survival

Trauma score	Percentage survival
16	99
15	98
14	96
13	93
12	87
11	76
10	60
9	42
8	26
7	15
6	8
5	4
4	2
3	1
2	0
1	0

Source: Champion, H. R., Gainer, P. S., Yackee, E. A progress report on the trauma score in predicting a fatal outcome. *J. Trauma* 26:927–931, 1988.

Table E.4 Glasgow Coma Scale

Sign	Finding	Value
Eye opening	Spontaneous	4
	To voice	3
	To pain	2
	None	1
Verbal response (arousal with voice or noxious stimulus)	Oriented	5
	Confused	4
	Inappropriate	3
	Incomprehensible	2
	None	1
Motor response (response to command or noxious stimulus)	Obeys command	6
	Localizes pain	5
	Withdraws from pain	4
	Flexion (decorticate posturing)	3
	Extension (decerebrate posturing)	2
	None	1

Body Surface Area Nomogram

Merrily A. Kuhn

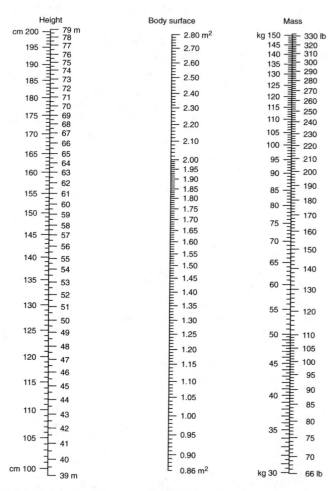

Figure F.1 Body surface area nomogram. (From *The Nursing Process and Fundamentals of Drug Therapy* (8th ed.). Summit, N.J.: Ciba-Geigy Pharmaceuticals, 1991.)

Cranial Nerve Function and Dysfunction

Diane Schwenker

Brain function	Cranial nerve and function	Conditions exhibited when damaged
Diencephalon	I. Olfactory—smell II. Optic—sight	Disruption of smell sensation; visual disturbances
Mesencephalon		
Relays impulses from higher to lower centers; contains auditory and optic centers; contains red nuclei	III. Oculomotor—pupil reaction, sight IV. Trochlear—sight	Coma; central neurogenic hyperventilation; no response to dolls' eyes/calorics*; decerebrate posturing; pupils midline/fixed
Pons		
Connects cerebellum and upper hemispheres; provides some control over involuntary respiration	V. Trigeminal—chewing and feeling in face VI. Abducens—sight VII. Facial—taste and crying VIII. Acoustic (cochlear branch)—hearing	Coma; apneustic breathing; flaccid posturing; no dolls' eyes; pinpoint pupils; no reaction
Medulla		
Connects brain to spinal cord; crossing of motor fibers; the centers for cardiac, vasomotor, and respiratory control are located here	VIII. Acoustic (vestibular branch)—balance IX. Glossopharyngeal—taste and gagging X. Vagus XI. Accessory—turning of head and shoulders XII. Hypoglossal—movement of tongue	Cluster breathing; flaccid posturing; coma; no dolls' eyes/calorics*; pinpoint pupils; no reaction

*Dolls' eyes or the oculocephalic reflex—a function of the medial longitudinal fasciculus, a pathway in the brainstem; side-to-side movement of the head results in coordinated eye movements away from the direction of head movement. Ice water calorics or the oculovestibular reflex—iced water irritation of an ear produces a nystagmus toward the stimulated ear; abnormal or absent responses indicate dysfunction in the brainstem.

Cardiopulmonary Monitoring: Values and Formulas

Jennifer Hebra

Parameter	Normal value	Formula
Cardiac output (CO)	4–8 L/min	Obtained value *or* HR × SV
Cardiac index (CI)	2.5–4.2 L/min/m²	$\dfrac{\text{CO}}{\text{BSA}}$
Pulmonary artery systolic pressure (PAS)	15–30 mm Hg	Obtained value
Pulmonary artery diastolic pressure (PAD)	5–15 mm Hg	Obtained value
Mean pulmonary artery pressure (MPAP)	10–20 mm Hg	Obtained value *or* $\dfrac{2(\text{PAD}) + \text{PAS}}{3}$
Pulmonary artery wedge pressure (PAWP)	4–12 mm Hg	Obtained value
Modified Fick equation	2.5–4.2 L/min/m²	$\dfrac{9.19 \times \text{BSA}}{\text{Hgb}(\text{Sa}_{O_2} - \text{S}\bar{\text{v}}_{O_2})}$
Stroke volume (SV)	60–135 mL/beat	$\dfrac{\text{CO}}{\text{HR}}$
Stroke volume index (SVI)	35–70 mL/m²/beat	$\dfrac{\text{SV}}{\text{BSA}}$
Systemic vascular resistance (SVR)	800–1400 dyn/sec/cm⁻⁵	$\dfrac{\text{MAP} - \text{CVP}}{\text{CO}} \times 80$
Mean arterial pressure (MAP)	65–105 mm Hg	$\dfrac{2(\text{DBP}) + \text{SBP}}{3}$
Central venous pressure (CVP)	2–6 mm Hg	Obtained value
Pulmonary vascular resistance (PVR)	30–100 dyn/sec/cm⁻⁵	$\dfrac{\text{MPAP} - \text{PAWP}}{\text{CO}} \times 80$
Pulmonary vascular resistance index (PVRI)	70–180 dyn/sec/cm⁻⁵	$\dfrac{\text{MPAP} - \text{PAWP}}{\text{CI}} \times 80$
Coronary perfusion pressure (CPP)	60–80 mm Hg	DBP − PAWP
Left ventricular stroke work index (LVSWI)	40–75 gm/m²/beat	SVI × (MAP × PAWP) × 0.136
Ejection fraction (EF)	60–70%	$\dfrac{\text{SV}}{\text{LVEDV}} \times 100$

Continued

Parameter	Normal value	Formula
Arterial oxygen content (CaO_2)	20 mL/100 or 20 vol%	$SaO_2 \times Hgb \times 1.38) + (PaO_2 \times (0.0031)$
Venous oxygen content (CvO_2)	15.5 mL/100 mL or 15.5 vol%	$(SvO_2 \times Hgb \times 1.38) + (PvO_2 \times 0.0031)$
Arterial oxygen delivery ($\dot{D}O_2$)	750–1100 mL/min	$CO \times CaO_2 \times 10$
Oxygen consumption ($\dot{V}O_2$)	200–250 mL/min	$CO \times 10 \times (CaO_2 - CvO_2)$
Mixed venous oxygen saturation ($S\bar{v}O_2$)	60–80%	$1 - \dfrac{\dot{V}O_2}{\dot{D}O_2}$ or Obtained value from oximetric pulmonary artery catheter
Respiratory quotient (RQ)	0.8*	$\dfrac{CO_2 \text{ production}}{\dot{V}O_2}$
Compliance	50–100 mL/cm H_2O	$\dfrac{\Delta \text{ tidal volume}}{\Delta \text{ inspiratory pressure}}$ or $\dfrac{\Delta V}{\Delta P}$
Minute ventilation (V_E); $\dot{V}$	5–10 L/min	$V_T \times \text{frequency} = V_E$
Ventilation/perfusion ratio in lung ($\dot{V}/\dot{Q}$)	0.8* 0.8 = dead spacing 0.8 = shunt-producing disorders	$\dot{V}/\dot{Q}$
Arteriovenous oxygen content difference	4–6 mL/100 mL	$C(a\text{-}v)O_2$
Tidal volume (V_T)	500 mL	Obtained value
Dead space/tidal volume ratio (V_{DS}/V_T)	0.55 L*	$\dfrac{V_{DS}}{V_T}$
Dead space (V_{DS})	1 mL/lb or 0.45 mL/kg (150 mL for average (adult)	$V_T \times \dfrac{PaCO_2 - PeCO_2}{PaCO_2}$
Alveolar–arterial tension gradient ($PAO_2 - PaO_2$; A-aO_2; A-aO_2 difference; or A-aDO_2)	5–20 mm Hg (>20 mm Hg = shunting)	$PAO_2 - PaO_2$
Shunted CO ($\dot{Q}_S$) + total CO ($\dot{Q}_T$)	5–10%	$\dfrac{\dot{Q}_S}{\dot{Q}_T} =$ $\dfrac{(PAO_2 - PaO_2) \times 0.0031}{(4.5 \text{ vol}\%) + (PAO_2 - PaO_2) \times 0.0031}$ This equation is best with an FIO_2 of 1.0, when shunt is < 30% and PaO_2 > 100 mm Hg
Arterial/alveolar oxygen content ratio	0.8*	$\dfrac{PaO_2}{PAO_2}$

*No units.
HR, heart rate; BSA, body surface area; Hgb, hemoglobin; DBP, diastolic blood pressure; LVEDV, left ventricular end-diastolic volume; SBP, systolic blood pressure; SaO_2, arterial oxygen saturation; $PeCO_2$, carbon dioxide tension in expired air collected over a 3-minute period; FIO_2, fraction of inspired oxygen.

Index